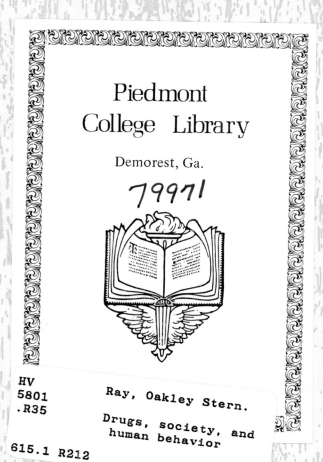

Drugs, society, and human behavior

Drugs, society, and human behavior

Oakley S. Ray, Ph.D.

Professor, Department of Psychology, Vanderbilt University;
Associate Professor, Department of Pharmacology, Vanderbilt University School of Medicine;
Chief, Psychology Service, Veterans Administration Hospital,
Nashville, Tennessee

With 35 illustrations

Reprinted with emendations, July, 1974

The C. V. Mosby Company

Saint Louis   1972

MS/S/B   9   8   7   6   5   4   3   2

3/28/77   Becker & Taylor 7.50

Consulting authorities

Chapter 1

Beverly A. Asbury
University Chaplain, Vanderbilt University,
Nashville, Tennessee

Carrol E. Izard, Ph.D.
Professor, Department of Psychology, Vanderbilt University,
Nashville, Tennessee

Martin Katahn, Ph.D.
Professor and Chairman, Department of Psychology, Vanderbilt University,
Nashville, Tennessee

Frank Lackner, Ph.D.
Associate Professor, Department of Psychology, Chatham College,
Pittsburgh, Pennsylvania

Chapter 2

Robert S. Brandt, LL.B.
Attorney at Law, Nashville, Tennessee

M. I. Gluckman, Ph.D.
Associate Director of Research, Wyeth Laboratories,
Philadelphia, Pennsylvania

William Langeland, Ph.D.
Director of Project Coordination, Wyeth Laboratories,
Philadelphia, Pennsylvania

Chapter 3

Lewis A. Bettinger, Ph.D.
Assistant Professor, Department of Psychology, Vanderbilt University,
Nashville, Tennessee

Chapters 4 and 5

William J. Kinnard, Ph.D.
Dean, School of Pharmacy, University of Maryland,
Baltimore, Maryland

Chapter 6

Herbert Barry III, Ph.D.
Professor, University of Pittsburgh School of Pharmacy,
Pittsburgh, Pennsylvania

Joel M. Cantor, Ph.D.
Consultant in Program Development, Center for Studies on
Narcotics and Drug Abuse, National Institute of
Mental Health, Chevy Chase, Maryland

Samuel C. Kaim, M.D.
Director, Alcohol and Drug Dependence Service, Veterans
Administration, Washington, D. C.

Chapter 7

Theodore Adams
Director, Editorial Services, American Cancer Society,
New York, New York

Chapter 8

John Adinolfi
Director, Technical Services, Pan-American Coffee Bureau,
New York, New York

John M. Anderson
Executive Director, Tea Council of the USA,
New York, New York

Chapter 9

William J. Kinnard, Ph.D.
Dean, School of Pharmacy, University of Maryland,
Baltimore, Maryland

Chapter 10

John M. Davis, M.D.
Professor, Department of Psychiatry and Associate Professor
of Pharmacology, Vanderbilt University, Nashville, Tennessee

Charles E. Goshen, M.D.
Associate Professor, Department of Psychiatry, Vanderbilt
University, Nashville, Tennessee

Leo E. Hollister, M.D.
Medical Investigator, Veterans Administration Hospital,
Palo Alto, California

Hans H. Strupp, Ph.D.
Professor, Department of Psychology, Vanderbilt University,
Nashville, Tennessee

Chapter 11

John Griffith, M.D.
Associate Professor, Department of Psychiatry, University of
California, San Diego, California

Chapter 12

Daniel M. Buxbaum, Ph.D.
Assistant Professor, Department of Pharmacology, Vanderbilt
University, Nashville, Tennessee

William R. Martin, M.D.
Chief, Addiction Research Center, National Institute of
Mental Health, Lexington, Kentucky

Chapters 13 and 14

Leo E. Hollister, M.D.
Medical Investigator, Veterans Administration Hospital,
Palo Alto, California

Richard Schultes, Ph.D.
Professor, Department of Biology, Harvard University,
Cambridge, Massachusetts

Chapter 15

Daniel M. Buxbaum, Ph.D.
Assistant Professor, Department of Pharmacology, Vanderbilt
University, Nashville, Tennessee

William R. Martin, M.D.
Chief, Addiction Research Center, National Institute of
Mental Health, Lexington, Kentucky

For the people who really turn me on:

Kathy
Steve
Debbie GRANT
Chris GRANT
Tom

... substances which act on the brain
mock at all obstacles which oppose their extension.
Their attraction grows slowly,
silently, but surely.

Phantastica
L. Lewin, 1931

PREFACE

In these times an author needs a fairly good reason to justify yet another book whose major theme revolves around human drug use. Quite simply, I hope to partially fill the void at the center of the triangle formed by the fields of pharmacology, psychology, and history. This book will not make you an expert in these areas, but the material should be of considerable value to the pharmacologist, the psychologist, and the social historian. The material presented here is a potpourri (some of my friends have suggested I use the term "hash") of the facts, attitudes, and opinions necessary to understand what psychoactive drugs do, how they do it, who uses them, and why.

A drug has no effect in isolation—the effect is always on an individual, a unique person in a particular environment. To comprehend the kinds of effects a drug can have on behavior, you must not only learn about the drug but also know much about the drug user and his society—now and in historical perspective. Drug use is very much part of our cultural history, and some of our scientific and technological progress has come as a result of the push for more and newer psychoactive drugs. An understanding of the history of our present drugs and our present drug use is essential to appreciate the changes now rapidly occurring.

Many people feel that the current increase in drug use (drug misuse?) is an unusual phenomenon—a new experience for our civilization. Some have suggested that this increased drug use is a cancer that can be removed from our life—through laws or education—without affecting the fabric of our society. Contrary to this belief, one of my conclusions is that the increase in drug use now seen in our country is an integral part of our developing culture, and to eliminate it will require major changes in some of our beliefs and attitudes—changes that many may not support.

Usually in a preface some mention is made of the groups that might be particularly interested in the book. Originally the book was aimed at a college population—for use in a course I teach entitled "Drugs and Behavior." In introducing that course, and now this book, I say that no prior information is needed. We're going to start from scratch and do two things. First, the material will cover all that most people need and want to know about drugs and drug use—legal and illegal. Second, enough background and basic material will be presented so that the reader will be better able to understand the whys and wherefores of new drugs as they come on the scene.

Referencing a book such as this is difficult. I have referenced quotes and also those facts and opinions that do not appear either in the already cited material or in one of the standard books in this area. A smattering of these standard references is listed at the end of the book. It should be clear that neither the form of presentation, the opinions, nor the conclusions represent the views of the Veterans Administration.

To protect myself and the reader from errors of fact and interpretation, I asked friends who are authorities in the various areas of this book to read and comment on the next-to-final draft of the chapters in their area of expertise. They made many valuable suggestions and I acknowledge here that they may have saved me from myself. However, their assistance does not constitute an endorsement of the chapters; since they have not seen the final draft, the errors, if any, are mine. These expert friends are listed on pages v to vii.

Special acknowledgement for making this book possible goes to four people. Barbara Brocker, as a library research assistant, found journals and books the librarians did not know existed. A good secretary is important, but mine, Elsie Marklin, was essential. Robert Barrett, my friend and colleague, made it possible for me to write. Many thanks. Perhaps some people naturally write coherent, well-organized sequences of sentences. I suspect most of us don't. You need a friend with a red pencil. I have a friend with an inexhaustible supply of red pencils and Nancy Leith had the task of translating this book into English from my native Greek. For Jim Korn, John Parascandola, Gerald Schaefer, Jeannette Landis, and all the others who helped, many many thanks.

Oakley S. Ray

CONTENTS

UNIT

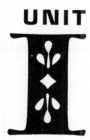

Introduction

1 Drug use: an overview

There'll be Bluebirds over THE WHITE CLIFFS OF DOVER
Tomorrow, just you wait and see
There'll be love and laughter and peace ever after,
Tomorrow, when the world is free
The Shepherd will tend his sheep, The valley will bloom again
And Jimmy will go to sleep, In his own little room again

> *The White Cliffs of Dover*

When the moon is in the seventh house
And Jupiter aligns with Mars
Then Peace will guide the Planets
And Love will steer the Stars
This is the Dawning of the Age of Aquarius . . .

Harmony and understanding
Sympathy and trust abounding
No more falsehoods or derisions
Golden living dreams of visions
Mystic Crystal Revelation
And the mind's true liberation

> *Aquarius*
> ©*1966, 1967, 1968 James Rado, Gerome Ragni, Galt MacDermot, Nat Shapiro*
> *and United Artists Music Co., Inc. All rights administered by United Artists*
> *Music Co., Inc., New York, New York 10019. Used by permission.*

In the year twenty-five twenty-five
If man is still alive.
If woman can survive they may find.
In the year thirty-five thirty-five
Ain't gonna need to tell the truth,
Tell no lies, Ev'rything you think do and say
Is in the pill you took today.

> *In The Year 2525*
> *Words and Music by Rick Evans*
> ©*Copyright 1968 Zerland Music Enterprises Ltd., New York, New York*
> *Used by permission.*

The increase in drug use and misuse can be viewed as a part of a rapidly developing biological revolution. It is not possible here to examine all the ramifications of the many rapid advances in the field of biology, but special note should be made of two of the broad issues.[1-4] First, it is no longer clear that all biomedical advances are seen as good for society. Until recently every step forward was clearly in the direction of solving a problem for which most people agreed a solution was needed. Now, certain advances are giving us the capability of accomplishing things that do not clearly solve one of society's problems.

This realization leads us directly to the second point. It is now obvious that the advances in biology and the biomedical fields have had very broad impact on our society— on our mores, on the way we view Man. Rather than just improving the quality of living that exists at the time of the breakthrough, these advances sometimes greatly change the character of our culture.

There have been many cultural changes that have resulted from some of the advances in the field of pharmacology. By reviewing these changes it is possible to set the scene for a consideration of our present use of drugs.

There have been literally hundreds of important drugs developed since the turn of the century.[5] The rate at which new compounds are being produced is now at a high point, and there is every indication that it will remain high, if not increase still more. In 1970 Dr. Stanley Yolles, then Director of the National Institute of Mental Health, predicted a one hundred-fold increase over the next 10 years in the number and type of drugs that would affect the mind.[6] Psychoactive drugs, chemicals that affect the mind, are and evermore shall be here to stay.

PHARMACOLOGICAL REVOLUTIONS

The first revolution is the one that brought the major communicable diseases well under control.[7] The use of vaccines, which began with Pasteur and Koch in the nineteenth century and is still continuing with the development of the rubella (measles) vaccine, has certainly had a major impact on our society. There are now thirteen established and effective vaccines. In 1954 there were over 18,000 cases of paralytic polio; in 1971 only nineteen cases occurred. The measles vaccine, first mass-produced in the United States in 1969, is 93% to 95% effective in preventing the disease in children. So it seems clear that another hurdle in the path of growing up is almost demolished. Students today don't know what a quarantine sign is—they've never seen one! Diphtheria and whooping cough are words that the pediatrician mumbles as he inoculates the baby. Protracted absence from school, long-term aftereffects from childhood disease, death of a young child—all these are no longer part of our culture, gone because of the development of techniques that can prevent most of the serious childhood illnesses.

The second pharmacological revolution resulted from the introduction of sulfa drugs, penicillin, and broad-spectrum antibiotic agents. Proved first in war, they continue to save and prolong lives in peacetime. This change in mortality and in the role of hospitals is ongoing. The increase in longevity (and thus the number of "senior citizens") and the utilization of hospitals as places to be treated and recover from illness are clearly shaping our economy and our politics (a la Medicare and Medicaid).

These two revolutions may be too pervasive and too close to home to impress anyone. This is not the case with the third pharmacological revolution: the advent of tranquilizers for the treatment of the mentally ill. (See Chapter 10.) The rapid development of tranquilizers in the early 1950's and the beginning of their widespread use in 1954 have resulted in many cultural effects. One of the most interesting, but little studied, cultural results was the realization that the tranquilizers are used for their effect on the mind, not on the body. The first two revolutions were aimed at restoring the physiological homeostasis that we call physical health. The tranquilizers introduced to the public the concept that drugs that act on the mind could be used to return one's mental health to normal. Not much was said about this different effect because mental illness was viewed as a disease, and tranquilizers were acting the *same way* an antibiotic did—to remove the disease!

The impact on our mental hospital population was more obvious. Between 1957 and 1967 there was a 33% decrease in the number of hospitalized schizophrenic persons in spite of an increasing population. The return of these schizophrenic individuals to the community and the prevention of hospitalization for others have had a major effect on the methods and models developed in the 1960's for the delivery of mental health services. The move to mental health centers and post-hospitalization programs is based on the fact that, with drugs, the major part of a treatment program can be accomplished outside a hospital. The singular effectiveness of tranquilizers, followed by considerable success with antidepressant agents in the late 1950's, clearly made chemotherapy the only effective procedure available for the treatment of severely disturbed individuals.

The fourth pharmacological revolution is still developing. Although its ultimate effect cannot be known now, some of its possible impact can be predicted with moderate confidence. This revolution is the development of the oral contraceptive. Still in preliminary stages are the "day-after" pill and sustained-release agents that would be effective for months or years. What additional impact these drugs, or oral contraceptives for males, will have cannot be predicted, but for the over 8 million American women now using oral contraceptives there has been a change in many attitudes and behaviors. How greatly the concept of "sex without worry" will accelerate certain trends in our society that were already obvious in the 1950's cannot be determined. It seems reasonable, though, that the demise of the family[8] as the basic unit of our social structure and the development of equal rights for women are both considerably advanced when concern over pregnancy is removed.

Of more interest here, however, is the fact that for the first time potent chemicals clearly labeled as drugs are being widely used by healthy people because of their social convenience. No longer are we eliminating infection to have a healthy body, nor are we reducing anxiety to have a better functioning mind. Now we are adding a drug to alter a healthy body and mind because of the convenience it offers in interpersonal contacts. This is a major shift in our thinking about drugs and is a result of, and a part of, our present credit card culture—instant pleasure!

There are two pharmacological revolutions that have been repeatedly predicted. One is the development of euphoriants. We have moved from drugs to cure the body, through drugs to cure the mind, to drugs that alter the body for our convenience and pleasure. The next step would be compounds that deliver the pleasure themselves. Why wake up in the morning and just feel good? Why not feel *really great*? Ecstatic! In 1949 one writer phrased it:

> And a time may come when people take Benzedrine in a suitably flavored drink for breakfast instead of coffee or tea, and before luncheon conferences instead of a cocktail. One day, maybe, we'll have to test students for Benzedrine before exams, the way we test race horses. It is doubtful that Benzedrine will ever be considered good form on the race track or in athletic events, but a time may come when, like liquor, it will be quite all right socially if you carry it like a gentleman.*

It may come. We are rapidly losing the Protestant Ethic that says you should enjoy life only after much hard work. With the development of drugs that are specific in their neural and behavioral effects, it is becoming possible to select the effect we want. As that happens we'll all turn on . . . easily, and regularly. Aldous Huxley foretold it in *Brave New World*,[9] and in a recent article[10] entitled *A Land of Lotus-Eaters?* it is observed that, in contrast to times past: ". . . everyone nowadays expects to be happy. Pills have come to be regarded as a means to do away with the everyday anxieties and pain. . . ."

Another drug revolution frequently mentioned is the development of chemicals that will increase our learning ability—smart pills![11, 12] If learning is, as it seems to be, dependent on the availability of certain neural connections in the central nervous system *and* on the effectiveness of those connections, then certain drugs should be potentially capable of increasing the efficiency of the neural

*From Lees, H.: Farewell to benzedrine benders, Collier's **124**:32, 1949.

connections that exist. Work with animals indicates that this is a real possibility.[13] Drug facilitation of learning in animals suggests that some (much, most?) of the variability in learning ability in humans may be eliminated. Interestingly, though, it may be the less bright that will be affected most by the drugs.

The social changes such a development suggests are immense. The one remaining legal basis for discrimination in this country is intelligence. The brighter people have the opportunity for education, better jobs, better salaries, and so on. If drugs could possibly make 80% to 90% of the population bright enough to benefit from a college education and to hold down high-level positions, how would we pick who gets the chance? Or would we see that everyone gets paid the same no matter what he does?

There are many revolutions in pharmacology that could be (and have been) predicted. No one knows, of course, what will happen, but the changes in social values and attitudes discussed here make it likely that there will be a very great increase in the use of psychoactive drugs by normal people in the next 30 years.[14]

DRUG-TAKING BEHAVIOR

In recent years there has been a tremendous increase in illegal drug use by individuals with healthy minds and bodies. These drugs are not used to improve physical health or to reduce symptoms of mental illness. How should we view this current upsurge in drug-taking behavior? What purpose does it serve? Why does it persist?

A neutral view suggests that this nonclinical drug-taking behavior can be seen as problem-solving behavior. Our society is searching for, and finding, new solutions to both old and new problems. Some of our difficulties develop because we have yet to reach an acceptable social standard on these new ways of solving problems. Finding a cultural norm in the area of drug use is particularly important since, as new drugs are produced, both the amount and pervasiveness of drug use will increase.

Why do people take drugs? Is drug taking a unique phenomenon? Are there no counterparts to it in our society? One thing that must

be understood is the fact that *drug taking is behavior!* As such it follows the same rules and principles as any other behavior, the most basic principle being that behavior persists when it either increases the individual's pleasure or reduces his discomfort. That is, people don't use just any old drug; they take only those that have *for them* either a positive, satisfying, pleasurable effect or those drugs that cause a decrease in their discomfort. And of those drugs that do increase pleasure or decrease discomfort, the particular ones selected must be acceptable within the individual's cultural group.

As with other behaviors, there are multiple causes underlying a person's drug-taking behavior. To look for a single reason for drug taking is to whistle in the wind. Studies with animals show that susceptibility to narcotic addiction is, in part, genetically determined, and strains of animals have been bred that are either very easy or very difficult to addict.[15] Similarly, strains of animals have been developed that prefer alcohol over water for drinking, although most animals will select water if given a choice.[16] There are suggestions that alcoholism in humans is partly based on the individual's heredity.

Drug taking (whether there is a genetic predisposition or not), like other behavior, is the result of a complex interaction of past experiences and present environment. It is possible to group some individuals together because of a commonality of history and environment and to predict whether or not they will probably use drugs as well as which class of drugs they will most likely use.[17, 17a, 17b] Drug taking has only recently been widely studied, so individual potential users cannot be readily identified. Groups of individuals can probably be selected who differ in their probability of drug use since there are some personality and background differences between those who use different classes of drugs.[18, 18a] Increasingly in the mid-1970's the trend is to multiple drug use: if it's available, try it![18b-d]

The primary point is that drug-taking behavior is not unique; it is like any other behavior. An appreciation of this goes a long way toward taking a rational look at current drug use. For example, a more common set of behaviors that approximates drug-taking behavior in motivation and effect is the "neuroses." Drug-taking behavior can be viewed as cut from the same cloth as neurotic behavior. The two have many similar characteristics, and possibly over the next several years some of the more traditional neurotic symptoms will gradually be replaced by drug taking. It may be that drug taking will just be superimposed on neurotic behavior, or vice versa. It follows that the same kinds of concern should be shown toward drug taking as toward neurotic patterns of behavior.

As is true of neurotic behavior, illegal drug taking offers the individual both benefits and disadvantages. The benefit is usually some short-term gain such as a more positive feeling or a decrease in discomfort. The disadvantages are multiple but more remote in time. For one, there is a decrease in the chance of reaching long-term, permanent solutions to the underlying problems. There is also, in our society, a probable decrease in the rewards an individual can obtain if he persists in repeated drug taking.

If this is a reasonable way of viewing drug taking, then the concern many people have about drug use should perhaps be shifted to include the fact that drug taking *may* have negative effects on the individual *only* when it becomes the dominant mode of problem solving. Taking drugs does solve immediate problems! It offers the individual short-term solutions. However, it may have adverse long-term effects either by preventing a better solution or by causing new problems to arise. In the case of some drugs, used in certain ways, it seems that adverse long-term effects are not only possible but almost inevitable for most people. (See Chapters 6 to 9 and 11 to 15.)

PSYCHOACTIVE DRUG EFFECTS

Thus far, the term "drug" has been used to indicate the generality of what has been said; the foregoing statements are true of all psychoactive drugs. There are so many kinds and classes of psychoactive drugs that to attempt to specify a few of them would be of little value. Are there any other general statements that can be made about psychoactive drugs—

those compounds that alter consciousness and affect mood? In fact, there are four basic principles that seem to apply to all of these drugs.

First, *drugs, per se, are not "good" or "bad."* There are no "bad drugs." When drug abuse is talked about, it is the behavior, the way the drug is being used, that is being referred to. The labeling of a particular use of a drug as an "abuse" requires the adoption of a particular set of values. All drugs, like most other things, can be used in ways that our society labels *bad* or *good.* These labels, though, have a way of shifting—sometimes gradually, sometimes rapidly.

This is not just a semantic matter. Some things can probably be labeled bad by everyone's standards: cancer, a tidal wave, and so forth. In most self-selected human behaviors there are both positive and negative factors to be considered before choosing to participate. Usually the more information available, the more the decision will be in line with what the individual really wants. You may agree to go for an automobile trip, taking a chance on becoming a statistic, but then change your mind when you see the car is in poor mechanical condition. You didn't want to take *that big* a chance!

Different factors will be given different weight by different people. Usually there are two phases in reaching a decision: is the behavior something that can even be conceived; if conceivable, do the advantages outweigh the disadvantages? Most 50 year olds cannot conceive of ever skydiving; it's an unthinkable thing. For many 20 year olds, however, it is something to be thought about, the pros and cons considered, and a real decision reached. To do this rationally, much information is needed.

The same is true with drugs. Using amphetamines under any conditions may be unthinkable and, since it's also illegal, labeled bad by some people. To many young people "using amphetamines" is a real possibility when the dose, the way the drug is taken, and the reason it's to be taken are brought into the picture. To label a drug "bad" categorically solves nothing and convinces no one.

A second basic, and often forgotten, fact

about psychoactive drugs is that *every drug has multiple effects.* Although a user may focus on a single aspect of a drug's effect, clearly we do not yet have compounds that alter only one aspect of consciousness. That a drug usually has many different effects on the individual using it might be expected from the fact that most drugs act at many different places in the brain.

This brings us to a third principle about psychoactive drug effects. *The effects of a drug depend on the amount the individual has taken.* This relationship between dose and effect works in two ways. By increasing the dose there is usually an accentuation of effects noticed at lower drug levels. Also, and frequently this is a more important relationship, at different dose levels there is often a change in the kind of effect, an alteration in the quality of the experience. Varying doses, then, can change not only the magnitude but also the character of the drug effect. Do certain dose levels constitute an abuse of a drug while other dose levels do not?

The fourth item of general relevance about psychoactive compounds is that *their effect, in part, depends on the individual's history and expectations.* Since these drugs act to alter consciousness and thought processes, the effect they have on an individual depends on what was there initially. The attitude an individual has can have a major effect on his perception of the drug experience. The fact that some people can experience a *real* high when smoking oregano and dry oak tree leaves—thinking it's good marijuana—should come as no surprise to anyone who has arrived late at a swinging cocktail party and found himself turned on after one martini rather than the usual two or three. It is not possible, then, to talk about many of the effects of these drugs independent of the user's attitude and the setting.

Reviewing some of the basic points before moving on to talk about society and the extent of psychoactive drug use, it seems well supported that the current increase in drug-taking behavior reflects (mainly) a general cultural change in the direction of beginning to see drugs as acceptable ways of solving problems. The answers drugs provide are usually only short-term solutions and may prevent the individual from finding a permanent, nondrug resolution to the problem.

Drugs have multiple effects that vary with the amount of the drug used and the personality of the user, as well as his expectancies about the effects of the drug. The reason people initially take drugs recreationally varies considerably but, at a very fundamental level, it is either to obtain a pleasurable experience or to reduce unhappiness. Whether or not a person decides to use drugs to solve problems depends on his background, his present environment, and the availability of drugs.

With respect to the last point, the availability of drugs is both a major and a minor item. If drugs were not available, obviously no one would be using them; thus, availability is at the very heart of the matter. Given, however, a culture in which many drugs and chemical substances are legally available and widely used, there will probably be a demand for, and the production of, additional illegal drugs. If drugs were the problem, the issue could be handled by shutting off the supply—a big job, perhaps one with undesirable social effects, but actually possible. The problem, though, is people, not drugs. Individuals are looking for rapid solutions to problems, and drugs are one of the options our society makes available.

CREDIT CARD CULTURE

There is a revolution under way. It is not like revolutions of the past. It has originated with the individual and with culture . . . It is now spreading with amazing rapidity, and already our laws, institutions, and social structure are changing in consequence.*

The present comes so quickly now that it's difficult to remember the past. To remember Pearl Harbor, Dunkirk and D-Day, the "real" Mrs. Miniver and not just the rose. To remember when General MacArthur was a pure hero—solid gold and 20 feet high. Adults who experienced these things grew up in a very different world from that of today. Not different just because we now have color television

*From Reich, C. A.: Reflections (the greening of America), The New Yorker **46:**42-46, September 26, 1970.

and MacDonald's and interstate highways and frozen pizza, but different in part because we have them. To be a child in the 1930's and 1940's was to grow up in a world that was predictable, but tough; a world that was black and white; a world where good guys clearly wore the larger cowboy hats.

Norman Rockwell was the Face of America and if Scattergood Baines did, once in a while, trick (he never cheated) someone, it was always one of the bad guys. *Everyone* read *The Saturday Evening Post* and/or *Collier's*. During World War II, the blue stars and the gold stars and the applause in the movie when the American flag appeared all made the country single-minded in purpose. Not now. Those days are long gone and may never return. If you do remember, you're not with it today, even though you may very much be an active participant in the current scene.

Out of that background came the man in the gray flannel suit who was determined to make up for lost time. These were the hard-working, nose-to-the-grindstone, quiet, young Americans who learned that we could have better living through chemistry and that progress *was* the most important product. College students in the 1950's were studied and described as "politically disinterested, apathetic, and conservative."[19]

When the rate of change in a society is slow, certain truths are self-evident and affect everyone's behavior. With moderate cultural movement the future is predictable. It is easy to feel secure extrapolating from where we are to where we will be in 10 to 20 or 50 years. With a predictable future you can make plans, follow through with them, and expect them to work out. As a guide to what you should plan for and educate for, you look to the past and see where society has been. With a slow rate of social change your personal and society's history are important in planning for the future.

The rate of social change has now been fueled to a high level by modern educational techniques and present technological capability. With a high rate of cultural change it is clear that the past is less relevant to the present than ever before. The future is less easily predicted from the past or the present.

A technological civilization has arrived and is having a major impact on human relationships.[20] Even though "the roots of the technocracy reach deep into our cultural past and are ultimately entangled in the scientific world-view of the Western tradition,"[21] it may be that technocracy will destroy those factors that brought it into being.

> The main feature of technological society is not merely rapid change, but, as its admirers have said, creative destruction. It not only destroys habits, beliefs, and institutions inherited from the past, but those which were created only yesterday. In a society where memory is an irritant because it impedes progress, concepts like "tradition" or categories like "the past" are mostly meaningless.*

Is there no stability anymore? In 20 years we may have the final answer. Without a doubt, the traditional institutions are no longer rocks. The churches are changing with their ecumenical movements, saying that those differences between churches that we used to teach are not really important. Similarly, the universities have decided to move into the community, to get involved, to become relevant. Since the expansion of funds for research and education in the 1950's, the halls of academe have become increasingly dependent on the federal dollar and thus, naturally, more responsive to federal needs and wants. Once the emphasis shifted from the university as a repository of thoughts and thinkers to a full-service bank meeting the needs of its supporters, it was destined to become less stable and more responsive to social pressures. Now, many universities are full-scale political arenas.

The family is also slowly following the dodo bird. In an agrarian society a family made a lot of sense and served a real purpose. Many young hands made it possible for the adult to handle more land and thus live better, so it was an advantage to have a large family. The children benefited too because in the family setting they could learn the roles and the skills

*From Schaar, J. H., and Wolin, S. S.: Education and the technological society, New York Review, October 9, 1969, p. 3. Reprinted with permission from The New York Review of Books. Copyright ©1969 NYREV, Inc.

they would need and use as adults.[8] Today? What does a child know about what his father does? What should he know? Why should he know anything? A child cannot participate in or even understand his father's work much of the time. As the number of working mothers increases—it's now 40%—the daughter will learn her adult role less and less from the mother. In home economics at school she'll learn what she needs to know about home-making, and in other courses they will teach her what she really needs to know to be an independent soul.

Hand in hand with the rapid rate of social change, we've undergone an information explosion. In science, the amount of information now doubles every 5 to 10 years, while in the early part of this century it took 50 years.[22] Probably of more importance is the information explosion everyone is experiencing as a result of new techniques in the mass media. Many people have commented on the influence the rapid transmission of information has had on the spread of certain kinds of social behavior, from fads to riots. As an example, the inter-university student radio communication system facilitated the spread of action and greatly strengthened the impact of student demon-strations following the Kent State shootings in the spring of 1970.

A more subtle result of the information explosion is of particular interest here. Because of the great amount of information we have available to us about everyone in public life, the young have no lasting, culturally integrated heroes.[23] Without heroes, without images to follow, boots to fill, people to respect, there is even less meaning to life. Knowing that public officials—potential heroes—are really politi-cians who have been merchandised like an antacid leaves little to believe in, except, perhaps, a consistently winning public rela-tions agency.

What can you believe in? If you can't trust the leaders, whom can you trust? You trust only those who have no particular bag. How do you show you've got nothing to gain, no big thing going? By being, by not having. By experiencing, by dropping out.

The world is no longer predictable; there are no more heroes. But the organization men of the 1950's and 1960's have made this an affluent society. This is another important determiner of the Aquarian and the hang-loose ethic. Because it is possible to live adequately with very little work (and if you've always had everything, it seems easier to give it up than if you have never had it), and because there is little training for achievement today, the Protestant Ethic is fast disappearing.[12, 19] Most middle-class adults grew into the economic, achievement-oriented people they are by being subjected directly and indirectly, consciously and unconsciously, to the Protestant Ethic. This belief in self-restraint, drive, and hard work as the way to get ahead and be happy is fast leaving the scene. Why work hard to have leisure time to enjoy life when you can work less, have more leisure time, and still survive?

The decline in the belief in the Protestant Ethic is, in part, based on the fact that at the same time an individual's personal future becomes more difficult to predict, and the likelihood of major upheavals in our culture increases, some things have become more pre-dictable for many people. The satisfaction of bodily needs is likely to become more and more sure as time goes on. That government will provide if you can't or won't is almost an axiom today. In addition, the graduated income tax and the narrowing of the range in the standard of living takes some edge off making it big for a lot of people. The number of college-educated taxi drivers must surely be at an all-time high. It is difficult to get involved and put in a lot of time getting ready for something that you may lose interest in. Or, even worse, the field may be an over-subscribed occupation by the time you are ready to work.

The Protestant Ethic is also diminishing because with each passing year the age at which puberty is reached decreases, while the age at which the individual leaves the youth category (the termination of schooling) in-creases. Each year, then, the period of social adolescence increases. The individual is treated as an adult in some respects, since physically he is an adult, and not in others— since he is still not emotionally or financially independent. The social adolescent is given many of the advantages of being an adult, but he doesn't have to work for them and he keeps the advantages of being young.[24]

Becoming an adult is a tricky business in the most stable of settings. Becoming independent and establishing a unique identity is especially difficult today. Social adolescence today is one big double bind, a period in which almost everything told to the youth is contradictory—double-edged. Be yourself—but don't let your hair grow down to your collar. Do what you want to do with your life, pick your profession—but don't pick your courses in school, they know best. Learn some responsibility—here's your allowance. Dress sexy, look sexy—but don't go all the way.

The young do learn some things. They do listen to the messages we send them every day. They're not rebelling against the establishment; they're outdoing the establishment. What the over-30 and over-40 groups are doing, the under-30 and under-20 groups are doing better! People wonder where the young get their ideas. People forget that the young are still learning rules to live by and forming basic beliefs about the way the world is and how it ought to be. The young get their ideas from the older generation, its ads, its behavior, whether the older generation knows it or not. A 40-year-old junior executive can watch one of the 1969 Peace Corps ads on TV—the take-off on "The Graduate" that ends with the phrase, "isn't there more to life than making money?"—and grunt that it's stupid or say that it's nice to help people but . . . , or he may simply ignore the ad and its message because it doesn't fit with what he believes. The 12 to 20 year old, though, doesn't have a lot invested in capitalism, in achieving, in making it. He may watch the ad and think—there must be more!

The magic word today is alienation. Alienation may be inevitable in a technologically oriented bureaucracy. Whether it is or not, clearly more and more people at all ages feel that they can no longer exert any influence on the social institutions that determine the options that are open to them in life. When an individual feels that his life is not predictable, partly because of groups and ideas beyond his influence and control, he has three options. He can drop out, as the hippies and many drug users have done. They are just saying: "If I can't help make the rules I'm to live by, I won't play your game. After all, you've been telling me for years in school and church and the mass media that I should think for myself. Why get up tight when I do?" Another option is taken by those who feel they know what changes they want. They don't just want a say in making the rules, they want certain rules—now! These are the social activists of the right and the left. Their aim is to establish certain premises as basic to the game, and they are willing to ruin the game if they can't have their way. The final group consists of the activists of the middle, those who try to initiate change within the system. The Peace Corps, the McCarthyites, the Robert Kennedy student workers all fit into this slice of the pie. There is, of course, a large silent majority at all ages, and the most that can be said of them is that they are at least satisfied enough with the status quo not to actively try to change it.

With no meaningful history and no foreseeable future, how can a person plan, why should he plan—what's there to grab hold of? The only thing to hold on to is the here-and-now, the immediate experience. And that's what it's all about today—the NOW generation. What's in the NOW?—experiences. What are experiences made of?—actions, sensations.

If you can't see the value of planning for the future, and if you live for the immediate experience, then anything that maximizes the experience—the sensations, the action—is good and true and beautiful. Drugs. Mysticism. Eastern religions. All have a primary emphasis on increasing one's capacity for experiencing. All of them are becoming increasingly important in the attitudes and behavior of today's youth. Even Christianity is undergoing a revival with the emphasis on inner experience. Youth rallies exhort the believers to "Turn on with Christ" and "Do your thing for God." Speaking in tongues is again in the land—and not just with the young.

There is even a movement in some areas from drugs to religion, but it is not the religion of the suburbs. Sometimes its relationship to the drug scene is clear.

Many of us were seeking thru drugs, and Eastern religious cults for truth and reality, but we found that the only way to the true and living God is thru our Lord Jesus Christ.*

In other cases there is a broader study of religion *as an experience* and its relationship to drug use and other cultural factors.

It has been our thesis that the model for understanding the campus apocalypse that best draws together the variety of activities in which students are involved is the religious model of the search for salvation. For the inward looking activities of drug use and sensitivity explorations, and for the fascination with the unusual in religions, the clearest explanation is that students are seeking to know themselves and one another as fully as possible, and to discover what it might be that unifies and brings together the disparate experiences of the young human being. They have turned to these things because more traditional patterns of growth and fulfillment afford little self-knowledge and tend to fragment rather than unite people, and because the institutions in which traditional paths to salvation are preserved have lost the seriousness of purpose that is required. For the most part, institutions concerned with growing up—church, school, family—have turned in upon themselves for self-preservation and have diminished thereby the sense of their own purpose. What these institutions have traditionally communicated to rising generations, students still want, but they feel that they have to seek it elsewhere.†

Being, not having, is a basic component of today's youth philosophy. You can *be* only if you've experienced—yourself, your environment, the world around you. The individualism in clothes, in actions, in thoughts, are all components of the Aquarian philosophy. Give to others as Aquarius the water-bearer gives; but first know yourself, be yourself, experience yourself, through drugs if necessary.

Is this attitude, this philosophy, this emphasis on the NOW, a cancer growing in society, a foreign body that doesn't represent the mainstream of our culture? Hardly. This grab-what-you-can-when-you-can approach to life is but one aspect of our credit card culture—instant pleasure! No need now to work and worry to earn your pleasure—like it, charge it! Why wait? Have it now, a small down payment and thirty-six easy monthly installments.

WHY DRUGS?

In view of the facts that our society has been rapidly moving toward a more comfortable life for more people, that there is a great increase in the amount of time we have available to do things other than try to survive, that these factors mean we are putting less pressure on our children to be like us, it should not be surprising that our culture is showing a considerable increase in the use of drugs and other asocial and antisocial behavior that is undermining the society of the 1930's and 1940's. This was brought out vividly in one study of college student drug use and the results summarized:

Use of drugs was more likely to occur among those students whose behavior, attitudes or values, and self-image were indicative of opposition to the traditional, established order. Such differences occurred regardless of those demographic characteristics of the students also related to drug use, such as sex, socioeconomic status, and religion.*

No single factor is the basis of all drug-taking behavior, and probably no individual's drug taking has only a single cause.[25] The search for an identity explains some drug taking, but there are many more reasons why young people take drugs. Illegal drug users take drugs, in part, for the same reasons legal drug users do: to reduce tension and anxiety, to remove fatigue or boredom, to influence mood, to change activity level, to facilitate social interactions, to feel good.

Some motivations for illegal drug use are probably different from those for legal use: curiosity—I wonder what would happen if? A particularly hazardous (stupid?) form of this is the "punch party." Everyone brings one of

---

*From Klenk, R.: The 23rd psalm, handout of the organization, "The 23rd Psalm Ministries," Nashville, Tennessee, 1970.
†Reprinted with permission. From Rogan, D. L.: Campus apocalypse: the student search today, New York, 1969, The Seabury Press, Inc., p. 140. Copyright 1969 by The Seabury Press.

*From Suchman, E. A.: The "hang-loose" ethic and the spirit of drug use, Journal of Health and Social Behavior 9:146-155, 1968.

each kind of pill he can find at home and puts them into a dry punch bowl. You close your eyes, reach in, take a pill, and down it with water. If there's no effect in 15 minutes, you take another pill from the punch bowl and continue until you get an effect, get sick, or the party's over.

There is no question that many young people try some drugs—like marijuana—because it's a fad and "all the kids are doing it," even though *not all* are doing it. This is reminiscent of the reason many people in earlier generations got introduced to alcohol in one of its forms.

In the antitechnological, antiscientific, religious-mystic individuals there may be a high incidence of drug use. Following the lead of Aldous Huxley and Timothy Leary, some people search for religious experiences through drugs. And, in fact, some probably find them there. Too few drug users appreciate Leary's statements that there are other, nondrug ways of assuring a religious experience. Drugs, for Leary, seem to be a shortcut, not the only way to a religious experience.

Last, but perhaps not least, illegal drug taking in the young sometimes occurs just to aggravate the parents.

> Speak roughly to your little boy,
>   And beat him when he sneezes;
> He only does it to annoy,
>   Because he knows it teases.*

Drug taking is an almost guaranteed way to upset parents since there are many aspects of drug taking that can bother them—it's illegal, it may harm the user, it's a rejection of social standards and mores, and, most importantly, it's a denial of the value and the meaning of the parents' life and way of living. Since many parents only live for the future through their children, the threat of losing this link to the future is particularly disruptive. This possibility has been vividly phrased:

> Why, one wonders, is the older generation so perturbed at the spectacle of their children experimenting with mind-expanding drugs? It is not simply a realistic concern for their welfare. If this were all, the older people would be equally concerned to prevent their children from acquiring the habit of overindulgence in alcohol and in cigarette smoking. I suggest that the real cause for this exaggerated concern is recognition of the fact that young people are deliberately challenging, and in many cases repudiating, the values which their elders have lived by; and it is this which we of the older generation find so hard to tolerate.*

DRUGS AND DRUG USE TODAY

If the credit card culture encourages drug use and drug use supports and extends the credit card culture and denies the Protestant Ethic as a philosophy of life while substituting the Aquarian and hang-loose ethic, there should be widespread use of psychoactive drugs today. And there is. In all, Americans spend over $30 billion each year for legal chemicals that alter consciousness, awareness, or mood.

There are four classes of commercially available and legal psychoactive drugs. The group of compounds most people think of as "drugs" are the prescription drugs. These are compounds that require a physician's prescription to purchase legally, and they comprise a large market. In 1970 $8.4 billion was spent for over 2 billion prescriptions. About 30% of all prescriptions are for drugs that act on the brain, making this class of compounds the most commonly prescribed group. Importantly, 70% of all prescriptions written today are for drugs unknown 20 years ago.

Another group of psychoactive agents are those called over-the-counter (OTC) drugs. These drugs are intended for temporary medication of minor illnesses and are considered safe for use without a physician's supervision if the instructions on the label are followed carefully. Unfortunately this is frequently not done, and the potential dangers of these drugs are not appreciated. As one example of the problem with these compounds, in 1972 in the United States over 8,000 children under the age of 5 were poisoned by aspirin, a decrease from 14,500 in 1969.

Over-the-counter compounds are a big busi-

*From Carroll, L.: Alice in Wonderland, London, 1865, The Macmillan Company.

*From Carstairs, G. M.: A land of lotus-eaters? American Journal of Psychiatry **125**:1576-1580, 1969. Copyrighted 1969, The American Psychiatric Association.

ness and getting bigger all the time. Over $4 billion was laid out in 1973 by the American consumer for this class of products.

The third class of mood- and consciousness-altering chemicals legally available in this country includes the social drugs: alcohol, caffeine, and nicotine. Some governmental control is exerted over the purchase of products containing alcohol and nicotine but, in spite of these restrictions, the social drug business is extremely large. Americans yearly spend about $25 billion on alcoholic beverages, $12 billion on cigars and cigarettes, and $2.5 billion on coffee, tea, and cocoa. For comparison with the dollar figures it may be noted that in 1972 Americans spent a total of $49 billion on public school education.

The last group of psychoactive compounds is quite different from the other agents that are manufactured and merchandised for their psychoactive effect. This final group includes many compounds and items sold for nondrug purposes that, under some conditions, do have effects on mood and awareness. Substances such as airplane glue, certain herbs like nutmeg, and the seeds from some morning glory plants all have been used for their psychoactive properties.

With drugs and other psychoactive agents readily available and a large amount of money spent each year on these compounds, it would be expected that a very high percentage of the population uses one type drug or another. Excluding the social drugs and those agents that are marketed for nondrug purposes, a good place to start looking at drug use in the United States today is your drug cabinet. Count the number of different drugs you have stashed away. It will probably surprise you—the leftover drugs from last winter's colds and other illnesses, plus the basic "necessary" drugs, plus... . A study by the Stanford Research Institute found that the average household had thirty drugs.[26] One out of five was a prescription item, but the other four were over-the-counter drugs that could be bought by anyone in any amounts. With many homes containing twenty to thirty different drugs, it should not be a shock that in 1971 56% of the adults in a national Gallup-type survey reported that at some time in their life they had used a psychoactive drug—that is, a drug whose primary effect is on the brain and on mood and/or consciousness.[26a] Perhaps more shocking is the finding that only 7% had reported using tranquilizers in the year 1957 while 27% admitted using them in the year 1967.[27]

In another study it was found that:

...Men...are most likely to report use of stimulants in their 30s, tranquilizers in their 40s and 50s, and sedatives from age 60 on.... Women...are most likely to report use of stimulants throughout the age period 21 through 39...frequent use of tranquilizers occurs most often among women in their thirties...With respect to sedatives, use patterns are similar for men and women—the proportion of frequent users increases steadily with advancing age.*

It is almost as if the 30- to 40-year-old group were trying to hold on to some of the zip and stamina they had in their twenties. The slings and arrows and tensions and anxieties of the middle-aged, 40 to 60, are not unexpected with the problems accompanying growing children and the attempt to establish oneself in a job. After 60 it might be that sedative use increases because the fun has gone from fighting and trying and, rather than just take the nervous edge off living, it is preferable to blot it out with drugs.

An interesting sex difference in drug use is that, in 1967, 53% of the population were women but they made 59% of the visits to doctors and accounted for 68% of all prescriptions for psychoactive drugs. It is not that females just generally require more medication. As the illness becomes more physical in nature the percentage of prescriptions issued to women is more in line with their visits to a physician.[28] The finding that more psychoactive drug prescriptions are issued to women than men is compatible with some other results, namely that about four times as many men as women are alcoholics and narcotic addicts. Similarly, there are three to five male suicides for every female suicide. It must be that there are differences in our society in

*From Manheimer, D., Mellinger, G., and Balter, M.: Psychotherapeutic drugs—use among adults in California, California Medicine **109**:445-451, 1968.

the way the two sexes seek relief from stress and anxiety.

Different religious groups also vary in psychoactive drug use, with Jews reporting the highest incidence—about 47%—and liberal Protestants, conservative Protestants, and Catholics, in that order, having fewer legal drug users.[27] This is consonant with reports that Jews have a higher incidence of neurosis but a lower rate of alcoholism than members of the other religious groups.

Drugs are obviously very much an essential part of modern medical practice. The question is whether drugs are overused. There is no clear answer but some findings are pertinent. A report from researchers at Johns Hopkins Hospital indicated that the average number of different drugs given a hospitalized patient without infection is eight, while those with infection received eleven different drugs— some receiving none, with others receiving as many as forty-two.[29] These results are in line with other studies reporting that patients on medical services average ten to fourteen different drugs during hospitalization. In a study of five Boston hospitals it was generally found that older patients received more drugs than younger ones and females more than males.[30]

The effect of so many drugs on a patient is not necessarily good. Of particular interest is the fact that there was a direct relationship between the number of drugs used in treatment and the number of adverse side effects from drugs. This relationship was reported at Tufts University in a study of a Boston hospital. The study involved 7,078 consecutive uses of drugs on 830 patients.[31] There were 405 adverse drug reactions—6% of the drug administrations resulted in a negative reaction in the patient! About 35% of the patients had at least one adverse side effect. "Twenty-six percent of the reactions were life threatening, and 12% led to prolongation of hospitalization." The single most important cause of the adverse reactions (22%) was the interaction between drugs given to the patient.

The negative aspects of medical drug use have been emphasized since some authorities are now raising the question of whether too many drugs are being used and whether they

are being used indiscriminately.[32] Some clinicians[32a] and researchers[32b] have suggested that many patients with emotional problems are undermedicated, not overmedicated. As with all such issues, until there are clear criteria there will be no final answer. It must be remembered that the use of the drugs that cause adverse reactions in a few have had therapeutic effect on many. The question is: can we use therapeutic drugs more wisely?

The illegal use of drugs is not as widespread as the use of legal drugs, although accurate estimates of illegal use are not available. The best estimates are that 14% of all adolescents and 16% of all adults had at least tried marijuana by 1972.[26a] In the same year the federal estimate of heroin addicts in this country was 550,000.[32c] One report suggests that there may be 100,000 heroin users in Harlem itself.[33]

There are many facts that could be marshalled to emphasize the fact that drug use is on the increase. Department of Defense officials state that about 25% to 30% of all United States servicemen, and perhaps 70% of those in Vietnam, have experimented with illegal drugs,[34] while in another report they show that the number of civilians rejected from the service because of drug use was 391 in 1964 but over 2,600 in 1969.[35] The number of people who have tried one or more of the potent illegal psychoactive agents has been estimated from one in a hundred to one in a thousand. Whatever the actual incidence of use of the illegal psychoactive drugs, it is increasing regularly and the age at which it occurs has decreased each year. As the incidence increases the number of negative reactions is bound to go up. This fact, plus the prevalent feeling that the use of drugs as a way of life is not desirable, has made many citizens of all ages up tight.

This public concern over drug use is reflected in two nationwide surveys completed in the spring of 1971.[36] Sixty-four percent of the individuals polled felt that the United States was heading in the wrong direction, and almost half were pessimistic about the future of this country. The people questioned believed that there was a real possibility of a social breakdown in the United States, and almost half felt that drug use was the major reason why the nation is on the wrong track.[37] A 1971 Gallup Poll found drug use to be considered the United States' third most pressing problem. Times change. By September, 1973, drugs were only sixth. Even so, about half of those polled felt the quality of life was deteriorating in America.

CONCLUDING COMMENT

The focus in this chapter has been on the general factors in our cultural and scientific history that have led us to where we are today—a nation of drug users. Throughout the remainder of this book that fact will be documented, and there will be an attempt to illustrate similar patterns of behavior in other times and with other drugs. It is not that our present condition is just another repeat performance of what has happened before—it isn't, there are important differences this time in the kinds of drugs, the potency of the drugs, and the way the drugs are taken. Drug use today is having more influence on the entire society than ever before. A historical approach is not a search for answers in the past to present problems. Rather it is to gain a full understanding of the present problem so that effective solutions can be found. Winston Churchill said it best:

The farther backward you can look, the farther forward you are likely to see.

PRECEDING QUOTES

1. Burton, N., and Kent, W.: The White Cliffs of Dover, New York, Shapiro, Bernstein & Co., Inc.
2. Ragni, G., and Rado, J.: Aquarius, New York, United Artists Music Co., Inc.
3. Evans, R.: In the Year 2525, New York, Zerland Music Enterprises, Ltd.

REFERENCES

1. Crick, F.: The social impact of biology. Cited in Nature 220:429, 1968.
2. Platt, J. R.: The step to man, Science 149:607-613, 1965.
3. Potter, V. R.: Society and science, Science 146:1018-1022, 1964.
4. Kinzel, A. B.: Engineering, civilization, and society, Science 156:1343-1345, 1967.
5. Davies, W.: The pharmaceutical industry, London, 1967, Pergamon Press, pp. 1-22.
6. Yolles, S. F.: The drug phenomenon, Journal of the American Pharmaceutical Association NS10(7):403-407, 1970.
7. Stafford, R. O.: The growth of American pharmaceutical biology, BioScience 16:675-679, 1966.
8. Morison, R. S.: Where is biology taking us? Science 155:429-433, 1967.
9. Huxley, A.: Brave new world, London, 1932, Chatto, Chatto, and Windus.
10. Carstairs, G. M.: A land of lotus-eaters? American Journal of Psychiatry 125:1576-1580, 1969.
11. Gattozzi, A.: Drugs and patients: evaluating chemicals that change human behavior. In Mental Health Reports 2, Public Health Service Publication No. 1743, February, 1968.
12. Klerman, G. L.: Drugs and social values, International Journal of Addictions 5(2):313-321, 1970.
13. McGaugh, J. L.: Drug facilitation of memory and learning. In Efron, D., editor: Psychopharmacology: a review of progress 1957-1967, Public Health Service Publication No. 1968, pp. 891-904.
14. Evans, W., and Kline, N., editors: Psychotropic drugs in the year 2000: use by normal humans, New York, 1971, McGraw-Hill Book Co.
15. Nichols, J. R.: Addiction liability of albino rats: breeding for quantitative differences in morphine drinking, Science 157:561-563, 1967.
16. Segovia-Riquelme, N., and others: Nutritional and genetic factors in the appetite for alcohol. In Popham, R. E., editor: Alcohol and alcoholism, Toronto, 1970, University of Toronto Press, pp. 86-96.
17. Blum, R.: Social and epidemiological aspects of psychopharmacology. In Joyce, C. R. B., editor: Psychopharmacology: dimensions and perspectives, Philadelphia, 1968, J. B. Lippincott Co., pp. 243-282.
17a. Friedlob, J. W.: The relationship between birth order and drug dependence, unpublished thesis for the master of science degree, The University of Tennessee, Knoxville, March, 1973.
17b. Louria, D. B., Lavenhar, M. A., and Sheffet, A.: The epidemiology of drug abuse with some comments on prevention, Adolescent Drug Abuse, February, 1973, pp. 11-21.
18. Robbins, L., Robbins, E. S., and Stern, M.: Psychological and environmental factors associated with drug abuse, Drug Dependence (National Institute for Mental Health) 5:1-6, 1970.
18a. Braucht, G. N., Brakarsh, D., Follingstad, D., and Berry, K. L.: Deviant drug use in adolescence: a review of psychosocial correlates, Psychological Bulletin 79(2):92-106, 1973.
18b. Thompson, R. E.: Pattern of multiple drug abuse among adolescents, letters to the editor, Pediatrics 49(1):152-153, 1972.
18c. Markham, J. M.: Mixing of illicit drugs is increasing as the spread of heroin addiction slows, New York Times, March 25, 1973.
18d. Pilot poly-drug treatment program, Drugs and Drug Abuse Education Newsletter 4(7), July, 1973.
19. Suchman, E. A.: The "hang-loose" ethic and

the spirit of drug use, Journal of Health and Social Behavior **9**:146-155, 1968.

20. Ruesch, J.: Technological civilization and human affairs, Journal of Nervous and Mental Disease **145**:193-205, 1967.

21. Rosayk, T.: The making of a counter culture, Garden City, N. Y. 1969, Anchor Books, p. 7.

22. White, D.: The challenge of change. In Biomedical communications: problems and resources, Annals of the New York Academy of Sciences **142**:405-414, 1967.

23. Fort, J.: The pleasure seekers, New York, 1969, The Bobbs-Merrill Co., Inc., pp. 212-213.

24. King, S. H.: Youth in rebellion: an historical perspective, Drug Dependence **2**:5-9, 1969.

25. Hollister, L. E.: Education versus legislation as a way of influencing patterns of drug use, talk given at the 8th Annual Meeting of American College of Neuropsychopharmacology, February, 1970.

26. Roney, J. G., and Nall, M. L.: Medication practices in a community: an exploratory study, research report, Menlo Park, California, 1966, Stanford Research Institute.

26a. Drug use in America: problem in perspective, Second report of the National Commission on Marihuana and Drug Abuse, March, 1973.

27. Parry, H. J.: Use of psychotropic drugs by U. S. adults, Public Health Reports **83**(10):799-810, 1968.

28. Balter, M. B.: The use of drugs in contemporary society, presented at the 14th Annual Conference Veterans Administration Cooperative Studies in Psychiatry, Houston, Texas, April 1, 1969; Highlights of the Conference, Washington, D. C., 1969, Veterans Administration.

29. Smith, J. W., Seidl, L. G., and Cluff, L. E.: Studies on the epidemiology of adverse drug reactions, V. Clinical factors influencing susceptibility, Annals of Internal Medicine **65**(4):629-640, 1966.

30. Seidl, L. G., and others: Studies on the epidemiology of adverse drug reactions, III. Reactions in patients on a general medical service, Bulletin Johns Hopkins Hospital **119**:299-315, 1966.

31. Borda, I. T., Slone, D., and Jick, H.: Assessment of adverse reactions within a drug surveillance program, Journal of the American Medical Association **205**(9):645-647, 1968.

32. Lasagna, L.: The diseases drugs cause, Perspectives in Biology and Medicine **7**:457-470, 1964.

32a. Kline, N. S.: The under-medicated patient, American Druggist, January 24, 1972, pp. 29-30.

32b. Balter, M., and Levine, J.: Character and extent of psychotherapeutic drug usage in the United States. Presented at the Fifth World Congress on Psychiatry, Mexico City, November 30, 1971.

32c. Statement of Dr. Jerome H. Jaffe, Director of the Special Action Office for Drug Abuse Prevention before the House Committee on Government Operations Special Studies Committee, May 1, 1973.

33. Hunsinger, S.: The search for solutions, Christian Science Monitor, August 26, 1970, p. 9.

34. Ashworth, G. W.: What is being done about it, Christian Science Monitor, July, 1970, p. 10.

35. PotPorri, If (monthly newsletter from the National Coordinating Council on Drug Abuse Education and Information) **3**(1):8, 1971.

36. Sixty-four percent in poll say U. S. is on wrong track, New York Times, July 9, 1971, p. 10.

37. Bartley, R. L.: Failure of nerve: message for today? The Wall Street Journal, April 12, 1971.

2 Regulation of drug use

I pledge to you that the new Attorney General will open a new front against the pill peddlers and the narcotics peddlers who are corrupting the lives of the children of this country.

> *Richard M. Nixon*
> *August, 1968*

Within the last decade, the abuse of drugs has grown from essentially a local police problem into a serious national threat to the personal health and safety of millions of Americans.

A national awareness of the gravity of the situation is needed; a new urgency and concerted national policy are needed at the federal level to begin to cope with this growing menace to the general welfare of the United States.

> *President Richard M. Nixon*
> *July, 1969*

The answer is not more penalties, the answer is information.

> *President Richard M. Nixon*
> *December, 1969*

...the deliberate procedures embodied in present efforts to control drug abuse are not sufficient in themselves. The problem has assumed the dimensions of a national emergency.... America's Public Enemy No. 1 is drug abuse.

> *President Richard M. Nixon*
> *June, 1971*

...the fundamental problem of drugs...gets down to why — why do people take them? There we find the fundamental challenge of our time...as a society comes to the point where there is negativism, defeatism, a sense of alienation, it is inevitable that younger people will give up. They will turn to drugs...

> *President Richard M. Nixon*
> *July, 1971*

17

With all the hubbub nowadays, it might appear that illegal drug use is a new phenomenon and that until a few years ago there were no laws governing the use of drugs. Nothing could be more wrong. In the United States, drug addiction became a major problem after the Civil War. There were probably three factors that contributed to widespread narcotic addiction in the last third of the nineteenth century. One was the invention of the hypodermic syringe in 1853. Although Sir Christopher Wren as early as 1656 had injected through the skin, the procedure was quite crude and involved first making a slit in the skin with a knife and then using a dull quill.

The hypodermic syringe was introduced to the United States in 1856 and was used on a large scale for the first time in the Civil War. Injecting morphine, the primary active ingredient in opium, gave near-immediate relief from pain. Morphine was used widely, and not always wisely, in the treatment of the two major afflictions in the Civil War—pain and dysentery. So many soldiers became addicted to morphine because of imprudent medical use that addiction was called the "soldier's disease" or the "army disease" in the years following the war.

The second development that contributed to an increase in narcotic addiction following the War Between the States was the importation of Chinese workers to help build the rapidly expanding railroads. The Chinese brought with them the habit of smoking opium. As always happens when a new pleasure is introduced into a society, the practice of opium smoking spread rapidly. A contemporary report in 1882 outlined the spread of opium smoking in San Francisco.

> The practice spread rapidly and quietly among this class of gamblers and prostitutes until the latter part of 1875, at which time the authorities became cognizant of the fact, and finding, upon investigation, that many women and young girls, as also young men of respectable family, were being induced to visit the dens, where they were ruined morally and otherwise, a city ordinance was passed forbidding the practice under penalty of a heavy fine or imprisonment, or both. Many arrests were made, and the punishment was prompt and thorough.*

This San Francisco act was the first ordinance in America forbidding opium-smoking, and in 1882 New York State passed a similar law aimed at opium use in New York City's expanding Chinatown.

The broadest impact on narcotic use in this country probably came from neither of these factors but instead from the widespread legal distribution of patent medicines. These patent medicines were dispensed by traveling peddlers and were readily available at local stores for self-medication. Sales of these patent medicines increased from $3.5 million in 1859 to $74 million in 1904. The names of these well-advertised cure-alls are no longer familiar—for example, Pierce's Golden Medical Discovery and Mrs. Winslow's Soothing Syrup—but some of the general names for agents popular then are still in use. Paregoric (a Greek word meaning soothing) is an elixir containing 1 grain of opium to 480 drops of alcohol; it was made a prescription drug only in June, 1972. Laudanum, which dates from about the year 1500, is the miracle drug every doctor uses in western movies and is even more potent. It contains 1 grain of opium for every 25 drops of alcohol.

As a result of these three factors—the hypodermic syringe, Chinese workers, and patent medicines—it was estimated that around the turn of the present century one individual out of every 500 in this country was physically dependent on some form of opium or its derivatives.

EARLY REGULATIONS

Although alcohol had been taxed (and thus controlled) since the early years of the republic, opium importation was not taxed until 1842. The tax levied against crude opium brought into this country for medical purposes fluctuated considerably up to about 1900. In the 1850's it became clear that most of the opium being imported was not for medical purposes but for smoking. In 1864 smoking opium was identified for the first

*From Kane, H. H.: Opium-smoking in America and China, New York, 1882, G. P. Putnam's Sons.

time as containing less than 9% morphine and was taxed separately. By 1890 the tax on smoking opium had increased to $12.00 a pound and the amount brought through customs decreased. When the tax was lowered in 1897, the amount of legally imported smoking opium increased again. Through all of these tax changes the amount of smoking opium actually brought into this country gradually increased. When import taxes were low, a large percentage of smoking opium entered legally. As taxes increased it became worthwhile to smuggle opium, and the amount entering legally decreased. The 1890 act also, for the first time, permitted only American citizens to manufacture smoking opium.

Within the boundaries of the United States there was increasing conflict between the steady progress of medical science and the therapeutic claims of the patent medicine hucksters. The alcohol and/or narcotic content of the patent medicines was also a matter of concern. One medicine, Hostetter's Bitters, was 44% alcohol while another, Birney's Catarrh Cure, was 4% cocaine. In October, 1905, *Collier's Magazine* culminated a prolonged attack on patent medicines with a well-documented, aggressive series, entitled "The Great American Fraud."[1] The American Medical Association, continuing the effort, reprinted the series and sold it for a nominal price to half a million Americans.

Responding to pressure from scientists and physicians President Theodore Roosevelt, in his annual message in December of 1905, recommended: "...that a law be enacted to regulate interstate commerce in misbranded and adulterated foods, drinks, and drugs."[2] In 1906 publication of Upton Sinclair's *The Jungle,* exposing the horribly unsanitary conditions in the meat packing industry, shocked Congress and America. It was the necessary straw that 5 months later, on the thirtieth of June, 1906, led to the passage of the Pure Food and Drugs Act, which prohibited the interstate commerce of adulterated or misbranded foods and drugs.

In defining the word "drug," the act referred to those compounds listed in the United States Pharmacopeia (USP) and the National Formulary (NF) and designated their drug standards as the legal basis for enforcing the law on adulteration. The United States Pharmacopeia, started in 1820, and the National Formulary, begun in 1888, are continually revised, nongovernmental compilations of the best available drugs. They also list established names and minimum standards for the listed drugs and their dosage forms. Beginning with the 1906 law, if a product used one of the USP or NF names it had to contain the ingredients listed in the USP or NF, and no listing of the ingredients was required on the label. If a medicine failed to meet these standards, the label had to clearly indicate what the product did contain.

It was the 1906 act that began the decline of patent medicines because, in the section on misbranding, the act specifically referred to alcohol, morphine, opium, cocaine, heroin, *Cannabis indica* (marijuana), and several other agents. Each package was required to state how much (or what proportion) of these drugs was included in the preparation. This meant, for example, that the widely sold "cures" for morphine addiction had to indicate that they in fact contained another addicting drug.[3]

The 1906 Food and Drug Act did not regulate imports of addicting drugs. That remained for the Opium Exclusion Act of 1909 to do. This 1909 act prohibited the importing of opium or its derivatives except for medical purposes and was regulated by the Secretary of the Treasury. Two items in this act are worthy of comment. The act only made it illegal to import opium for nonmedical use; it was not illegal to use or manufacture opium for nonmedical purposes. Second, there was a 2-month delay between the enactment of the bill (February) and when it went into effect (April). In this 2-month period over 100,000 pounds of smoking opium were brought into this country, although in the entire calendar year of 1908 only 147,000 pounds had been imported.

NARCOTIC RULES AND REGULATIONS, 1914 TO 1970

The basic narcotic control law in the United States until May of 1971 was the Harrison Act of 1914. In 1914 for the first time dealers and dispensers of narcotics (opium, cocaine, and their derivatives) had to register annually with the Treasury Department's Bureau of Internal Revenue, which was also charged with enforcement of the law. Physicians, dentists, and veterinary surgeons were named as potential lawful distributors if they registered. This was not a punitive act, penalties for violation were not severe, and the measure contained no references to users of narcotics. The Harrison Act specifically supported the continued legality of the 1906 and 1909 laws and was primarily aimed at regulation and control of the narcotic drug traffic. In 1914 it was estimated that about 200,000 Americans—one in 400—were addicted to opium or its derivatives. The Harrison Act was the first step toward making it impossible for addicts to obtain their drugs legally. The result was the development of an illicit drug trade that charged users up to fifty times more than the legal retail drug price.

Two decisions by the United States Supreme Court were important in this period in making it more difficult for the addict to obtain drugs legally. In the Webb case, decided in 1919, the court declared that it was not legal for a physician to prescribe narcotic drugs to an addict for the purpose of maintaining his use and comfort. That is, narcotics could not be administered just to keep the user from developing withdrawal symptoms.[4] The 1922 Behrman case went one step further, declaring that a narcotic prescription for an addict was not legal even if the narcotic drugs were prescribed as part of a cure program.[5] In brief, these two Supreme Court decisions said there was no legal way for an addict to continue his habit at any level. The addict was forced to look for his drugs in the illegal market.

Partly in response to this growing illicit market, Congress passed the Jones-Miller Act of 1922, which more than doubled the maximum penalties for dealing with illegally imported narcotics to $5,000 and 10 years' imprisonment. This act limited imports to *crude* opium and coca leaves for medical purposes and established the Federal Narcotics Control Board to initiate an active program against smugglers. Included also was the stipulation that the mere possession of illegally obtained narcotics was sufficient basis for conviction. In 1924 another act prohibiting importing opium for the manufacture of heroin was passed. (It should be mentioned that as a result of this law and an early amendment, it is illegal to possess heroin in the United States except for research purposes. Any heroin supply has thus been clearly obtained illegally.) In 1925 the Supreme Court reversed itself. In the Linder case it declared addiction an illness and said it was legal for a physician to prescribe narcotics for an addict if it was part of a curing (that is, elimination of the addiction) program.[6]

Around 1930 several changes with lasting impact were made in the American handling of illegal narcotic use. Narcotic addiction in this period became a major problem for federal prisons. In 1928 individuals sentenced for narcotic drug–law offenses made up one-third of the total prison population. Interestingly, since this was during prohibition, this number was twice as many individuals as those imprisoned for liquor-law violations.[7] Responding to pressure for action, in 1929 Congress established two narcotic farms for the treatment of persons addicted to habit-forming drugs who had been convicted of breaking a federal law. Included among the habit-forming drugs, in addition to opium and its derivatives, were Indian hemp (marijuana) and peyote (of which mescaline is the active agent). A social definition of an addict was used in this Revenue Act of May 29, 1928:

> Any person who habitually uses any habit-forming narcotic drug as defined in this chapter (of this Act) so as to endanger the public morals, health, safety, or welfare, or who has been so far addicted to the use of such habit-forming narcotic drug as to have lost the power of self-control with reference to his addiction.

Two farms were established—one in Fort Worth, Texas, for all males west of the Mississippi River, and the better-known institution at Lexington, Kentucky, for males east of the Mississippi and females from all over the country. The Lexington facility opened in 1935 and generally held about 1,000 patients, two-thirds of whom were prisoners. Although it was a Public Health Service Hospital, with an internationally famous narcotic research facility, the Lexington farm was primarily a prison. In 1967 the National Institute of Mental Health took over the hospital and developed a modern rehabilitation program. In February, 1974, the treatment units (but not the research facility) became part of the Bureau of Prisons to be used for federal prisoners with a history of drug abuse.

In addition to establishing the two narcotic farms, in 1930 Congress took several actions that culminated in the formation of a separate Bureau of Narcotics in the Treasury Department. This bureau assumed all the duties that had previously been the responsibility of the Federal Narcotics Control Board and continued in operation until April, 1968, when it became part of a new group, the Bureau of Narcotics and Dangerous Drugs in the Department of Justice.

The Commissioner of Narcotics, the head of the Bureau of Narcotics, was appointed by the president. Harry Anslinger was the first commissioner and he remained in that position until 1962 when he retired. Mr. Anslinger had a background in foreign service and was regularly reappointed by new presidents just as was FBI Director, J. Edgar Hoover. As Hoover had great impact on federal criminal and espionage laws, Anslinger became a personality, nationally and internationally, who exerted considerable influence on narcotic legislation for the period of his tenure. He was tough-minded in the area of drug use and early in his career led the fight that resulted in the passage of the Marijuana Tax Act of 1937. In 1956 he was one of the individuals responsible for the passage of the Narcotic Drug Control Act, which included the death penalty for anyone selling heroin to a person under 18. He commented on that particular provision by saying: "I'd like to throw the switch myself on drug peddlers who sell their poisons to minors."[8]

It should be clear that these laws, which were concerned with regulating the importation and manufacturing of drugs, were primarily aimed at the opiates and cocaine. In the 1930's another drug problem began to occupy the public eye—marijuana. Marijuana had been smoked in this country for many years and caused little excitement, but in the early 1930's its use increased and spread widely throughout the southwestern and south central states. Originally carried into the United States by Mexican laborers, marijuana became common among the lower socioeconomic groups, and newspapers and police began to associate its use with crime. In the mid-1930's the use of marijuana moved to the eastern seaboard and up the Mississippi River. Supported by Anslinger, the police, and newspapers, public outcry reached such a level that in 1937 Congress passed the Marijuana Tax Act. By requiring payment of a tax on all marijuana transactions, it was hoped to regulate (that is, eliminate) the importation and use of marijuana. But, as was true with narcotic control laws, the law failed to be effective. In 1969 the Supreme Court declared punishment for nonpayment of the tax unconstitutional. Marijuana was still controlled by the narcotic laws and was legally considered to be a narcotic until May, 1971.

An interesting event in the growth of our domestic narcotic control laws occurred in 1942 with the passage of the Opium Poppy Control Act. Until this law there was no basis for controlling the cultivation of the opium poppy in the United States! The Opium Exclusion Act of 1909 regulated imports, and the Harrison Act of 1914 was concerned with producers of narcotic drugs. This 1942 act required that growers of the opium poppy be licensed by the Secretary of the Treasury.

The background and contents of the Poppy Control Act are nicely summarized in a letter from the Secretary of War Henry Stimson to Senator Walter George, Chairman of the Finance Committee, in November, 1942, supporting enactment of the bill.

Opium poppy seeds do not contain narcotics and are widely used for flavoring and decorating bakery products, such as bread and rolls. Such seeds heretofore have been imported freely from European countries in considerable quantities. Due to war conditions, this product is no longer available for commercial use. Considerable impetus to the growing of poppies in this country has followed the domestic shortage of seeds, with the resulting danger of the spreading of illicit distribution of poppy stems and pods, from which a morphine solution used by addicts for the satisfaction of their cravings may be produced by the simple process of boiling. . . .

Accordingly, the War Department favors encouraging the domestic production of the opium poppy, not only for the purpose of providing sufficient quantities of narcotics but for the production in commercial quantities of poppy seeds for flavoring and decorating bakery products. It is not believed wise, however, to encourage production of the opium poppy at the risk of spreading drug addiction. Proper legislative safeguards and controls are deemed essential. It is believed that these are adequately provided for by the proposed legislation.

Individual rights to grow poppies in private flower gardens or in public botanical gardens for ornamental purposes would be protected by section 9 (c) of the bill, which provides that none of the prohibitions contained in the measure shall apply to such growers.*

The Opium Poppy Control Act was signed by President Franklin D. Roosevelt December 11, 1942.

With the end of World War II and the resumption of easy international travel, the illegal narcotic trade resumed and increased in volume every year. In 1951 Congress passed the Boggs Amendment to the Harrison Act, which ushered in a hard-line attitude toward illegal drug use including marijuana. This amendment established minimum mandatory sentences for all narcotic and marijuana offenses. It also prohibited suspended sentences and probation for second offenses.

This more stringent enforcement attitude continued and was reflected in a report by a subcommittee of the Senate Judiciary Committee in 1955.[9] The subcommittee stated that drug addiction was responsible for 50% of crime in urban areas and 25% of all reported crimes and found drug addiction to be one of the ways Communist China planned to demoralize the United States. With this background it is easy to understand that the 1956 Narcotic Drug Control Act raised the mandatory minimum sentence for conviction

*From Senate Report No. 1764, 77th Congress, 2nd Session, November 30, 1942.

of a violation of the narcotic laws. More importantly, this act prohibited suspended sentences, probation, or parole for all narcotic offenses *except* a first conviction for possession. Under this law a convicted seller or distributor of illegal narcotics had to be jailed. In most federal cases an individual who possessed a "large amount" of narcotics or marijuana was presumed to be a seller and was treated as such. This law also made execution possible for a pusher selling heroin to someone under 18.

It must be remembered that according to the Harrison Act and other federal narcotic laws it is not a crime to be an addict. Nor is the fact that someone is an addict with no legal source of narcotics adequate evidence for prosecution and conviction under federal laws. Several states did make addiction a crime, however, and instituted action to charge addicts under these laws and sometimes place them in treatment programs. In the 1962 Robinson case, in which an addict appealed his conviction, the Supreme Court declared it unconstitutional to call addiction a crime.

Partly in response to the developing World Health Organization program that was responsible for monitoring world production and medical needs of the opiates and partly to tighten internal controls on legal narcotics, the Narcotics Manufacturing Act was passed in 1960. This act licensed all medical narcotic drug manufacturers and made it illegal to manufacture or attempt to manufacture narcotic drugs unless registered. In addition annual quotas were established for the purchase and manufacture of these drugs.

To further increase controls but not to interfere with good medical practice, in 1962 the Bureau of Narcotics set up a four-part system for classifying drugs containing narcotics. Controls were tightened further in 1969, but this system was eliminated in the 1970 law when both narcotics and dangerous drugs were combined in a single five-part classification.

DRUG ABUSE CONTROL AMENDMENTS OF 1965

The early 1960's saw not only an increase in illegal drug use but also a shift in the type of drug being used illegally. The trend was for the new drug users to be better educated and to emphasize primarily drugs that alter mood and consciousness. In this period some university hospitals in large cities reported that up to 15% of their emergency room calls involved individuals with adverse reactions from illegal drugs. Responding to the need for better controls over the manufacturing and distribution of certain legal and illegal compounds (the so-called dangerous drugs), Congress passed the Drug Abuse Control Amendments of 1965.

These laws excluded narcotics and marijuana and brought three new classes of drugs under federal control. The act specifically names the barbiturates and the amphetamines as being controlled and further states that derivatives of these drugs can be designated as controlled by the Secretary of Health, Education and Welfare. The third group of compounds was broader and included any drug that the Secretary of Health, Education and Welfare named as having *a potential for abuse because of its stimulant or depressant or hallucinogenic effects*. In 1968 when the federal drug control system was reorganized, the authority of the Secretary of Health, Education and Welfare was given to the Attorney General.

In determining whether a drug is hallucinogenic, the FDA was to consider whether it causes hallucinations, illusions, delusions, or an alteration in:

1. Orientation with respect to time or place
2. Consciousness, as evidenced by confused states, dream-like revivals of past traumatic events, or childhood memories
3. Sensory perception, as evidenced by visual illusions, synesthesia, distortion of space and perspective
4. Motor coordination
5. Mood and affectivity, as evidenced by anxiety, euphoria, hypomania, ecstasy, autistic withdrawal
6. Ideation, as evidenced by flight of ideas, ideas of reference, impairment of concentration and intelligence
7. Personality, as evidenced by depersonalization and derealization, impairment of conscience and of acquired social and cultural customs*

*Depressant and stimulant drugs, Part 166, Title 21, Code of Federal Regulations, Food and Drug Administration, January, 1966.

It should be noted that through this act the FDA also brought under control the two chemicals, lysergic acid and lysergic acid amide. These compounds are starting points for the manufacture of LSD and, beginning in 1964, methods of producing LSD from these compounds had been published in the underground press.

The major control over the stimulants and depressants arose from two separate provisions of the act. One was that prescriptions for any of the stimulant or depressant drugs controlled by this law could not be filled or refilled more than 6 months after issued nor could the prescription be refilled more than five times. The second provision tightened the manufacturing and distribution of stimulants and depressants by requiring all who make or handle the controlled drugs to register with the federal government and to keep a record for 3 years of where their drugs are obtained and to whom they are sold.

Penalties for convictions under this act were originally imprisonment up to 1 year and a $1,000 fine for a first offense, and up to 3 years and $10,000 for subsequent convictions. A special provision, though, made the penalties much greater for anyone over 18 who was giving controlled drugs to someone under 21. These maximum penalties were increased in 1968 in an amendment that also made it possible for the court to suspend sentence for a first conviction of possession and to erase the conviction from the record if there is no violation during a mandatory 1-year probationary period.

In the initial regulations implementing the 1965 amendments, the Native American Church, a religious organization of Indians of the Southwest, was exempted from certain parts of the act dealing with hallucinogens. The peyote cactus, which contains mescaline, an hallucinogen, is used in their religious ceremonies and has been for many years. This exemption was readily given because earlier California had restricted the use of peyote and in 1962 and 1963 had convicted members of the Native American Church for violation of the state law. The American Civil Liberties Union appealed the conviction on the grounds that it violated religious freedom. In 1964 the Supreme Court of California reversed the conviction on the basis that peyote was a major part of their religious ceremonies and a cornerstone of their religion.

This 1964 decision was not a blanket statement that any drug used in religious ceremonies would be exempt from regulation. In a 1967 court decision involving Dr. Timothy Leary, earlier judicial decisions in this country were cited in which it was clear that certain religious acts could be controlled if they posed a threat to public safety. In the Leary case the court decided that the use of hallucinogens constituted a threat to society and, also, that marijuana was not essential to the practice of Hinduism![10]

COMPREHENSIVE DRUG ABUSE PREVENTION AND CONTROL ACT OF 1970

One of the last bills the Senate and the House of Representatives approved before adjourning for the 1970 election recess was H.R. 18583, the *Comprehensive Drug Abuse Prevention and Control Act of 1970*, signed on October 27, 1970, by President Richard M. Nixon. That ended a legislative process that began in July, 1969, when the President sent a message to Congress on the drug problem and followed it the next day with a proposed drug control act.

The political process began even before that, in the spring of 1969, when the administration began disclosing bits and pieces of its proposed drug legislation. The proposals were liberal and emphasized education, research, and rehabilitation. The concepts were applauded by biomedical professionals but received little support in Congress where the members were more concerned about law and order! As a result, the administration's emphasis shifted, and the proposals outlined in July, 1969, were conservative and emphasized law enforcement rather than education or treatment.

Scientists and health professionals concerned with the national problems of drug use, research, and rehabilitation were almost unanimous in their rejection of the ideas and philosophy expressed in the administration's proposals. These negative reactions resulted in a softening of the administration's position during the fall of 1969, but the real debate developed in the spring and summer of 1970 over Senator Thomas Dodd's bill, which was introduced in the Senate in January, 1970.

The Dodd bill primarily emphasized enforcement and received administration support. Concern over the possible enactment of a law enforcement measure as *the* response to the drug problem resulted in considerable political activity by professional and scientific organizations. These groups led the drive for increased funds and freedom in the areas of drug research and rehabilitation. Not until 1972 when private foundations pledged $15 million to establish and maintain the *Drug Abuse Council* was there a focal point for nongovernment thinking, planning, and leadership in the area of drug abuse. More perspective is necessary before the effects of various influences on drug legislation can be adequately evaluated, but it is obvious that any lobby is bound to.have more effect than no lobby at all.

Although the Dodd bill passed the Senate, it was the House bill that finally was adopted almost unchanged by the Senate and signed by the President. The law became effective .on the first of May, 1971, and since it is the present law of the land some of the provisions will be presented in detail. As has been true in the past the administrative regulations established to carry out the provisions of the act and the court decisions regarding the law will have considerable influence on the actual implementation of the 1970 Drug Abuse Law. Appreciate also that laws are regularly amended. In March, 1973, for example, the President proposed greatly increased penalties for selling heroin or morphine.

The Comprehensive Drug Abuse Prevention and Control Act of 1970 almost lives up to its title. It is comprehensive since it repeals and replaces or updates all of the previous laws concerned with both the narcotics and dangerous drugs. Even the Opium Poppy Control Act of 1942 is gone, the "bread and rolls" being remembered in this law only by the excluding phrase: "...except the seed..."! The law specifically states that the drugs controlled by the act are under federal jurisdiction whether involved in interstate commerce or not. The law does not eliminate state regulations; it just makes clear that federal enforcement and prosecution is possible in any illegal activity involving the controlled drugs.

The law deals with prevention and treatment of drug abuse by appropriating funds for expanding the role of Community Mental Health Centers and Public Health Service Hospitals in the treatment of those who misuse drugs. Funds are made available to assist public and private nonprofit institutions that develop programs for the treatment and rehabilitation of drug-dependent persons. It authorizes the Secretary of Health, Education and Welfare to develop educational material and to establish and conduct drug education workshops for professional workers as well as for the public schools.

A liberalizing aspect of the law is that the Secretary of Health, Education and Welfare is directed to work with professional associations to develop guidelines that will detail the methods—including presumably the use of narcotics—that can be used to treat narcotic addicts. Such guidelines would handle a problem never really resolved, even though the 1925 Linder decision said that a physician could use narcotics in treating addicts if the objective was a cure, that is, gradual decrease in the amount of narcotic needed.

The special status of marijuana and marijuana users is evident throughout the law. Of particular note is the fact that the law establishes a *Commission on Marijuana and Drug Abuse.* The Commission was instructed to complete a comprehensive summary on the medical, legal, and sociocultural aspects of marijuana and marijuana use and to submit a final report with "recommendations for legislative and administrative actions" within 2 years. The report arrived in March, 1973, and was praised for its comprehensiveness.[10a]

The control aspects of the bill were the most debated portions, and several basic philosophical, ethical, and legal issues are resolved (!) by the law. First is that this is a law to control drugs directly rather than through excise taxes. Enforcement authority was moved to the Department of Justice from the Treasury Department. To implement the

emphasis on enforcement, the law authorized 300 new agents. By 1973 there were about 1,500 agents.

A second major issue with which the law deals is the separation of enforcement of the law from the scientific evaluation of the drugs considered for control. The Attorney General is responsible for the administration of the control aspects of the law, but the Secretary of Health, Education and Welfare makes the final decision on which drugs should be controlled. This separation of enforcement from the scientific and medical decision of what should be controlled was a major victory for those arguing for a sane drug law.

In determining whether a drug should be controlled the Secretary of Health, Education and Welfare must consider the following factors:

1. Scientific evidence of its pharmacological effect, if known
2. The state of current scientific knowledge regarding the drug or other substance
3. What, if any, risk there is to the public health
4. Its psychic or physiological dependence liability
5. Whether the substance is an immediate precursor of a substance already controlled under this title

In addition the Secretary should use any relevant scientific and medical considerations in:

1. Its actual or relative potential for abuse
2. Its history and current pattern of abuse
3. The scope, duration, and significance of abuse

After specifically excluding "distilled spirits, wine, malt beverages, or tobacco" the law established five schedules of drugs that must be updated and published regularly. Table 2-1 summarizes the characteristics and penalties for illegally selling drugs in each of the five schedules.

There are several different aspects of control contained in this law. This law reformulated some of the restrictions on drug prescriptions found in earlier acts. No prescription for a Schedule II compound can be refilled, but in an emergency a Schedule II

Table 2-1. Summary of drug schedules and penalties for violation of the Comprehensive Drug Abuse Prevention and Control Act of 1970 (as of July 1, 1974)

Schedule	Potential for abuse	Medical use	Production controlled	Examples	Maximum penalties for illegal	
					Manufacturing distribution	Possession
I	High	None	Yes	Heroin, marijuana, THC (tetrahydro-cannabinol), LSD, mescaline; generally, opiates, opium derivatives, and hallucino-genic substances	Narcotics— 1st offense 15 yrs./$25,000/3 yrs.* 2nd and more offenses 30 yrs./$50,000/6 yrs.	1st offense 1 yr./$5,000 2nd offense 2 yrs./$10,000 For first offense probation may be given. Penalties for possession are the same for all schedules.
II	High	Yes	Yes	Morphine, cocaine, methadone, secobarbital, amobarbital, pentobarbital, meperidine, methaqualone, all amphetamine type stimulants	Nonnarcotics— 1st offense 5 yrs./$15,000/2 yrs. 2nd offense 10 yrs./$30,000/4 yrs.	
III	Some, less than drugs in I and II	Yes	No	Nonamphetamine type stimulants; some barbiturates, some narcotic preparations, diazepam (pending), chlordiazepoxide (pending)	1st offense 5 yrs./$15,000/2 yrs. 2nd offense 10 yrs./$30,000/4 yrs.	
IV	Low, less than drugs in III	Yes	No	Barbital, chloral hydrate, meprobamate, phenobarbital	1st offense 3 yrs./$10,000/1 yr. 2nd offense 6 yrs./$20,000/2 yrs.	
V	Low, less than drugs in IV	Yes	No	Compounds, mixtures, and preparations with very low amounts of narcotics; dilute codeine and opium compounds	1st offense 1 yr./$5,000/none 2nd offense 2 yrs./$10,000/none	

*Maximum prison sentence/maximum fine/mandatory probation period after release from prison.

drug can be dispensed on an oral prescription. Prescriptions for substances in Schedules III and IV cannot be refilled more than five times and not at all more than 6 months after written.

A statistic frequently appearing in the congressional debate on this law was that 8 billion doses of stimulant drugs are manufactured in this country each year and about half find their way into illegal distribution channels.[11] The best story about the looseness of the existing laws and the laxness of distributors concerned the regular large shipments of amphetamines to an address in Tijuana, Mexico. One problem: the address was nonexistent and if it had existed it would have been the green of the eleventh hole of the Tijuana golf course!

To curtail this type of activity the law requires (as did the 1960 and 1965 laws) annual registration of everyone who manufactures, distributes, or dispenses any controlled substance. Researchers must also register. The law states that the Attorney General shall determine the quantity of substances in Schedules I and II needed for medical, scientific, research, and industrial use and then limit production of these compounds and assign quotas to the various companies manufacturing these drugs. All registrants must keep a complete record of all controlled substances—whence it came, whither it goest—and retain the record for at least 2 years. Every 2 years beginning May 1, 1971 each registrant—manufacturer, distributor, pharmacy, or other—must make a complete inventory of his existing controlled drugs. There is little doubt that these measures will drastically decrease the amount of legitimately produced drugs that are funneled into the illegal market. The impact on the use of these drugs remains to be seen.

Use of drugs does not decrease just because one source is eliminated. The 1914 Harrison Act, which made it difficult for addicts, was responsible for the development of the illegal drug trade as we know it today. It may be that the primary effect of the 1970 law will be to shift drug users to illegally manufactured drugs and not result at all in a decrease in drug use.

Another major change in the federal drug laws is apparent in the fact that there is now *no federal mandatory sentence for a first offense of illegal possession of any controlled drug.* A first offense of illegal possession of a controlled drug or ". . . distributing a small amount of marijuana for no remuneration . . ." can be punished by a year's imprisonment and/or a fine of $5,000. In lieu of this the court can place the individual on probation for up to 1 year. If there is no probation violation the charge is dismissed, the conviction erased from the individual's record, and, for every legal purpose, the conviction never existed. This erasing of the conviction (and the return of rights that would be lost if the conviction were allowed to stand) can only occur once. Not only can the conviction be vaporized, but (a la *1984*) if the individual

is not over 21 the court, if asked to, will have all public records relating to the arrest, trial, and conviction destroyed. From a legal point of view the individual is then restored to his prearrest status and can legally deny under oath that he was ever arrested on such a charge.

Obviously the law is becoming less stringent in its dealings with the possessor and user. Some have suggested that this is a result of the drug scene moving swiftly into white suburbia. "Since sons and daughters of prominent persons—including senators—started getting busted for crimes previously associated with lower-class blacks, compassion for marijuana criminals was sure to arise."[12] The real pressure and penalties must be brought against the professional peddlers and pushers. Their operations must be shut down before they ruin all of our children. These are the same sentiments expressed in San Francisco in the late nineteenth century that resulted in the anti–opium-smoking laws.

Three classes of individuals have severe penalties placed on them by the 1970 law. One group consists of those individuals over 18 who distribute a controlled drug to an individual under 21 years of age. If convicted the individual receives twice the penalty for a first offense and three times the penalty for a second or subsequent offense.

Aiming at the illegal drug entrepreneur, this law mentions specifically "continuing criminal enterprise" and "dangerous special drug offenders." An individual is engaged in *a continuing criminal enterprise* if he violates this law in conjunction with five or more other people to whom he is an organizer or holds ". . . other position of management . . ." and from whom he receives substantial income. Conviction under this section of the law has a first offense penalty of not less than 10 years and not more than $100,000, while a second offense is not less than 20 years and not more than $200,000. For either a first or second offense life imprisonment can be the sentence, and the government can confiscate all profits and property resulting from the enterprise. Neither probation nor a suspended sentence can be given an individual under this category.

A United States attorney may identify an individual as *a dangerous special drug offender* if in violating this law an individual acted as a supervisor to three or more people, received a substantial portion of his income from dealing in controlled substances, or has been convicted on drug charges twice within a 5-year period and was imprisoned at least once. The information supporting this identification is above and beyond any used in a trial to prove guilt and is additional material to be used by the judge only in determining the appropriate sentence for the convicted individual. The law provides for a sentence of up to 25 years.

Between the enactment of the Comprehensive Drug Abuse Prevention and Control Act in late 1970 and mid-1971, public and political awareness of illegal drug use increased greatly. Much attention centered on Congressional investigations into the widespread use of heroin by Americans in Vietnam. In part because of the extent of drug use in the military the President established a new *Special Action Office for Drug Abuse Prevention*. This was formalized by Congress in March, 1972, for a period not to exceed June 30, 1975. This agency was given broad powers for "overall planning and policy" and establishing "objectives and priorities for all federal drug abuse prevention functions." The director was given control over *all* expenditures of federal funds in the areas of drug abuse treatment, rehabilitation, education, and research. Most of these functions will be placed in the newly established (September, 1973) National Institute on Drug Abuse. The problems of enforcing federal drug laws were handled separately and resulted in a proliferation of agencies. In July, 1973, all enforcement activities were consolidated into the Drug Enforcement Administration of the Justice Department.

INTERNATIONAL REGULATION OF NARCOTICS AND OTHER DANGEROUS DRUGS

Beginning with an 1833 treaty with Siam, the United States recognized the need for agreements with other countries on the opium trade. In 1887 Congress passed an act to execute an agreement between China and the United States that forbade importation of opium to the United States by Chinese nationalists and also forbade American citizens from engaging in the Chinese opium trade.

Awareness of the larger international nature of the narcotic problem increased slowly, and it was President Theodore Roosevelt who called the First International Opium Congress that was held in Shanghai, China in 1909. This Congress was attended by representatives of the United States, Great Britain, France, Germany, Austria-Hungary, The Netherlands, Persia, Portugal, Russia, Italy, Siam, Japan, and China. One of the results was the 1912 Hague Conference in the Netherlands where the thirteen nations represented agreed, loosely, to regulate domestic sale and use of the opiates. Overall, however, the conferences did little more than focus world attention on the narcotic problem.

After World War I international control of the growth, manufacture, and distribution of the opiates was assumed by the League of Nations. From a preliminary meeting in 1921, several agreements developed, the most noteworthy being the 1931 convention in Geneva attended by representatives of fifty-seven nations. This convention established rules for limiting production and regulating the distribution of narcotic drugs.

In 1948 the United Nations designated the World Health Organization as the agency responsible for the international control of narcotics. The World Health Organization has been quite active, and present international control is based on the 1961 Single Convention on Narcotic Drugs, which has been made a treaty obligation by over sixty countries. This 1961 agreement consolidated all eight previous international agreements on narcotics and became internationally effective in 1964. In 1967 it was ratified by the Senate and became a treaty obligation of the United States.

The operating arms of this agreement are two United Nations agencies with headquarters in Geneva. One, the Commission on Narcotic Drugs, is responsible for regularly updating and revising international agreements on narcotics. In early 1971 the Commission held a conference on controlling the international shipment of drugs such as hallucinogens, barbiturates, and amphetamines. In February the delegates approved the Convention on Psychotropic Substances, which requires government authorization for international shipments of hallucinogens and brings under control the production and distribution of other dangerous drugs. The treaty would supersede national laws and go into effect when ratified by a majority of the parliaments of the members of the United Nations. It will apply to the United States only if approved by the Senate.

The second agency, the International Control Board, has the mandate to monitor and regulate the legal production, stores, and needs of narcotics for the world. It is not an enforcement agency and can only try to negotiate cutbacks in production when supply seems to outrun demand. The actual value of the Board seems to be in keeping a reasonably good record of where legal narcotics come from and where they go. A special drug abuse fund was established by the United Nations in April, 1971, to initiate new, as well as to increase present, international efforts in treatment, prevention, and other aspects of the problem of drug use and misuse.

The international involvement of the United States does not end with its participation in these agreements. The United States also has narcotic agents operating in areas where controlled drugs are produced and distributed, such as Istanbul, Marseilles, Bangkok, Mexico City, and Hong Kong. These agents cooperate generally with local enforcement groups but are primarily concerned with stopping shipments and disrupting organizations that are linked with the American illegal market.

FEDERAL REGULATION OF NONNARCOTIC AND NONDANGEROUS DRUGS

In the last half of the nineteenth century there was considerable agitation at the state level for legislation to regulate the purity of drugs and to control the therapeutic claims made for medicines. Strongly supported by the American Medical Association and the American Pharmaceutical Association, founded in 1848 and 1852 respectively, state laws spread and by 1900 forty-five states had antiadulteration laws.

Federal regulation of nonnarcotic drugs progressed more hesitantly. In 1848 Congress passed the National Drug-Import Law in response to incoming shipments of drugs that were mislabeled, adulterated, and of general poor quality. The law authorized rejection of drugs that did not meet medical standards of quality and purity. Because unqualified political appointees were used as inspectors, the law was never effectively enforced.

In 1906 the Pure Food and Drugs Act brought the government full force into the drug marketplace, and subsequent modifications have built on this act. This act defined a drug as "any substance or mixture of substances intended to be used for the cure, mitigation, or prevention of disease." Of particular importance, it developed, was the phrasing of the law with respect to misbranding. Misbranding referred *only to the label, not to general advertising*, and covered "any statement, design, or device regarding . . . (a drug), or the ingredients or substances contained therein, which shall be false or misleading in any particular." The law was used successfully to force some patent medicine labels to tone down their therapeutic claims. The first contested case under the law was won by the government against a headache remedy named Cuforhedake Brane-Fude!

In 1911 government action against a claimed cancer cure on the grounds that the claim was false and misleading was contested by arguing that the law applied only to the ingredients and not to therapeutic claims. After this position was upheld by the Supreme Court, Congress passed the 1912 Sherley amendment that forbade therapeutic claims that were both "false and fraudulent." Even this was not enough because a 1922 case involving a tuberculosis cure was ruled not to be a fraudulent claim because it was truly believed to be effective by its manufacturer. Considering its ingredients of raw eggs, turpentine, ammonia, formaldehyde, and mustard and wintergreen oils, the claim was at least false, if not fraudulent.

As more and more cases were investigated it seemed clear to the Food and Drug officials that many of the violations of the 1906 law were unintentional and caused primarily by poor manufacturing techniques and an absence of quality control measures. The Food and Drug Administration began developing assay techniques for various chemicals and products and collaborated extensively with the pharmaceutical industry to improve standards. The prosperous 1920's, coupled with a friendly Republican administration and increasing scientific knowhow, resulted in many voluntary changes by the drug industry that improved manufacturing and selling practices.

The depression of the 1930's and increased competition for business, plus the election of a Democratic administration not overly friendly with big business, disrupted many of the working agreements between government and industry. FDA surveys in the mid-1930's showed that over 10% of the drug products studied did not meet the standards of the United States Pharmacopoeia or the National Formulary. These findings contributed to the development of new regulations incorporated into the 1938 Food, Drug, and Cosmetic Act.

This 1938 act contained many provisions that changed the role of the FDA in drug control. One of the provisions resulted from the fact that in 1937, 107 people, primarily infants, died following treatment with the drug "Elixir of Sulfanilamide." The 1930's had seen an expansion in the use of sulfa drugs—agents potently effective against certain disease-causing microorganisms. Most sulfa products could not be used with infants because the dosage form was tablet or pill, but the prescription drug "Elixir of Sulfanilamide" was a palatable liquid widely used with infants. Following the death of these children it was shown that the liquid, diethylene glycol, in which the sulfanilamide was dissolved caused kidney poisoning. *There was no government requirement that a manufacturer show that a drug was safe before*

marketing a new product! The concerns the government had up to this time were that a drug be properly labeled and/or meet United States Pharmacopeia or National Formulary standards. The only basis on which the government could stop the sale of "Elixir of Sulfanilamide" was that it was mislabeled—it contained no alcohol and a true elixir does.

Congress, appalled by the fact that a drug could kill but not be taken off the market for that reason, included in the 1938 amendments a requirement that manufacturers test a drug for toxicity. The safety of drugs was controlled by the requirement that before a new drug could be introduced in interstate commerce, a "new drug application" (NDA) had to be submitted by the company to the FDA. The FDA would determine whether the NDA met certain specifications in the regulations and, if it did, the application was allowed to "become effective." The specifications to be met included submission of "full reports of investigations which have been made to show whether or not such drug is safe for use." Note especially that the FDA does not *approve* the drug or make statements about its safety. The FDA only says that the new drug application has met certain requirements. Between 1938 and 1962, about 13,000 new drug applications were submitted to the FDA and about 70% were allowed to become effective.

The requirement that drug manufacturers present evidence showing a product to be safe is one of the three basic rules now governing the marketing of a new drug. In 1906 it was established that *a drug has to be pure and accurately labeled.* Since 1938 a *drug also has to be safe.* Only since 1962 is it a requirement that *a drug also has to be effective.* The 1938 amendments also stipulated that drug labels give adequate directions for use but added that the FDA could exempt drugs from that requirement on the basis that it was "not necessary for the protection of public health." If a drug was exempt from this direction-for-use requirement, it could be sold only on prescription and had then to carry the label: "Caution: to be used only by or on the prescription of a physician." The wording was later changed to: "Caution: federal law prohibits dispensing without prescription."

There was much confusion over what was to be termed a prescription drug until the Humphrey-Durham Amendment of 1951. It clarified the issue by setting up three classes of prescription drugs: (1) those that must be labeled, "Warning: may be habit forming" (the narcotic drugs); (2) those determined by the FDA to be unsafe because of toxicity unless administered by a physician; and (3) new drugs. Only then could the FDA effectively control which nonnarcotic drugs needed to be pre-scribed by a physician. The restriction seems only moderately successful since a 1973 study found that retail pharmacists honored fake prescriptions 56% of the time![12a]

In the late 1950's Senator Estes Kefauver began a series of hearings investigating high drug costs and marketing collaboration be-tween drug companies. As the hearings pro-gressed there was some involvement of the committee with the regulation and control of drugs, but it was the thalidomide disaster that gave the 1962 amendments their particular flavor and ensured their passage. It is clear that if thalidomide had been evaluated under the controls outlined in the 1962 amend-ments, its effects on fetuses would have been determined.

There are three important features in these 1962 amendments including one that requires advertisements for prescription drugs to con-tain a summary of information about adverse reactions to the drug. Also, prior to market-ing, every new drug has to be shown effective for the illnesses mentioned on the label or brochure accompanying the drug. Last, drugs marketed between 1938 and 1962 (that is, those that were safe but of unknown effective-ness) had to be evaluated by the FDA and re-moved from the marketplace if they were shown to be ineffective.

The requirement that there be an evalua-tion of the effectiveness of drugs introduced between 1938 and 1962 was a major task. In that 24-year period 237 companies had sub-mitted NDA's for 4,349 formulations of 2,824 drugs for which they made over 16,000 therapeutic claims. It has been estimated that for each of these 4,349 new formulations

there were probably about five identical products on the market covered by each NDA. Thus, although only 4,349 formulations were involved, there may have been over 20,000 new products between 1938 and 1962. Of these about 15% were over-the-counter com-pounds, the remainder being prescription drugs.[13]

In 1966 the Food and Drug Administration contracted the task of evaluating these formu-lations to the National Academy of Sciences National Research Council. The Council es-tablished panels of medical and scientific experts in thirty areas to study the therapeutic claims of these drugs. In the fall of 1967 the panels began sending final reports to the Food and Drug Administration, with the last being forwarded in 1969.[14]

Overall, about 15% of the formulations were found to be *ineffective* for their claimed therapeutic values. Since there are multiple claims made for most drugs and each thera-peutic claim was evaluated separately, some drugs will be approved for certain uses but not for all of their previous claims. To remain on the market these drugs will have to submit NDA's containing claims about effectiveness only for the approved uses. If they wish to extend the number of therapeutic uses, then additional information must be forwarded to FDA.

The advisory panels also classed drugs as *"probably effective"* (7%) and as *"possibly effective"* (35%)—both classifications suggest-ing that there is some evidence of the com-pound's effectiveness but not enough for it to be finally approved. If the manufacturer wants to continue marketing these formula-tions, he must submit NDA's with information supporting the therapeutic claims. These applications must be submitted within 12 months on "probably effective" drugs and within 6 months for those classed as "possibly effective."

It is necessary to pause a moment to make clear what the present status is on drug labels, drug advertising, drug safety, and drug effectiveness. The 1906 federal law was con-cerned only with what the label said about the drug, not what was said in general ad-vertising. A cancer cure could be advertised as such in newspapers and magazines and, as long as the label did not claim curative powers and did describe the ingredients accurately, no federal law was violated.

The 1938 act said that, henceforth, a manufacturer had to show that a drug was safe before it could be introduced into interstate commerce. The drugs already on the market at that time were presumed to be safe and were not required to prove their safety. The 1962 act clearly stated that a drug had to be shown to be both safe and effective before introduction to the public. It also required the 1938-1962 drugs to be evaluated for effectiveness. Nothing was said about drugs already on sale before 1938. This means that there may be products legally sold today that are neither safe nor effective. Furthermore, these laws are concerned only with interstate commerce. A drug manufactured and sold within a single state does not come under these laws but is subject to the individual state regulations. Recently there have been attempts to include these drugs on the basis that *the ingredients* moved in interstate commerce.

The FDA does not have jurisdiction over advertised claims for nonprescription drugs. This is the concern of the Federal Trade Commission (FTC), which was established in 1914 to guard against unfair business practices. Since 1938 it has not been necessary for the FTC to show that advertising impaired competition before it could move against "unfair or deceptive acts or practices." The burden of proof does rest with the FTC and a claim can be made in newspaper, magazine, radio, and television advertising until the FTC proves in court that it is not a legitimate claim.

In 1954 the FDA and FTC formally entered into an agreement that gave "primary responsibility for preventing misbranding of foods, drugs, devices, and cosmetics to the Food and Drug Administration; primary responsibility with respect to the regulation of the truth or falsity of all advertising (other than labeling) of such products being assigned to the FTC." A 1968 agreement updated the liaison and essentially said that the FTC will use the FDA's data in acting on advertising of over-the-counter products and that the FDA has responsibility for the advertising of prescription drugs.[15]

A July, 1967, regulation by the FTC clearly indicates the interrelationship between FTC's actions and FDA's control over drugs. This regulation states that it is a violation of the Federal Trade Commission Act if an advertisement for a drug "contains any representation with respect to efficacy or safety which contradicts, or in any manner exceeds, the warnings, statements, or directions for use appearing on the label or in the labeling of such product." In short, if the FDA won't let you say it on the label, don't say it in your advertising.[16]

The FDA has recently expanded its regulatory power in this area. In October, 1971, the FDA initiated a policy on prescription drugs that requires that their labels and advertisements must include adverse conclusions reached by the National Academy of Sciences National Research Council.

REGULATIONS CONTROLLING THE MARKETING OF A NEW DRUG

To translate the 1962 law on the safety and effectiveness of a new drug, the FDA has established certain regular procedures and standards that must be met by the pharmaceutical house that hopes to market a drug. As does the consumer of legal drugs, the pharmaceutical industry has a considerable stake in these FDA requirements. Developing a compound to the point where it can be marketed is a long and expensive procedure for the drug company. It has been estimated that of every 3,000 new compounds produced by the chemists working for a drug company, only twenty prove to be safe enough in animal studies to be tested in man. On the average, only one of these twenty is marketed for general clinical use.[17]

It is not only new drugs that must be evaluated by the FDA but also a new use for an established drug. A drug may prove to be effective for a group of conditions and be passed by the FDA for sale as a treatment for those conditions. If the company finds the drug is also effective for a different group of conditions, it must submit the new information to the FDA and may not advertise the drug as effective for the new conditions until permitted by the FDA. A similar situation occurs when a new form of a drug is introduced, for example, a sustained-release form; the FDA requires that it be handled as a new drug.

The FDA formally enters the picture only when a drug company is ready to study the effects of a compound in humans. At that time the company supplies to the FDA a "Notice of Claimed Investigational Exemption for a New Drug" (IND). This IND must include the composition of the drug, its source if a biological preparation, and complete manufacturing information. At this time the manufacturer is required to submit all his information from preclinical (before human) investigations, including the effects of the drug on animals. The principle purpose of this preclinical work is to establish the safety of the compound.

As minimum evidence of safety, the animal studies must include acute, one-time administration of several dose levels of the drug to different groups of animals of at least two species. There must also be studies where the drug is given regularly to animals for a period related to the proposed use of the drug in man. For example, a drug to be used chronically requires 2-year toxicology studies in animals. Again two species are required. The method of drug administration and the form of the drug in these studies must be the same as that proposed for human use. (Requirements for new oral contraceptives are different from, and more stringent than, those presented here.)

In addition to these research results, the company must submit a detailed description of the proposed clinical studies of the drug in man. Information on the physicians who will conduct the clinical studies must also be submitted so that the FDA can evaluate their competency. In addition to the credentials on the clinical investigators, the FDA requires that it receive copies of all information given to the investigators about the drug.

The company must also certify that the human subjects will be told they are receiving an investigational compound and that the subjects will sign a form stating that they know

they are to receive such a compound and that this is acceptable to them. Finally, the company must agree to forward annually a comprehensive report and to inform the FDA immediately if any adverse reactions arise in either animals or humans receiving the investigational drug.

If the FDA authorizes the use of the drug in humans, the company can move into the first phase of clinical investigation. In Phases I and II the drug is given to healthy volunteers to determine a safe dose range of the compound and also its absorption, metabolism, and excretion in humans. Usually only a few individuals are used under well-controlled conditions. Frequently the individuals studied are prisoners because their living conditions can be well controlled and because they are eager to be paid volunteers.[18] Phase II studies must also include a small number of diseased patients.

Only after the safety of the drug is established in Phases I and II can Phase III be started. Phase III is quite extensive and involves administering the drug to individuals with the disease or symptom for which the drug is intended. If the compound proves effective in Phase III, the FDA balances its possible dangers against the benefits for the patient before releasing it for sale to the public. When the drug is marketed, the company must send reports on its use and effects to the FDA every 3 months for the first year, every 6 months for the second year, and every 12 months for the third and following years.

CONCLUDING COMMENT

In two areas of drug control the federal government has recently made major new commitments. Until the impact of these moves is clearly felt, it is useless to predict future directions. The 1970 Drug Abuse Law for the first time emphasizes the sociocultural aspects of drug use and abuse by making possible leniency toward the occasional illegal drug user while increasing penalties for those who regularly profit from illegal drug sales. In the area of legal drug use the FDA and FTC are expanding their influence in an attempt to reach a point where the consumer is protected from dangerous or ineffective agents but is still assured of a continuous supply of new and better drugs from the pharmaceutical industry. Only time will tell whether these new directions are practical, long-term changes that can be maintained.

No status remains quo very long today. Even though the 1970 Drug Abuse Law practiced and preached tolerance and understanding for drug users and a crackdown on professional illegal drug dealers, not everyone was satisfied. Some argue for the removal of criminal penalties (but not legalization) for all drug use.[19] Others argue that all drugs used for recreational purposes should be legalized and controlled the same as alcohol.[20] In September, 1973, New York State enacted "get tough" drug laws for all drug dealers, for example, selling 1 ounce of a narcotic meant a life sentence with at least 15 years in prison.[21] Other evidence suggests (!) that having strict laws on the books does not necessarily decrease drug use or sales.[22]

The pendulum swings. Nothing works for long. Only when concerns over drug use and drug users are expressed in the context of all of our society's values, problems, and hopes will we know what laws need to be enacted and enforced.

PRECEDING QUOTES

1. From acceptance speech at Republican National Convention, Miami Beach, Florida, August 8, 1968. In Vital Speeches **34**:22, 1968.
2. From message to Congress on the drug problem, July 14, 1969. Entire message in U. S. News and World Report, July 28, 1969, p. 60.
3. From statement to state governors at a White House Conference on Drugs on December 3, 1969. In U. S. News and World Report, December 15, 1969, p. 38.
4. New York Times, June 18, 1971, p. 22; Time, June 28, 1971, p. 20.
5. Drugs and defeatism...U.S. decadence–what Nixon said, U. S. News and World Report, July 19, 1971, p. 37.

REFERENCES

1. Adams, S. H.: The great American fraud, Collier's, six segments from October, 1905, to February, 1906.
2. Congressional Record **40**:102 (Part I), December 4, 1905, to January 12, 1906.
3. The best condensed reference to the federal drug laws is Handbook of Federal Narcotic and Dangerous Drug Laws, Superintendent of Documents, Washington, D. C., 1969, U. S. Government Printing Office, or latest edition. The only way to really appreciate and understand these laws is to read them as well as the Congressional hearings and debates prior to the enactment of the laws.
4. 249 U.S. 96, 99 (1919).
5. 258 U.S. 280 (1922).
6. 268 U.S. 5 (1925).
7. Schmeckebier, L. F.: The bureau of prohibition, Service Monograph No. 57, Institute for Government Research, 1929, Brookings Institute. Cited in Narcotic Drug Laws and Enforcement Policies, King, Rufus: Law & Contemporary Problems **22**:122, 1957.
8. U. S. News and World Report **41**:22, 1956.
9. Senate Committee on the Judiciary: The illicit narcotic traffic, Senate Report No. 1440, 84th Congress, 2nd Session, 1956.
10. Handbook of federal narcotic and dangerous drug laws, (ref. 3), pp. 72-73.
10a. Drug use in America: problem in perspective, second report of the National Commission on Marihuana and Drug Abuse, March, 1973.
11. Congressional Record—House, September 24, 1970, p. H9170.
12. A little less illegal, New Republic **161**:11, 1969.
12a. Glass, A. A., Goodman, K. G., and Hinkley, S. W.: Project script: a study of prescription fraud vulnerability, Bureau of Narcotic and Dangerous Drugs, U. S. Department of Justice, 1973.
13. Biomedical News, January, 1971, p. 8.
14. Hampshire, G. D.: The NAS-NRC drug efficacy study: a peer review, FDA Papers **3**:4-7, 1969.
15. FDA Papers **2**(2):18-19, 1968.
16. Sweeny, C. A.: Liaison agreement, FDA Papers **2**(2):18, 1968.
17. Drug searches draw on best of two worlds, Medical World News **6**:46, 1965.
18. Adams, A., and Cowan, G.: The human guinea pig: how we test new drugs, World, pp. 20-24, December 5, 1972.
19. Stachnik, T. J.: The case against criminal penalties for illicit drug use, American Psychologist **27**:637-642, 1972.
20. Szasz, T. S.: The ethics of addiction, Harper's Magazine, pp. 74-79, April, 1972.
21. Farber, M. A.: Opinion remains divided over effect of state's new drug law, New York Times, August 31, 1973.
22. A perspective on "get tough" drug laws, The Drug Abuse Council, Inc., May, 1973.

UNIT

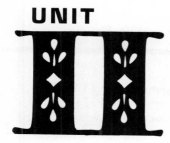

II

Fundamentals

3 Nervous system

...the influence of three great scientists has been with me as I have
striven to given a coherent account of synapses, which we may regard as
the key structures of the nervous system. . . . Ramon Y Cajal whose
achievement was to show that the nervous system was made up of
independent structures, the neurones . . . Sherrington who linked
this structural separateness with neuronal integration by the concept of
the synapse . . . Dale who was the leader in developing the theory of
chemical transmission across synapses . . .

> *The Physiology of Synapses*
> *Nobel Laureate Sir John Carew Eccles, 1964*
> *Berlin-Göttingen-Heidelberg: Springer, 1964*

...the human nervous system still remains the better computer in some
respects . . . Undoubtedly the most impressive feature of the human
brain is its flexibility and the comparatively enormous variety of
programmes that can be packed into an instrument occupying less than
half a cubic foot, and consuming only some 15 watts.

> *The Uncertain Nervous System*
> *B. Delisle Burns, 1968*

...the higher mental functions are complex, organized functional systems
that are social in origin . . . have a wide, dynamic representation
throughout the cerebral cortex . . . are formed in the process of social
contact and objective activity by the child . . . (and) have as their basis
relatively elementary sensory and motor processes.

> *Higher Cortical Functions in Man*
> *Aleksandr Romanovich Luria, 1966*
> *Translated by Basil Haigh. Basic Books, Inc., Publishers, New York, 1966*

Psychoactive drugs have many actions. Some we experience as pleasant, some as unpleasant, some bizarre, some as natural as warm apple pie. Whatever the experience, it results from an action on the information-processing systems of the body. A detailed analysis of these systems is not necessary, but an overview is essential to appreciate where drugs act and why and to begin to understand how they can influence consciousness, mood, and feeling.

Complex organisms such as man can survive only if they continually adapt and adjust themselves to the changing environment. Both the internal (inside the body) and the external (outside the body) environments have important effects on the well-being of the individual. It is necessary to maintain the physiology and biochemistry of the body within certain limits, and man is equipped with many self-adjusting systems to keep body functions within these limits. The term for these self-adjusting characteristics is *homeostasis*.

To maintain homeostasis the body needs to carry out three types of functions. First, it must be able to monitor the activity of the internal and external environments, that is, to sense changes and constancies in those environments. Second, information about the environments must be integrated with memories of previous features of the environment. Third, when the processing of old and new information is complete, there must be a way for the necessary adjustments of the body to be carried out.

In man there are two information-processing systems, each with certain characteristics, capabilities, and qualities that make it uniquely suited for its particular role in maintaining homeostasis. These two systems are the *nervous system* and the *endocrine system*.

The nervous system is a combination electrical-chemical system with several distinctive functions. It is designed to monitor relatively specific changes in the environments, to carry information about these changes along distinct routes to a specific processing center, and to do these things rapidly. Communications in the nervous system are both specific and

fast, reaching a speed of 200 miles per hour at times in man.

The endocrine system is a chemical system and has a role that complements and, in part, underlies the nervous system. In contrast to the nervous system, it is slower and more diffuse in terms of both what elicits a response and how the response occurs. The endocrine system is responsive to a wide range of not clearly defined changes in both environments. Much of the output from this system has effects on all the cells of the body, and as such has a pervasive effect. Some parts of this system, though, are sensitive only to restricted changes in the internal environment and have quite discrete effects. The endocrine system does not have a pathway used only for the transmission of its information, since the complex molecules that carry the information of the endocrine system are secreted into the bloodstream to be carried to the places where they are to have their primary effect. Speed of information transmission is slow in the endocrine system (blood circulation time is about 60 seconds in humans) when compared to the nervous system.

It is accurate to say that the endocrine system is more involved in setting base levels from which the nervous system functions, but it is not a complete statement since these two systems are interrelated and affecting one affects the other. Because they primarily play different roles and are quite different anatomically and physiologically they are usually studied separately. Since our concern is with the psychoactive drugs, which primarily have their effects through actions on the nervous system, only the nervous system will be outlined here.

FUNDAMENTALS

The basic unit in the nervous system is a specialized cell called a *neuron*. There are about 11 billion separate neurons in man, and since the end of the nineteenth century it has been clear that the nervous system is not continuous like the circulatory system. Information moves from one neuron to another only across a specialized gap of 0.00002 millimeter, called a *synapse*.

A neuron has three parts that are important in information transmission. *Dendrites* receive information that is then carried along the thread-like *axon* to the *terminals*. The length of a neuron is almost completely determined by the axon, which may vary in man from much less than a millimeter in the brain to a few feet when connecting the spinal cord to the toe. The diameter of axons varies some but is rarely larger than 20 microns in man. There are many dendrites collecting information and many terminals, but a neuron has only a single axon. The terminals of one neuron end close to dendrites of other neurons, and this terminal-dendrite area is the synapse. Information movement in a neuron is from dendrite to axon to terminals. From the terminals of one neuron information moves via the synapse to the dendrite of the next neuron. Dendrites may also receive information from specialized cells called *receptors*, which are the windows to the inside and outside world for the nervous system. Receptors change one form of information — light, sound, carbon dioxide concentration, and the like — into electrical activity, which is the way information is carried in neurons.

The nervous system is electrical in that information is carried from dendrites along axons to terminals as an electrical pulse. Usually, this information is actually a series of pulses, with each pulse lasting about 1/500 of a second and having an amplitude of 1/10 volt. The electrical pulses are little affected by most drugs. However, the pulse is generated because of certain characteristics of the neuron's cell wall, and some drugs do influence information processing by acting on and changing the cell wall.

At the synapse information is *not* transmitted electrically. It was only in the 1940's that the evidence became overwhelming that electrical pulses did not jump the synaptic gap but instead caused a release of chemicals from the terminals. These chemicals move across the synapse and cause electrical changes in the dendrite of the next neuron. The dendrites of a single neuron may have many synapses, up to 10,000, with terminals of many neurons. If enough synapses in a dendrite are active at about the same time, an electrical pulse is initiated in the axon, which then travels to its terminals. The sequence of information movement in the nervous system is summarized in Fig. 3-1.

The chemicals released from the terminals are called *neurotransmitters*, and the best evidence now is that only one kind of chemical is released from each cell. There are four chemicals almost all authorities accept as neurotransmitters: acetylcholine, noradrenaline, dopamine, and serotonin. There is still controversy over whether there are more neurotransmitters. Most psychoactive drugs exert their actions via their effects on these neurotransmitters.

The exact way in which neurotransmitters bring about changes in the dendrite is not yet known, but the place on a dendrite where a transmitter has its effect is called a *receptor site*. It is established that both the electrical characteristics and the structural configuration of the neurotransmitter must conform to those of the receptor if the electrical activity of the dendrite is to be affected. The standard analogy is to a lock and key. The receptor, the lock, is such that various chemicals, keys, may occupy it, but only one — the specific neurotransmitter — normally unlocks it, that is, causes a change in the electrical activity of the dendrite.

The receptor site is still hypothetical, but much research attempts to specify the characteristics it must have for the nervous system to function as it does. Appreciate the fact that a synapse in the brain is only

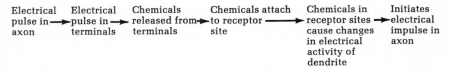

Fig. 3-1. Sequence and mode of information movement in the nervous system.

about 0.5 square micron in area—a square inch could contain 63 billion. Within this 0.5 square micron there must be many receptor sites since each electrical impulse may release a million molecules of the transmitter. These molecules must move across the gap, occupy a molecular-sized receptor site, and have their effect in about a millisecond. It may be helpful to realize that the acetylcholine molecule is only about 10 square angstroms; a square inch could contain 62.5 trillion of the molecules.

Within the nervous system integration of information occurs in the dendrite. If certain conditions are met, an impulse is initiated and travels down the axon. Functionally, this is one of two types of synapses and is called an *excitatory synapse*, since the neurotransmitter acting at the receptor sites makes it likely that an electrical impulse will travel along the axon. There are also inhibitory synapses, which are similar except that the chemicals released affect the dendrite to make it less likely that an impulse will be initiated in the axon.

The final output from a dendrite, pulse or no pulse in the axon, will depend on what type of synapses are active, how many of each type, and how frequently they are active in a brief period of time. Phrased a little differently, the dendrite acts as a gate at each step of information processing. No matter how many neurons carry information to a dendrite, there are only two possible outputs: an electrical pulse in the axon or no electrical pulse.

Therefore, no matter what effect a drug has on synaptic transmission, it should be clear that at the level of the neuron there are basically only two things that can happen to a neuron. It can be made more excitable— that is, easier to elicit an electrical impulse in the axon—or less excitable. It is a combination of what a drug does to these synaptic processes, where it does it, and for how long that determines what effects a drug will have.

Many psychoactive agents have their action by affecting the production, storage, or deactivation of the neurotransmitters. Normal functioning of the nervous system depends on the regular manufacturing of neurotrans-

mitters in neurons, their release as a result of an electrical impulse, and their breakdown or deactivation after they have had their effect on the dendrite. By changing one of these processes information transmission is modified or blocked.

The receptor site is the place where drugs act that mimic or block the neurotransmitters. Some drugs have electrical and spatial characteristics similar to the transmitters so that they can occupy the receptor and activate it—they open the lock! Other agents prevent transmitters from having an effect because they occupy but do not activate the receptor site.

NEUROTRANSMITTERS

Although it is only probable that *acetylcholine, noradrenaline, dopamine,* and *serotonin* are neurotransmitters in the brain, it is well established that acetylcholine and noradrenaline are neurotransmitters in other parts of the body. These chemicals are manufactured and stored in the neurons that release them. To understand how drugs disrupt these processes, it is necessary to know something about the manufacturing and storing process.

Manufacturing complex molecules in the body is frequently accomplished in several steps, with each step adding to or taking away some part of the existing molecule. The particular action at each step is accomplished by a molecule called an *enzyme*. An enzyme acts as a catalyst, that is, a substance that makes possible a chemical reaction but does not itself get used in the reaction. If one of the enzymes involved in building a neurotransmitter is destroyed or prevented in some way from having its effect, then the supply of the neurotransmitter will eventually decrease and drop below the amount necessary for normal functioning of the neuron. The same process is utilized in the deactivation of a neurotransmitter. Specific enzymes change the transmitter to a molecule that is no longer active at the receptor site. In some cases the enzymes further modify the molecule so that it can readily be excreted. Blocking the activity of a deactivating enzyme may result in a prolongation or intensification of the action of the neurotransmitter.

The manufacture of noradrenaline is a four-step process and begins with the amino acid phenylalanine. Fig. 3-2 shows the chemical structure,* name of the molecule, and the name of the active enzyme at each step. Note especially that dopamine is the step just before noradrenaline, so this series of biochemical transformations manufactures two neurotransmitters.

The step changing noradrenaline to adrenaline has been included because, under some conditions, the chemical adrenaline is released from the adrenal gland into the bloodstream and it then acts at the same receptor sites as noradrenaline. The deactivation processes of dopamine, noradrenaline, and adrenaline are quite complex and will not be detailed here. It must be mentioned that there are two primary enzymes involved, monoamine oxidase (MAO) and catechol-O-methyl transferase (COMT), but in normal functioning the adrenergic transmitters leave

---

*Throughout this book the standard convention will be used in showing chemical structures of ring-shaped (closed) molecules. Although the atoms joined together are carbon atoms (C) and each has a hydrogen (H) atom attached to it, neither the carbon nor the hydrogen atoms are indicated. Thus

This is a benzene ring. When a hydrogen atom is replaced with another atom or atoms, then the new atoms are shown. When only one hydrogen in a benzene ring is replaced with any atom or group of atoms, then the unit is called a *phenyl*. When two hydroxyl groups (OH) are substituted on a benzene ring, the structure is called a *catechol*:

It should be noted that both dopamine and noradrenaline are catechols, and since they have an amine group, NH_2, attached they are frequently referred to as *catecholamines*.

---

the receptor site and are taken up again in the terminals to be reused.

The synthesis of serotonin is simpler than that of noradrenaline. Beginning with the essential amino acid tryptophan, it takes only two steps to build serotonin. Fig. 3-3 shows the synthesis of serotonin as well as its deactivation. Deactivation is not complex, and excretion in the urine of the end product provides an easy way to monitor the deactivation of serotonin.

Acetylcholine formation and breakdown is the simplest of them all. Starting from choline and acetic acid, acetylcholine is formed directly and its deactivation is readily accomplished as shown in Fig. 3-4.

Neurons that release acetycholine are termed *cholinergic* and noradrenaline-, dopamine-, and serotonin-releasing neurons are called, respectively, *adrenergic, dopaminergic,* and *serotonergic.* Most frequently, a system of neurons that serves a specific function is made up of one type of neuron. Usually acetylcholine acts as an excitatory neurotransmitter, serotonin is probably an inhibitory transmitter, while noradrenaline and dopamine can be either excitatory or inhibitory, depending on the place of action.

PRELUDE TO THE NERVOUS SYSTEM

The combination of individual neurons into a smoothly functioning mechanism that carries information from the environment to the brain and then, sometimes, back out to muscles or glands is a remarkable achievement. To simplify the task of understanding the way in which the nervous system works, it is usually divided into two parts. Protectively enclosed in the skull and vertebral column are the brain and spinal cord, which together are called the *central nervous system* (CNS) and which form the major integrating system of the body. A second integrating system is the *autonomic nervous system* (ANS), which forms a ladder-like network of nerves along each side of the vertebral column. This ladder and clusters of terminals and dendrites connects with the spinal cord at each vertebra.

Dividing the entire nervous system of the body into the central nervous system (CNS)

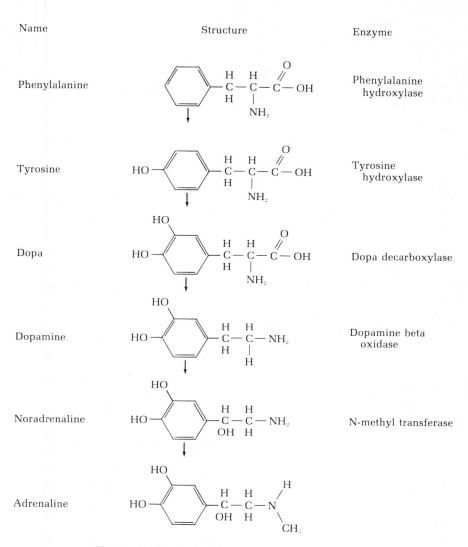

Fig. 3-2. Synthesis of adrenergic neurotransmitters.

and the autonomic nervous system (ANS) is a convenience, but it is not completely honest since part of the ANS is in the CNS and some of the outputs from the CNS travel via the ANS to muscles and glands. The two systems have unique enough characteristics to make it meaningful to separate them for the purpose of discussion, but it must be realized that the systems are intimately related in many of their functions. Briefly, the ANS is primarily concerned with the regulation of visceral functions and the maintenance of a stable internal environment, while the CNS functions to integrate incoming information from the internal and external environments and then sends out information to muscles and glands.

AUTONOMIC NERVOUS SYSTEM

The ANS is primarily a motor or output system and has most of its synapses outside the CNS. This point is important since there are many chemicals that cannot enter the CNS and thus have effects only on the ANS. The

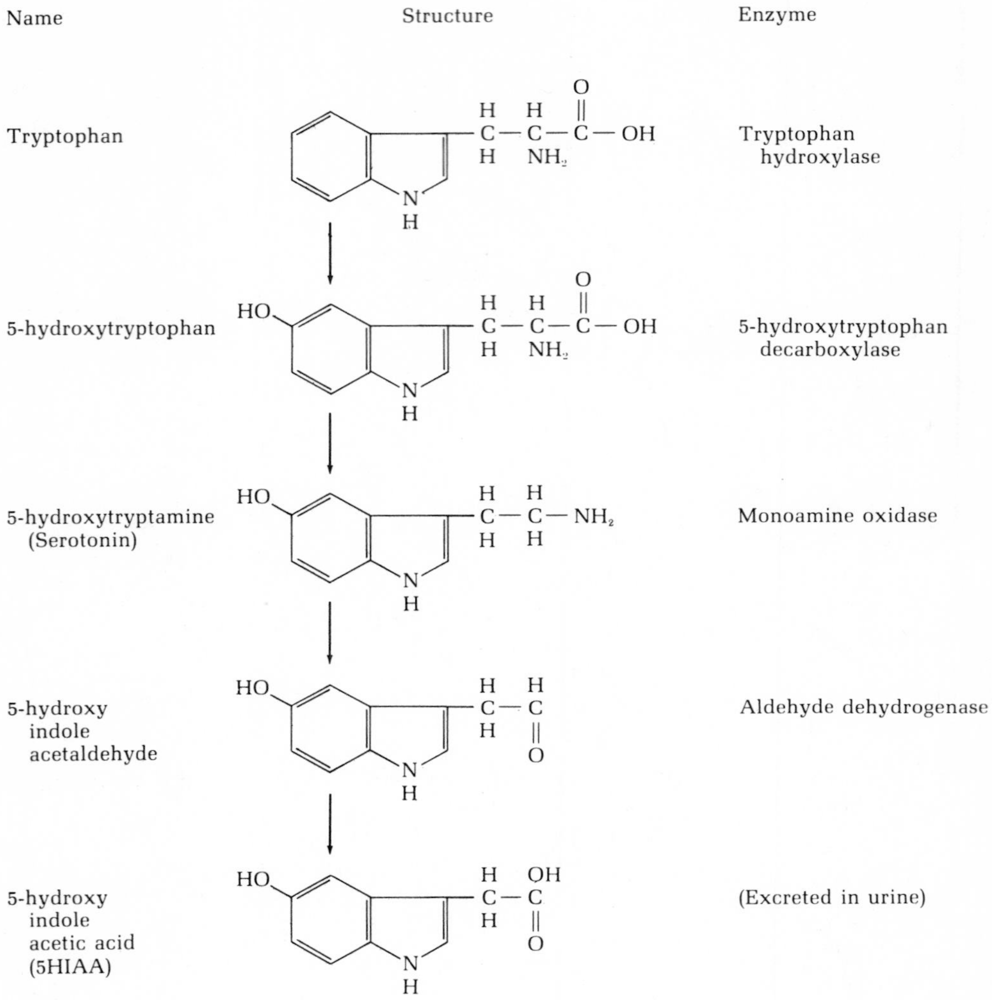

Name	Structure	Enzyme
Tryptophan		Tryptophan hydroxylase
5-hydroxytryptophan		5-hydroxytryptophan decarboxylase
5-hydroxytryptamine (Serotonin)		Monoamine oxidase
5-hydroxy indole acetaldehyde		Aldehyde dehydrogenase
5-hydroxy indole acetic acid (5HIAA)		(Excreted in urine)

Fig. 3-3. Synthesis and deactivation of serotonin.

ANS is meaningfully divided into two units, the *sympathetic* and the *parasympathetic systems*, which have generally opposite effects on an organ or function. Both systems send neurons to most visceral organs as well as to smooth muscles, glands, and blood vessels.

Since the control of most visceral functions and the circulatory and glandular systems is via the ANS, there are many examples that could be given of opposing sympathetic and parasympathetic effects. A few of the most relevant are given in Table 3-1. The sympathetic system is quite diffuse and undifferentiated in its actions compared to the parasympathetic system. The sympathetic division of the ANS functions principally to mobilize the organism for action, while the parasympathetic system generally operates to maintain ongoing production of necessary materials via the digestive system.

Of particular interest is the fact that in the parasympathetic system synapses at each structure being affected are cholinergic, while the sympathetic synapses at the same structure are adrenergic. When blood levels

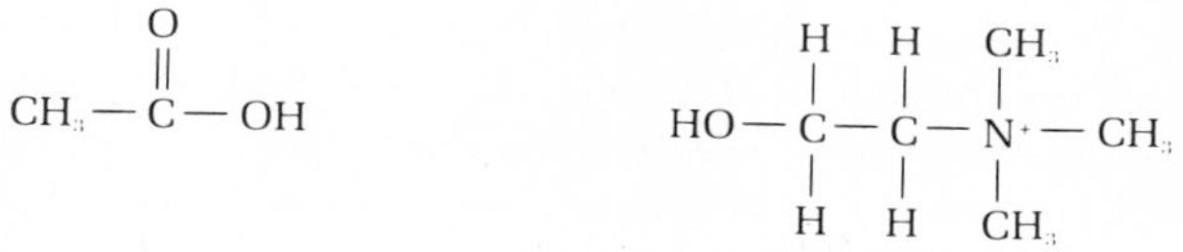

$$CH_3 - \overset{\overset{\displaystyle O}{\|}}{C} - OH$$

Acetic acid

$$HO - \overset{\overset{\displaystyle H}{|}}{\underset{\underset{\displaystyle H}{|}}{C}} - \overset{\overset{\displaystyle H}{|}}{\underset{\underset{\displaystyle H}{|}}{C}} - \overset{\overset{\displaystyle CH_3}{|}}{\underset{\underset{\displaystyle CH_3}{|}}{N^+}} - CH_3$$

Choline

In presence of choline acetylase and energy
are combined into

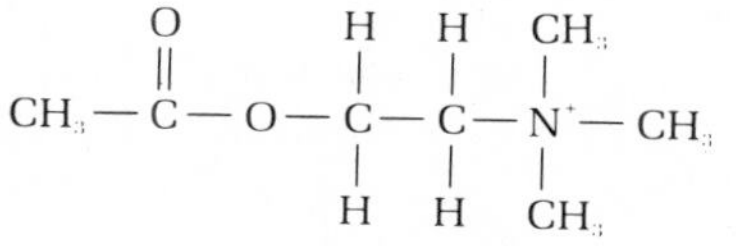

$$CH_3 - \overset{\overset{\displaystyle O}{\|}}{C} - O - \overset{\overset{\displaystyle H}{|}}{\underset{\underset{\displaystyle H}{|}}{C}} - \overset{\overset{\displaystyle H}{|}}{\underset{\underset{\displaystyle H}{|}}{C}} - \overset{\overset{\displaystyle CH_3}{|}}{\underset{\underset{\displaystyle CH_3}{|}}{N^+}} - CH_3 \qquad \text{and} \qquad H_2O$$

Acetylcholine   Water

In the presence of choline esterase, acetylcholine is broken
into choline and acetic acid.

Fig. 3-4. Acetylcholine formation and breakdown.

Table 3-1. Sympathetic and parasympathetic effects on selected structures

Structure or function	Sympathetic reaction	Parasympathetic reaction
Pupil ot eye	Dilation	Constriction
Heart rate	Increase	Decrease
Breathing rate	Fast and shallow	Slow and deep
Stomach and intestinal glands	Inhibited	Activated
Stomach and intestinal wall	No motility	Motility
Sweat glands	Secretion	No effect
Skin blood vessels	Constriction	Dilation

of adrenaline rise or when drugs are given that mimic the action of noradrenaline, the result is the same as if the sympathetic nervous system had been activated. These sympathomimetic effects are important in considering the actions of many drugs, since most drugs do have an effect on the ANS. Sometimes these are more important than the effects on the CNS.

CENTRAL NERVOUS SYSTEM

The brain and spinal cord make up the central nervous system (CNS), but since the spinal cord functions primarily to carry information to and from the brain, it will not be mentioned further. The human brain is a wondrous structure that contains about 10 billion neurons and weighs 3 pounds. It is an integrating and storage device that is not yet equalled by the largest computers. Even though the brain is much slower than a computer in its operations and in processing each bit of information, the brain has the advantage in being able to handle more channels of information simultaneously.

The functions of some of the parts of the brain will be detailed because they have particular importance for the study of drug actions and for understanding the effects of drugs on behavior. The *reticular activating system* is in the area where the spinal cord connects with the brain. It modulates incoming sensory information and outgoing motor impulses and regulates the degree of arousal and alertness an individual shows. The *hypothalamus* is located near the bottom of the brain and is integrator of information from many sources as well as being the control center for the autonomic nervous system. The hypothalamus is also the primary point of contact between the nervous system and the endocrine system. The *medial forebrain bundle* is a collection of axons of neurons coursing along both sides of the hypothalamus and is the anatomical focus of pleasure. The *periventricular system* is another collection of nerve fibers. These fibers are acted on by the medial forebrain bundle; this fiber system seems to be the substrate for punishment. Several clusters of neurons above and to the sides of the hypothalamus form the *basal ganglia*, which are the primary control centers for involuntary motor movements such as those involved in posture.

The *cerebral cortex* is the most complex structure in the animal kingdom and is the part of the brain that gives man his special uniqueness among animals. It almost completely surrounds the rest of the brain and lies just inside the skull. It is responsible for the analysis of incoming information and for the initiation of voluntary motor behavior. In the cortex the center for speech has been identified as well as areas for sensation and movement. These six parts of the brain will be briefly discussed, some general rules about brain functioning will be mentioned, and, finally, some possible mechanisms for drug actions will be suggested.

Reticular activating system

The reticular activating system (RAS) is very old phylogenetically and is characterized as being an area that receives inputs from all the sensory systems as well as from the cerebral cortex. The RAS is multisynaptic and sends many axons throughout the brain. Being multisynaptic means that information moving through this structure must cross many synapses, and thus it is particularly susceptible to influence by drugs.

One of the primary functions of the RAS is to control the arousal level of the brain, especially the cerebral cortex. The RAS is stimulated following input to any sensory system and sends impulses to many parts of the cortex. The RAS initiates impulses in the neurons there and thus prepares the cortex to receive further information via the sensory pathways. When the cortex has been activated by the RAS the organism is behaviorally aroused and the nervous system is active and alert to environmental stimuli.

The RAS receives electrical impulses from the sensory systems through *collaterals,* which are branches of the sensory neurons. Input into a sensory system, then, sends impulses directly to the appropriate receiving area of the cortex and also to the RAS. Both paths are essential if the individual is to be aware of the stimulus. Information arriving at an unaroused cortex is equivalent to no information, and arousal without sensory input to the cortex results in an alert person without anything to be alert about!

The RAS seems to be predominantly adrenergic. High blood levels of adrenaline or noradrenaline result in its activation and thus activation of the cerebral cortex. Compounds that are sympathomimetic activate the RAS, while compounds that disrupt adrenergic synapses decrease the responsiveness of the RAS to sensory input.

Hypothalamus

The hypothalamus is probably best described as the structure that primarily controls the autonomic nervous system and therefore functions to integrate information from the body that is relevant to the maintenance of the organism. The hypothalamus is composed of pairs (one in each side of the brain) of nuclei, which are clusters of the dendrites of neurons, serving a common function. Some of these nuclei monitor blood levels of various chemicals, and if the blood level goes outside the normal range, the hypothalamic neurons send impulses to appropriate control centers to restore normal levels. The hypothalamus is also the interface between the nervous system and the endocrine system and acts to adjust the release of hormones to the homeostatic needs of the body.

The hypothalamus is an area with a rich blood supply, and because of this fact many drugs first enter the brain in high concentrations at this structure. The initial effects of these drugs are frequently autonomic ones, with changes in consciousness and mood developing more slowly as drug levels increase in the areas of the brain controlling those experiences.

Medial forebrain bundle

For years hedonists have talked about and sought the locus of pleasure, but it was not until 1954 that the specific brain systems were discovered that seem to form the physiological substrate of pleasure and reward. The details of this system, the medial forebrain bundle (MFB), are only slowly being uncovered, but two things are clear. First, animals and humans will perform work to have the neurons in this system activated electrically via a permanently implanted electrode. Electrical activity in the system seems, then, to act as a reward. Second, humans report that activation of this band of neurons is experienced as pleasurable, and there is evidence that stimulation in this area will counteract feelings of depression.

The function of this system in humans is not well understood and its relationship to natural stimuli that result in pleasurable feelings, such as food and sex, is not known. The suggestion has been made that psychosis is related to abnormal functioning of the MFB. This has not been shown directly, but drugs that calm the agitated psychotic person also decrease the reward value of electrical stimulation of the MFB. Another hypothesis is that the level of electrical activity of the MFB is the decisive factor in determining general mood level and clinical depression. Again, most drugs that affect clinical depression also affect the reward value of electrical stimulation in this area, with those agents that reduce depression making the MFB more sensitive to direct stimulation.

Periventricular system

One of the long-standing questions in philosophy has been whether negative feelings and unhappiness are only the absence of good feelings or whether there is an active process involved. A question moves into the scientific realm when techniques become available for answering it. Paralleling the discovery and explanation of the characteristics of the medial forebrain bundle there has been investigation of the punishment or aversive collection of fibers called the periventricular system (PV).

In both the reward and the punishment systems there are two kinds of effects that must be kept clear, although they may have the same physiological basis. One effect is the experience, the feeling that accompanies electrical stimulation of these systems. A second effect is that which these neural paths have on the other aspects of behavior. There have not been many studies in which humans have been electrically stimulated in these brain areas. The procedure is obviously very experimental, so caution must be used in accepting the results. It does seem clear, however, that the feelings and emotions an individual experiences are drastically different when these two systems are electrically stimulated.

Stimulating the reward system brings forth expressions of pleasure and satisfaction, while periventricular stimulation is followed by strong verbalization of discomfort. Similarly, MFB stimulation increases behavioral activity while a slowing or stopping of behavior seems related to PV activation. Pharmacologically, the best evidence is that adrenergic synapses dominate the reward system while the inhibitory PV system seems to be mostly cholinergic. The two systems may be related functionally so that activation of the MFB inhibits the inhibitory PV system. Inhibition of an inhibitory system results in a release of the neural fibers normally inhibited, and this results in activation.

Basal ganglia

The basal ganglia consist of a group of nuclei that form a secondary motor system. The primary motor system originates in the motor area of the cerebral cortex and controls voluntary movements. It is in the cortical motor area that electrical impulses originate when an individual decides to make a behavioral response. The basal ganglia are concerned with the nonvoluntary, nonconscious adjustments of the skeletal muscles that maintain posture and muscle tone.

The basal ganglia are mentioned here for two reasons. One is that damage to this secondary motor system sometimes results in a syndrome called Parkinson's disease.

This disorder is characterized by postural rigidity and a decrease in facial expressiveness and tremors. Recent work suggests strongly that dopamine is the neurotransmitter in this area, and some cases of Parkinson's disease have been successfully treated by the administration of the drug L-dopa, which is the precursor to dopamine.

The second reason for identifying these ganglia and their functions is that one of the undesirable effects of the phenothiazine drugs used in the treatment of psychotics is the appearance of Parkinson-like symptoms. Frequently these symptoms are so severe that they must be controlled by the administration of an additional drug.

Cerebral cortex

The cerebral cortex is a structure weighing about 1 pound. It contains the dendrites and axon terminals of 9 billion neurons, their supporting cells, and blood vessels. The cerebral cortex is the brain structure that has changed most from other animals to man; a much higher percentage of the brain is devoted to the cortex in man. The human cerebral cortex has become so large that it folds over on itself in many places and almost completely covers the other parts of the brain. A side view of the brain would show only the cortex and some of the other brain centers.

The cerebral cortex can be divided into receiving areas, output areas, and association areas. The receiving areas, those to which neurons from the various senses send information, and the output areas are clearly affected by some psychoactive agents. The sensory areas and their sense organs are connected in very specific ways so that receptors responding to a particular stimulus characteristic always terminate in the same general area of the cortex. Any drugs that affect the electrical activity in the receptors or the connecting neurons or the synapses in the pathway from receptor to cortex will thus affect that specific stimulus quality.

The part of the cortex that has changed most in the evolutionary process is that area called the association cortex. In large part, the proportion of the cerebral cortex that is association cortex is a good index of the extent to which an animal is not under the direct influence of the environment. The association areas do not directly receive inputs from the environment nor do they directly initiate outputs to muscles or glands. These association areas may function to store memories or control complex behaviors or . . . much is unknown but it is clear that some of the psychoactive drugs disrupt the normal functioning of these areas.

A QUICK REVIEW

The nervous system is the primary site of action for psychoactive drugs. Individual neurons are the building blocks that are functionally but not structurally joined to transmit information. Information is carried within a neuron as an electrical impulse, and this intraneuronal activity is little affected by most drugs.

The functional connection between neurons is the synapse. Complex molecules called neurotransmitters carry information from one neuron to another. Most psychoactive drugs influence the functioning of the nervous system by modifying the production, release, action, or breakdown of these neurotransmitters. The type of effect a drug will have depends on the neurotransmitter with which it interacts, the form of such interactions, where in the nervous system that neurotransmitter is found, and what function that area of the nervous system serves.

It is possible to spend a lifetime worrying about the bits and pieces that go to make up the nervous system and still have almost no idea about how the brain works. The capabilities that neurons have set limitations on what the brain can do and how it can function, but these limitations are so broad as to be almost meaningless. The true, fantastic potential of the brain becomes clear only as its processes and operations, not just its parts, become known.

TOWARD AN UNDERSTANDING OF DRUG EFFECTS ON COMPLEX PROCESSES

The autonomic effects of drugs can be fairly readily understood since there is much knowledge about the anatomy and biochemistry of the autonomic nervous system. Similarly, when a drug acts on a sensory system input, there is at least a partially acceptable neural basis for the drug experiences. With more complex behaviors and experiences, a complete physiological explanation of a drug's effects becomes impossible since neither the neuroanatomical locus nor the biochemical processes involved are known.

One approach to understanding psychoactive drug effects on complex behaviors is to study the general ways in which the cerebral cortex functions. Another method is to analyze those aspects of behavior that in part determine the effects of drugs. Briefly, there are modes of central nervous system functioning that are consistent no matter what drug is being used. Similarly, there are some aspects of behavior that influence the effects of all drugs.

Principles of nervous system functioning

To understand the role of the cerebral cortex in determining psychoactive drug effects, four rules must be remembered. One is that the cortex varies continually in its state of arousal, that is, its receptivity and sensitivity to incoming information. Sleep is a condition of low arousal, alertness, and responsiveness to environmental changes. In conditions of intellectual activity and emotional stress the cortex is "activated," alert and responsive to electrical pulses coming to it. The level of arousal is primarily controlled by the reticular activating system, and inputs from the senses go both to the reticular system and to the cerebral cortex.

A second rule is that any electrical activity in a sensory area is experienced and interpreted by the individual as coming from the receptors that normally feed into that sensory area. For example, electrically stimulating the visual cortex directly with an electrode is experienced as flashes of light, or geometric figures are "seen." The experience of a sensation does not depend on where the electrical activity comes from but rather on the part of the cerebral cortex that receives the electrical pulses. To go one step further, *all experience, thoughts, and feelings are nothing more than electrical activity in some part of the brain.* By modifying the electrical activity of neurons in the central nervous system, psychoactive drugs influence and modify experience, thoughts, and feelings.

The third rule is that once information arrives at a sensory receiving area, it then goes to memory areas. The incoming information has meaning only if it coincides with some information in the memory storage area. For incoming impulses to be understood they must not only arrive at the correct sensory area but also be transmitted to the correct memory area. Location of the memory areas is not well known, but probably both cortical and subcortical portions of the brain are involved. Since impulses from a sensory area must travel to a memory area, it may be that this type of organization is the basis for certain drug effects. With some drugs there seems to be interaction between the senses, and inputs to the visual system may be experienced as both a visual and an auditory experience. This could occur if impulses leaving the visual cortex are incorrectly processed (because of the drug) and sent to both the visual and auditory memory areas.

A fourth rule is that many of the functions of the cerebral cortex are carried out by inhibiting or suppressing other parts of the brain or of the cortex itself. In the process of maturing, both physically and psychologically, one role of the cortex seems to be to inhibit some behaviors and thoughts. The inhibition seems to be an active process, so that when the inhibition is removed the ideas and behaviors reappear. This occurs in some kinds of organic brain damage where the cortex is physically incapable of functioning normally, and inhibited behaviors, thoughts, and emotions appear. The same phenomenon occurs with some drugs when the functioning of the cortex is disrupted so that it temporarily ceases its inhibitory role. This fact is one of the reasons for the wide range of effects reported with some psychoactive drugs—what appears depends in part on what was inhibited originally.

Behavioral determinants of drug effects

Behavior is the final output of a complex and incompletely understood nervous system. It results from both past and present inputs to that system. Even though the underlying processes are not clear, it is possible to relate the actions of drugs to at least five dimensions of behavior.

Three behavioral dimensions that are clearly different, but perhaps highly related, are level of abstraction, level of complexity, and level of learning. The more abstract and the more complex the behavior, the more likely it is to be changed following ingestion of a drug. Abstract ideas and complex motor or thought patterns probably are more susceptible in part because they are less well learned than simpler or more concrete behaviors. With a particular task the probability of disrupting it with a given dose of a drug decreases with an increase in the degree of learning. Some behaviors are probably such well-learned habits that very little this side of a coma will disrupt them.

One way of viewing these dimensions is to consider what the neural basis might be. For complex behaviors there must be a lengthy sequence of neural events, all of which must be correct if the behavior is to be intact. In abstract ideas there may be a large number of essential associations (neural connections) if the level of abstraction is to be constant. When there are many elements in a situation, all of which are necessary for complete functioning, there is a greater probability of a drug disrupting at least one step of the neural activity than if there were only a few component parts. In the same vein, an increase in level of learning may improve synaptic functioning or increase the redundancy of the neural patterns that underlie the behavior. Either of these changes would result in a decrease in the ease with which a given drug dose could modify the behavior.

The other two behavioral dimensions relating to the actions of drugs are concerned with motivational aspects of the behavior. Motivation may vary with respect to both type and level. Motivation for a particular behavior might be positive or negative. That is, the behavior may primarily be moving toward or approaching a particular kind of stimulus. It is expected that this behavior would be physiologically based in a normally functioning medial forebrain bundle. Or the behavior may be oriented toward avoiding or escaping from some event. The periventricular system is the physiological substrate underlying this negatively motivated behavior. Some drugs do have different behavioral effects, depending on the type of motivation governing the behavior.

Motivation level seems also to be an important factor in predicting the effect of a drug on behavior. It seems likely that as the motivational level increases there will be an increase in the amount of electrical activity in the motivational systems. This may be the result of more frequent pulses in the same neurons or of the same frequency of pulses in more neurons. In either case, the predicted effect would be increased electrical activity in the motivational systems, and the data support the prediction: as the motivation level of a behavior increases, it becomes more difficult to disrupt the behavior with drugs.

CONCLUDING COMMENT

The preceding factors point out very well the difficulty involved in talking about specific drug effects when the drugs do not act on parts of the nervous system that have built-in functions. All of these behavioral factors refer in some way to the history of the individual. As the history changes, so will the behavioral effects of the drug.

Psychoactive drugs act on the nervous system. To the extent that the actions are on those parts and processes of the nervous system that have built-in, specific functions, the effects of a drug can be predicted. As the behaviors studied become more dependent on factors in the individual's personal history, the exact effects of a drug become less predictable.

PRECEDING QUOTES
1. Eccles, J. C.: The physiology of synapses, New York, 1964, Academic Press, Inc., p. v.
2. Burns, B. D.: The uncertain nervous system, London, 1968, Edward Arnold Ltd., p. 15.
3. Luria, A. R.: Higher cortical functions in man, New York, 1966, Basic Books, Inc., pp. 34-36.

Prelude to pharmacology

A desire to take medicine is, perhaps, the great feature which distinguishes man from other animals.

Sir William Osler, 1891

I firmly believe that if the whole materia medica as now used could be sunk to the bottom of the sea, it would be all the better for mankind — and all the worse for the fishes.

Oliver Wendell Holmes, 1860

Adverse reactions to drugs are part of the price we pay for more effective remedies. Unless a drug can modify or repress biological processes it will be impotent in treatment, but if it can do so it is bound to cause adverse effects from time to time. Those who say that nothing but the complete safety of drugs will suffice demand the impossible, and were their clamour to be taken seriously therapeutic stagnation would result.

Sir Derrick Dunlop, 1970

. . . never before in its history has medicine had so many useful, effective drugs on hand; and never before has there been such promise of even better ones to come.

Walter Modell, 1963

In considering the ways in which a drug can act and the numerous factors that influence the effectiveness of a drug, it is necessary to push headlong into the complex science of pharmacology. The field of pharmacology has a long past but, as a science, it has a short history. Although the earliest clear record of a compendium of drugs is about 1500 B.C., according to some authorities the modern era of pharmacology did not begin until the work of Francois Magendie (1783-1855). American pharmacology begins even later, with John J. Abel (1857-1938) as the father.

An early connotation of the Greek word "pharmakon" was of a harmful substance—something to be eliminated. However, pharmacology is now defined as the study of the interaction of chemical agents with living material. Those interactions whose effects are harmful are generally relegated to the specialty area called *toxicology*. Another specialty area, the most active field in pharmacology, and one that cuts across all of its research areas, is pharmacodynamics. *Pharmacodynamics is concerned with studying the mechanism of action of drugs*. It deals with the problem of how a drug has its effect on the living organism. Chapter 5 is in large part a discussion of pharmacodynamics.

The specialty area that is probably most familiar to the reader is that of pharmacy. Pharmacy is "the art and science of preparing from natural and synthetic sources suitable and convenient materials for distribution and use in the treatment and prevention of diseases."[1] Today's retail pharmacist serves more as a check on a physician's prescriptions than as a compounder of drugs. Over 98% of all drugs prescribed are already formulated—that is, compounded and manufactured in a convenient dosage form—and a pharmacist need only count the tablets or measure the total amount prescribed. The advantage, however, to having a knowledgeable second person monitor both the physician's and the patient's use of today's potent drugs is clear.

The word "drug" comes from the French "drogue" meaning dry substance. It reflects well the condition of many of the early herbs used for the treatment of various illnesses. The classic story of a plant making the transi-tion from folk remedies to the mainstream of science and therapeutic usefulness is illustrated by digitalis. A folk remedy for the treatment of dropsy was a combination of many herbs plus an extract from the purple foxglove plant (*Digitalis purpurea*, purple finger, because of its shape and color). William Withering studied the remedy and reported in 1785 that the purple foxglove was effective in reducing the excessive body fluids in some types of dropsy. In 1799 J. Ferrior pointed out that the primary action of digitalis was on the heart, and the drug continues to be a basic therapeutic agent in cases of congestive heart failure. Drugs of natural origin are still found in about 50% of prescription drugs and about 40% of over-the-counter preparations.

In the science of pharmacology, *a drug is any substance, other than food, that by its chemical or physical nature alters structure or function in the living organism*. Drugs can be classified in many ways ranging from their chemical structure, to their effects on biochemical, physiological, or behavioral systems, to their social uses. The drugs in this book have been primarily categorized into socially meaningful clusters of compounds and then subgrouped on the basis of their chemical structure.

CATEGORIZING DRUGS

Physicians, pharmacologists, chemists, lawyers, psychologists, and users all have drug classification schemes that best serve their own purposes. A compound such as amphetamine might be categorized as an anti-appetite agent by many physicians since it reduces food intake for a period of time. It might be classed as a phenylethylamine by a pharmacologist since its basic structure is a phenyl ring with an ethyl group and an amine attached. The chemist wastes no time and says flat-out that amphetamine is 2-amino-1-phenylpropane. To the lawyer amphetamine may only be a drug of abuse falling in Schedule II of the 1970 federal drug law, while the psychologist may say simply that it is a stimulant. The user may call it a diet pill or an upper. The important thing to remember is that any scheme for categorizing drugs has meaning only if it serves the purpose for which the classification is being made.

Hopefully, some appreciation of the social meaning of the uses of drugs can be conveyed here as well as an understanding of the scientific basis of their use. Toward that end, socially and scientifically meaningful groupings are used in this book. A listing of the major classes of compounds in this scheme can be seen by looking at the Table of Contents. A brief survey of these classes and the rationale behind the classification may be helpful in following the unfolding story of drugs. It should be clear that this classification is only for psychoactive drugs, chemicals that alter experiences and mood.

There are some drugs—chemicals affecting living organisms—that few people think of as drugs. These *nondrug drugs* include alcohol and caffeine, a depressant and a stimulant, as well as those compounds that can be picked up at the friendly supermarket such as aspirin, antihistamines, and antacids. The single most important factor about all these compounds is that they are readily available without prescription and thus are not usually considered to be drugs.

The general grouping of *psychotherapeutic agents* seems to be widely accepted—these are the drugs used in psychiatric medicine. These compounds are prescribed when the symptom of illness is a disruption of the interaction between an individual and his environment. The drugs that reduce either the disruption or the reaction to the disruption are discussed together. At least two social characteristics distinguish these agents: they are used therapeutically to treat "mental disturbances," and they rarely fall into the category of abused drugs. Other therapeutically useful drugs are widely known and grouped together because they frequently are abused and their medical use is for the treatment of minor problems such as obesity and insomnia!

Although nearly everyone knows that the *opiates*, morphine and heroin, can have considerable therapeutic value, these drugs are generally not viewed as therapeutics. Rather, these narcotics are seen as the hard drugs, the drugs used by addicts and the ones peddled by the Mafia. In a very real sense these drugs are unique both socially and scientifically.

The *hallucinogens* form a separate class in our social thinking and the associations are almost automatic: hallucinogens—psychedelic—hippies—marijuana. To group drugs such as LSD and marijuana together and still clearly separate them does justice to the scientific data as well as the social scene.

Clearly, as time changes, so may the rational way to categorize drugs. The biochemical actions and the physiological effects do not change, but the relevance and implications for society of these effects may change considerably from one generation to another. Over 40 years ago a now-classic categorization of drugs was accomplished by Lewin primarily on the basis of social, behavioral, and experienced effects.[2] This is still a useful scheme, and contrasting it to the one used in this book will help provide a glimpse of the broad picture of drug classification. Lewin combines some drug groups differently than is done here, and tranquilizers and mood modifiers were unknown in 1931.

Lewin divided the centrally acting drugs into five groups and placed them in a circle as indicated in Fig. 4-1. By arranging them this way he brought home the fact that many drugs have multiple effects and thus fit into more than one group.

The *excitants* are compounds that cause behavioral and central nervous system

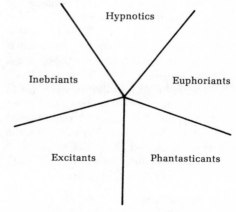

Fig. 4-1. Lewin's classification of centrally acting drugs.

stimulation. A naturally occurring agent in this group is caffeine, which is found in coffee and tea, while the amphetamines are good examples of synthetic excitants. All the drugs in this group have as their primary effect an activation of the central nervous system that results in behavioral arousal and stimulation.

The *inebriants* are those drugs that cause intoxication, in the social sense. The initial effect of these compounds is behavioral excitement but it is soon followed by distortions in perception and thought that accompany behavioral depression. Alcohol, a natural product of fermentation, is included in this class, as is the synthetic compound ether.

The *hypnotics* are divided into two major categories, but all are agents that cause amnesia and/or confusion and result in a state of consciousness that eliminates reality. Sedatives and anesthetics are included here, with the barbiturates perhaps the best example. In Lewin's classification this group also contains the delusional agents such as atropine.

The *euphoriants* are drugs that act to eliminate perception of the present world by replacing it with one in which the individual experiences no problems. Opium and its derivatives are naturally occurring substances that have just such effects, and a number of synthetic opiates such as methadone can act similarly.

The *phantasticants* are not an off-Broadway group but rather those drugs that replace the present world with an alternative world— one that is equally real, but different. Lewin separates these agents from the delusional hypnotics on the basis that with these drugs there is an awareness of "both realities." Both the drug-induced and the nondrug world can be attended to at the same time, and there is memory for the drug-induced reality after the drug effect diminishes. Peyote, a cactus of southwestern United States, is a naturally occurring phantasticant, while LSD is a well-known synthetic drug in this group.

NAMING OF DRUGS

Classifying drugs is a necessary first step in discussing the individual drug and its actions. The second step is the naming of drugs. When individual agents are discussed it becomes clear that the answer to the question of "what's in a name?" is "plenty," especially if it's a brand name! Although "a rose by any other name would smell as sweet," that may not be true of drugs. Commercially available compounds have several kinds of names—a brand name, a generic name, and a chemical name.

The *chemical name of a compound gives a complete chemical description of the molecule* and is derived from the rules of organic chemistry for naming any compound. Chemical names of drugs are rarely used except in a laboratory situation where biochemists or pharmacologists are developing and testing new drugs. Chemical names of drugs are given here only when the structure of a chemical is shown. There are several sets of rules for naming chemical structures. The most commonly used rules in the United States are those of *Chemical Abstracts* and those of the International Union of Pure and Applied Chemistry (IUPAC). Structures shown in this book are generally named using the *Chemical Abstracts* system, although a few have been named by IUPAC where that system's name is more common.

Much more commonly used by scientists is the simpler generic (or nonproprietary) name of a drug. Generic names are the official (that is, legal) names of drugs and are listed in the USP and NF. The generic, or nonproprietary, names of chemicals are standardized by representatives of the American Medical Association, the American Pharmaceutical Association, the U. S. Pharmacopeial Convention, Inc., and the Food and Drug Administration. This group, known as the United States Adopted Name Council (USAN), has certain principles for assigning generic names to structures. Of primary importance in considering generic names are two facts: *a generic name specifies a specific chemical structure,* and *generic names are in the public domain.* The last point means they can be freely used by anyone and are not protected by trademark laws, clearly differentiating them from brand names.

The brand name of a drug specifies a particular formulation and manufacturer of a generic product. A brand name is usually quite simple and as meaningful (in terms of the indicated therapeutic use) as the company can make it. The over-the-counter compound Compōz and the prescription drug Vesprin, for example, certainly aren't stimulants. Vesprin is a tranquilizer and the name alone almost makes you feel more relaxed, associating to it a quiet evening and vespers. Compōz, sold as a sleep aid and sedative, makes some people think of relaxation and smooth, easy experiences in life. However, brand names are controlled by the Food and Drug Administration and overly suggestive ones are not approved.

When a new chemical structure, a new way of manufacturing a chemical or a new use for a chemical is discovered, it can be patented. Patent laws in this country protect for 17 years and, after that time, the finding is available for use by anyone. Brand names, however, are copyrighted and protected by trademark laws. These laws indefinitely restrict the use of the brand name to the original copyright holder.

Since a patent permits manufacturing control for only 17 years, it is understandable that companies would seek other means to control the sale of the drug for a longer period of time. This is accomplished by advertising drugs under their brand names to physicians, not only through advertising in journals but also by direct contact of company representatives. According to some estimates, pharmaceutical houses spend about $4,500 a year per physician in this area of selling.[3]

Since brand names are more familiar to physicians and easier to use, nearly all prescriptions are written using brand rather than generic names. In 1969 less than 10% of the prescriptions were written using generic names. In that same year a list of the 200 leading drugs, which accounted for 66% of all prescriptions, included only sixteen generic names.[4] The name used on the prescription is important since forty-four states have anti-substitution laws. These laws make it illegal for a pharmacist dispensing drugs to substitute any drug for the one written on the prescription. If the physician writes a brand name, then that product must be given to the patient.

Use of brand names is a vital issue to the pharmaceutical companies, as well as to the consumer and the government. Partially as a result of physicians using brand rather than generic names, drug companies regularly show about twice as much profit each year (18%) as companies of equivalent size in other manufacturing fields. Such profit results from the higher price of the brand name product when compared to the same chemical sold under the generic name. Sometimes the price difference is considerable, several hundred percent, but a more realistic estimate of the average increased cost at the consumer level is 5% to 8%.[3]

Before leaving the general problem of the names of drugs one other term must be mentioned. Frequently in reports of arrests involving drugs the term "legend" drug is used. *Legend drugs are drugs that are available only on prescription.* Each container of these drugs must have on it the legend: "Caution: federal law prohibits dispensing without prescription." The legend drugs include many that are not psychoactive, such as the antibiotics, and the use of the term "legend drugs" seems to be restricted to the marketing and legal area.

Generic-brand name controversy

For 17 years a company that has discovered and patented a product can manufacture and sell it without competition. When the patent expires the discovery is free game for any manufacturer and, if the drug has been a money-maker, it is quite likely that new companies will develop the capability to produce the "same" drug. However, at this point a question arises—if the drug is chemically identical by Food and Drug Administration standards, is it the therapeutic equivalent?

A drug is initially released for sale by the Food and Drug Administration only after it has been shown to be safe and effective for the condition it is used to treat. This clearance is obtained by the original producer of the drug. The heart of the brand-generic conflict is whether it can be assumed that drugs manufactured to Food and Drug Administration standards by new companies do not have to go through the necessary pre-clinical and clinical trials to demonstrate safety and effectiveness.

A drug can be effective only if it is delivered to those cells where the drug acts. Almost all drugs reach the area where they are to act via the bloodstream, and any factors that influence a drug's ability to be absorbed by the bloodstream will influence its effectiveness. To separate out some of the factors involved in determining the equivalence of two drugs, three concepts have come into wide use recently.

The concept of *chemical equivalence* is fairly clear. Chemical equivalents are those drugs that contain essentially identical amounts of the identical active ingredients in identical dosages and that thus meet present Food and Drug Administration physiochemical standards. *Biological equivalents* are those drugs that, when administered in the same amounts, provide the same biological or physiological availability of the drug to the body tissues. The biological availability, or bioavailability, is usually assessed by determining the levels of the drug in the bloodstream.

Clinical equivalents are chemical equivalents that, when given in the same amounts, result in the same therapeutic effect. Thus, two drugs can be chemically equivalent but not be clinically equivalent. Whether biological equivalence is tantamount to clinical equivalence is not yet decided, but it seems likely. The primary factor involved in determining whether chemical equivalents have the same bioavailability is related to the way the drug is finally prepared for use. What would seem to be minor factors such as the hardness of the tablet of the drug and the solubility of the drug capsule become critical in determining the extent to which a drug can be absorbed into the bloodstream. If the drug does not reach the bloodstream there is little chance it can have an effect.

In 1970 the Commissioner of the Food and Drug Administration, Dr. C. C. Edwards, summed it up when he stated:

> It has become increasingly apparent that drug products which purport to be equivalent and which may satisfy chemical and other analytical tests of equivalence, may not be therapeutically equivalent. We believe the key to the problem lies in what we refer to as bio-availability. We have found that comparable bioavailability frequently does not exist for products that are otherwise, so far as currently available methods are concerned, identical. We are not fully aware of the extent of the problem, but know that it exists particularly in tablet or capsule dosage forms.*

A case history of a brand-generic conflict involves Terramycin, the Charles Pfizer Company's brand of oxytetracycline. Terramycin was discovered by Pfizer researchers in 1949 after screening over 100,000 samples of earth (hence the name "terra") and was a highly successful antibiotic. In 1967, when the patent ran out, several companies began producing oxytetracycline, which is the generic name for Terramycin and which was the chemical equivalent according to Food and Drug Administration tests. Considerable money was involved since the cost to the patient for Terramycin was about 30¢ a capsule while oxytetracycline was half that price. The Pfizer Company decided to study blood levels in groups of patients receiving Terramycin or the various brands of oxytetracycline.[5]

The Food and Drug Administration certified the chemical composition, amount, and purity of each of the generic brands and of Terramycin and all were equivalent. Following equal amounts of each drug, the blood levels of the drug in patients receiving the different brands were anything but equivalent. None of the generic brands gave blood levels (and thus "bioavailability") as high as Terramycin. The drugs produced by eight manufacturers resulted in blood levels too low to be acceptable and the Food and Drug Administration called in 40 million capsules by those producers. The sales field was left to Terramycin and two generic forms of oxytetracycline that did yield adequate blood levels. A similar story could be related for the Parke-Davis antibiotic Chloromycetin. In controlled studies

---

*From Edwards, C. C.: The FDA's views on generic equivalence and drug quality, Pharmacy Times 36(6):48, 1970.

it was shown that some generic brands of chloramphenicol did not give therapeutically effective blood levels of the drug.

There are these and other well-documented cases where a generic compound did not produce the same bioavailability as the brand name product, but examples are hard to find. The mountain-out-of-a-molehill concept was supported by the Final Report of a Department of Health, Education and Welfare task force of authorities from the drug industry, medical schools, and government, which concluded:

> . . . on the basis of available evidence, lack of clinical equivalency among chemical equivalents meeting all official standards has been grossly exaggerated as a major hazard to the public health.*

The government is still doing studies to determine the bioavailability equivalence of many widely used drugs. Whether such equivalence exists will perhaps be debated for many years. In 1973 the FDA said "It is not possible to specify at the present time the frequency with which lack of equivalence in bioavailability of chemically equivalent formulations may occur." No matter. In mid-1974 the United States required, when possible, the use of generic rather than brand names for *all* drugs bought from federal funds. This would include prescriptions covered by Medicare and Medicaid.

The expectation of an expanding market for generic drugs is being matched by American ingenuity. Trade magazines now contain advertisements to the effect: Buy your generic drugs from XYZ Company—a name you can trust and your assurance of quality! Perhaps a new era is about to dawn where brand names will be obsolete but all drugs will be prescribed by the generic-company name! This is progress? After all is said and done, until bioavailability is shown for generic agents, the prudent course is to utilize brand name compounds since, in the words of a Food and Drug Administration spokesman: ". . . it is evident that manufacturing procedures *can have* an effect on the availability for absorption of an orally administered drug. . . ."[6]

*From Task force on prescription drugs, final report, Washington, D. C., 1969, U. S. Department of Health, Education and Welfare, p. 31.

NONSPECIFIC FACTORS IN DRUG EFFECTS

Would that life were so simple that the effect of psychoactive drugs could be predicted by their level in the blood. With compounds such as the antibiotics, there is good evidence that blood levels are highly related to therapeutic effectiveness. This is readily understood since these drugs have very clear specific effects on the invading microorganisms responsible for the disease. If the drug is delivered to the area of the infection, it acts so that the body can reduce the disease process. Since the critical problem is getting the drug to the infected area, monitoring blood levels of the drug gives good evidence of the effectiveness of the product.

As will be discussed in a later chapter, there is no evidence that a similar causative agent exists for the mental disturbances. The psychoactive drugs appear to have their effect by altering patterns of neural functioning. Since these drugs act by altering function, it follows that the effects will in part depend on the activity that is already present. Another consideration in understanding the actions of these drugs is that they are frequently used to affect moods, feelings, and the individual's reactions to changes in his environment. These kinds of changes can also be brought about by nonchemical means, and this fact must be always considered when evaluating the effects of psychoactive drugs.

The bases for the effects of a psychoactive drug are usually divided into two groups. One group consists of those molecular, physiological, and biochemical changes that result from specific chemical characteristics of the drug and the cells or chemicals with which it interacts. Thus a basis for the effects of atropine in the body is the occupation of the acetylcholine receptor site by atropine. One specific effect resulting from this is the cessation of the flow of saliva and a drying of the mouth and throat. This effect will occur regardless of whether the patient believes it will happen, whether he knows he is receiving a drug, whether he likes his doctor, or whatever. *The specific effects of drugs are caused by physiobiochemical actions of the drug*, which depend only on the drug's reaching the site of action and a normal body chemistry.

The second group of causes for a drug's effect has only recently been widely studied and is termed nonspecific factors; "nonspecific" means merely that these effects of the drug are not based on its chemical activity. These nonspecific factors are those that reside in an individual with a unique background and a particular perception of the world. In brief, the nonspecific factors can include anything except the chemical activity of the drug and the direct effects of this activity. For example, a good trip or a bad trip from pure LSD seems to be dependent in part on the personality and mood of the user prior to taking the drug. In part, the kind of trip experienced depends on what the user expects to experience. The expectation is a nonspecific factor with respect to drug actions since it influences the experienced effect of the drug, but not the chemical activity of the drug.

Since the expectation of a drug effect can influence the effect that is experienced by the user or seen by an observer, most of the acceptable drug research with humans is carried out under *double-blind* conditions. In a double-blind experiment, neither the physician nor the patient knows whether the patient is receiving a drug or an inert substance—a *placebo*. When neither the patient nor his doctor knows if a drug is being used, a better evaluation can be made of the drug's specific effect on the symptoms. Another factor is necessary for a study to be considered adequately controlled. The patients should be assigned randomly to the drug and the placebo groups. A meaningful study of the effects of a drug can best be accomplished if patients are randomly assigned to groups and double-blind conditions are met.

However, even a double-blind study does not provide a pure evaluation. One investigator[7] studied the differential effects of two mild tranquilizers on anxiety in a group of patients of general practitioners. Neither the patient nor the physician knew which drug was being used and, *prior to the start of medication*, both the physician and patient had to indicate whether they were optimistic, indifferent, or pessimistic about the outcome of treatment. After 2 months, regardless of the drug used, patients for whom the doctors

were optimistic showed a 50% reduction in symptoms, while those patients for whom the physician had been pessimistic showed only a 20% decrease. Optimistic patients showed a 45% reduction in their anxiety symptoms while the patients pessimistic about outcome showed a symptom drop of only 35%.

It may simply be that the physicians were good predictors of treatment outcome, but other studies have also shown that the effectiveness of drug treatment compared to placebo varies in part with the attitudes of the physician. In general, authoritarian, extroverted physicians who believe in the effectiveness of drug treatment have higher patient improvement rates than do physicians with contrasting characteristics, regardless of whether or not the study is double-blind.[8]

Perhaps more impressive are those studies relating patient variables to improvement under drug and/or placebo administration. One report[9] compared the responses of neurotic outpatients receiving either minor tranquilizers or placebos during a 4-week treatment period. Several patient characteristics were related to clinical improvement following drug or placebo treatment. Of the patients with high intelligence, 77% improved with drug while only 44% improved with placebo. With low-intelligence patients improvement was the same whether thay had received drug or placebo—about 70%. In the same vein more patients with high initial anxiety improved under drug (69%) than with placebo (39%), but with initial low anxiety 79% improved with placebo and 65% with drug. The amount of improvement was greatest for those patients who reported high feelings of adequacy irrespective of whether they received drug or placebo. Other studies have suggested the importance of additional patient personality characteristics as determinants of response to psychoactive drugs and placebos.[10] Although many studies have tried to show a consistent relationship between particular personality traits and response to placebo, there is no convincing evidence. The only characteristic that appears regularly as a predictor of response to placebo is a high level of anxiety.[11]

Several interesting results come from a

large federally funded research program[12] designed to evaluate the effectiveness of several potent antipsychotic agents in reducing symptoms of hospitalized schizophrenic patients. In this nationwide study it was found that the drugs were consistently more effective than the placebo in reducing symptoms. The studies also indicated that female patients showed more improvement to the drug treatment than males, but less improvement to placebo than did males. Another differential response was that Negroes and Caucasians responded equally to drug therapy, but the Negroes responded more to the placebo than did the Caucasians.

Perhaps the major implication in this study was that, when using potent antipsychotic phenothiazines in acutely psychotic patients, there were *no* treatment effects that could be attributed to the many existing differences among the hospitals where the study was conducted. From this and other studies it seems that:

> ...the non-specific effects are important for *small treatments* and *small illnesses* ...If we have effective treatments, non-specific effects cease to be a practical problem...In the milder illnesses the personality of the patient, his environment, and his problems are factors which play a part not only in the treatment but also in the illness as well ...*

The quote states very well what seems to be the consensus of the work done in this area. When there is a relatively ineffective treatment, or if the illness is one reflecting nonorganic abnormal patterns of neural functioning rather than an illness resulting from an organic change, then nonspecific placebo effects may be important in determining the course of the illness. When the illness has an organic basis and when the drug's chemical actions result in specific effects on the organic basis, then nondrug factors become irrelevant.

Nowhere has it been said that the psychoactive drugs don't have very specific physiochemical actions. This might be inferred from the preceding section, but it would not be true and represents incomplete understanding. Psychoactive drugs do have specific effects. Because the underlying brain mechanisms are not known, no one is certain which drug effects are important for certain changes in mood and thinking to occur.

A final quote adequately expresses the general thrust of this section.

> The more the response system being measured involves cortical processes such as awareness, consciousness, and subjective feelings, the greater will be the role of nonspecific factors influencing drug response.*

General mechanisms of drug actions in neural systems

There are three general kinds of interactions a drug can have with a neuron that change the functioning of the neuron. A drug may interact with specific receptors at a synapse and thus alter synaptic functioning. Another possibility is that a drug may interact with one of the enzyme systems involved in the production or deactivation of a neurotransmitter. A final mechanism of action, and the one most poorly understood, is that a drug may act on the entire neuron membrane in such a way as to alter its normal functioning. In every case, however, the drug has an action that modifies neural functioning and thus disturbs the normal communication of information in the nervous system.

The way in which transmitters and receptors interact to cause electrical changes in the dendrite is not fully understood. That an agent must have particular structural and electrical characteristics in order to occupy the receptor has been established. One theory of receptor action suggests that the electrical change that occurs lasts as long as the transmitter occupies the receptor. The analogy is to an organ in which a tone is emitted as long as the note is held down. More likely, though, is the belief that the electrical changes occur only when the receptor is first occupied, that is, there

---

*From Hamilton, M.: Discussion of the meeting. In Rickels, K., editor: Non-specific factors in drug therapy, Springfield, Illinois, 1968, Charles C Thomas, Publisher, p. 134.

*From Fisher, S.: Nonspecific factors as determinants of behavioral response to drugs. In DiMascio, A., and Shader, R. I., editors: Clinical handbook of psychopharmacology, New York, 1970, Science House, Inc., p. 35.

is action only as a result of the combining, not of the occupation. Analogously, a piano key must be struck repeatedly if the tone is to persist.

There are then two characteristics of a drug molecule that influence its action at the receptor. One is its electrical and structural characteristics—can it occupy the site at all and will it excite the receptor or just occupy it. The second characteristic is the affinity of the drug for the receptor. That is, does the molecule occupy the receptor and remain there, or does it exit and permit another molecule or itself again to reoccupy it?

Even a minor discussion of the question of a drug fitting a receptor would take us far afield. The area of structure-activity relationships is large, and no overall generalizations have emerged. It is clear, though, that some agents mimic the postsynaptic action of a transmitter very well, while others are effective in blocking the action of transmitters by occupying the receptor site but not activating it.

Between these two extremes of drug actions there are many degrees of activity, and some relate to the matter of a drug's affinity for a receptor site. Nicotine can be mentioned as an example. It clearly mimics acetylcholine at first, causing stimulation of some cholinergic fibers, but later causes a depression of activity in the same fibers. It has been proposed that this biphasic effect of nicotine results from its occupying the acetylcholine receptor and thus exciting it, but then continuing to occupy the site and preventing other molecules from combining, thus blocking any further stimulation of the neuron. Nicotine, some evidence shows, has a much stronger affinity for the site than the normal transmitter and also is not deactivated as rapidly as the normal transmitter.

One comment must be made about a particular aspect of structure-activity relationships, namely, the direction in which molecules will rotate polarized light. Some molecules exist in two forms, chemically identical but differing in whether they rotate polarized light to the right (dextro) or left (levo). The magnitude of the rotation is the same, only the direction differs. These two forms have been found to be mirror

images (optical isomers) of each other and this is the basis for the difference in direction of the rotation of polarized light.

Of relevance here is the fact that one of the isomers is usually much more active physiologically than the other. Probably only when the chemical structure has a specific form can the drug occupy a receptor site. Usually the left (levo) rotating, or l, isomers are more active than the d (right, dextro) forms. This characteristic of a drug is indicated by using the letter d or l before its generic name.

The second mechanism by which a drug can have its effect is through interacting with one of the enzyme systems involved in information processing. These are usually enzymes involved in building neurotransmitters or in deactivating them. To understand the possible ways in which these enzyme-drug interactions can occur, it is necessary to appreciate what enzymes do.

Enzymes are necessary catalysts for manufacturing, dividing, or altering complex molecules. They are usually quite singular in their actions, and some function by combining certain atoms and molecules into new specific molecules having definite roles in the overall metabolism of the cell. Other enzymes act by breaking down molecules either into their more usable component parts or at least into molecules that are physiologically less active. The molecules on which an enzyme normally acts are called the *substrate* for that enzyme. The outcome of the substrate-enzyme interaction is the *end product*. A drug can clearly change the end product by affecting either the substrate or the enzyme.

In some cases the drug forms a better substrate for the enzyme than the usual substrate and in this way impairs the normal manufacturing of transmitter substances. Sometimes a drug acts by forming a bond with an enzyme, thus preventing the enzyme from acting. No matter which interaction occurs, normal neural functioning is impaired.

Drugs that act on neural membranes at other than receptor sites exert effects in one of several ways. They may act on one of the transport systems in the membrane or directly on the general physiochemical makeup of the membrane. Alcohol and the barbiturates are good examples of drugs that exert their action by altering the structure and permeability of the entire membrane. Changing cell membrane permeability changes the electrical difference across the membrane and thus affects the overall excitability of the neuron. The most familiar agent that acts on a transport system in the cell membrane is the naturally occurring hormone *insulin*. The presence of insulin is necessary for glucose to be transported into body cells so it can be utilized for energy. In the absence of insulin, as in a diabetic person, the glucose remains outside the cell and the body starves in spite of an adequate diet. Some drugs act on the presynaptic axon terminals and cause a release of the neurotransmitter. The physiologically active amphetamines act in this way. Other drugs affect the same area to prevent the reuptake of the adrenergic transmitter. Both cocaine and amphetamine seem to have this effect.

Dose-response relationships

Perhaps the most fundamental concept in understanding drug actions is the dose-response curve and phenomena associated with it. In simple terms the *dose-response curve*, mentioned in Chapter 1, *refers to the fact that as the amount of the drug administered is varied, there may be a change in a monitored behavior.* A basic point is that since the effects of a drug can be studied on many behaviors or responses, there are many different dose-response curves.

Drug effects arise from the collective effects of many molecular interactions. The more drug molecules there are at the site of action, the more interactions there can be and the greater their collective effects may be. There is always a minimum number of molecular interactions required before the result of their collective effects can be measured. When an effect is seen, it is called a threshold response, and the dose of the drug administered is called the threshold dose.

With an increase in the amount of drug given, there is an increase in the collective effect of the molecular interactions and thus of the response being monitored. At some point molecular interactions are occurring

at the most rapid rate possible; the addition of more drug does not then increase the response. This, in essence, is what a dose-response curve is. At some low dose (few drug molecules) there is an observable effect on the response system being monitored. This dose is the threshold and, as the dose of the drug is increased, there are more molecular interactions and a greater effect on the response system. At the point where the system shows maximal response, further additions of the drug have no effect.

In some drug-response interactions, the effect of the drug is all-or-none, so that when the system does respond, it responds maximally. There may, however, be variability in the dosage at which individual organisms respond, and, as the dose increases, there is an increase in the percentage of individuals who show the response. The relationship between the change in the response system and the dose of the drug is shown in Fig. 4-2. Each of the graphs is a dose-response curve and indicates the relationship between the amount of drug administered and a particular measure of the response being monitored. Three different types of measures are used, and they all indicate the same basic relationship.

Previously, mention was made that, as the drug dose increased, sometimes new response systems are affected by the drug. This fact suggests that some response systems have higher drug thresholds than others or that they are less accessible to the drug. Fig. 4-3 shows a dose-response curve that is reasonably accurate in indicating the relationship between the dose of LSD that an individual takes and the changing response systems affected or (and it's impossible to know now which is correct) the increasing effect on a single response system.[13]

In the rational use of drugs there are four questions about drug dosage that must be answered. First, what is the effective dose of the drug for a desired goal? For example, what dose of morphine is necessary to reduce pain 50%? What amount of marijuana is necessary for an individual to feel euphoric? How much aspirin will make the headache go away? The second question is, what dose

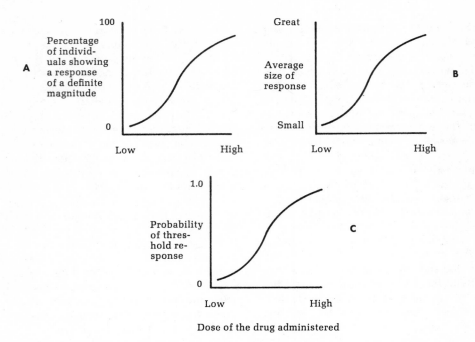

Fig. 4-2. Relationships between drug dose and a single response system.

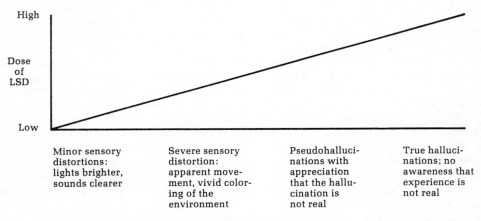

Fig. 4-3. Relationship between dose of LSD and changes in sensory experiences.

of the drug will be lethal to the individual? How much of the drug is necessary to kill a person? Combining those two, what is the safety margin—how different are the effective dose and the lethal dose? Finally, at the effective dose level, what other effects, particularly adverse reactions, might develop? Leaving aside for now this last question, a

discussion of the first three deals with basic concepts in understanding drug actions.

In any biological system there is considerable variability; response to drugs is no different. Some individuals will be very sensitive to a drug and show the desired effect at low dose levels. Others will be quite resistant and the desired effect of the drug will be reached

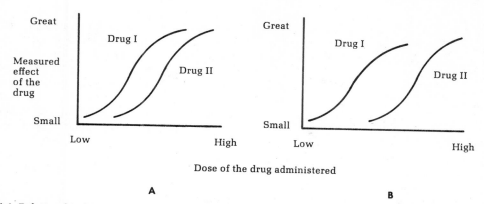

Fig. 4-4. Relationship between the measured effect of two drugs at varying dose levels. In **A,** drug I is more potent than drug II, that is, less of drug I than of drug II is needed to obtain a given effect, but both drugs have the same maximum effect. In **B,** drug I is more potent but drug II can give greater effects.

only after high doses are administered. Between these sensitive and resistant individuals there is usually an increasing percentage of effective responses as the dose of the drug is increased. This relationship was shown in Fig. 4-2, A.

The basis for this variability is not well understood, but there are many factors involved ranging from those determining the absorption of a drug from the digestive tract to the activity of the drug metabolizing enzymes in the liver. The importance of genetic factors in rate of drug metabolism has been clearly demonstrated, and there are active research programs going on in this field of pharmacogenetics.[14]

The *effective dose* (the dose that is effective in causing a particular effect) is abbreviated *ED,* and a number is attached to indicate the percentage of individuals who show the desired effects at a particular dose level. The term ED 50 means that at the indicated dose level, 50% of the people or animals showed the desired response. The ED 1 is a dose level at which the effect is observed in only 1% of the individuals, while the ED 99 is the dose at which 99% of the individuals showed the effect.

The *lethal dose, LD,* is determined in the same way; what percentage of the animals at each dose level die within a specified period of time? The *safety margin* refers to the dose difference between an acceptable level of effectiveness (ED 50? ED 90?) and the

LD 1. For most psychoactive drugs there is a considerable range between the dose giving the desired effect and a lethal dose. For some experimental anticancer compounds there is a small margin of safety.

Since most of the psychoactive compounds have an LD 1 well above the ED 95 level, the practical limitation on whether or not, or at what dose, a drug is used is the occurrence of side effects. With increasing doses there is usually an increase in the number and severity of side effects, those effects of the drug not relevant to the treatment. If the number of side effects becomes too great and the individual begins to suffer from them, the use of the drug will be discontinued or the dose lowered, even though the drug may be very effective in controlling the original symptoms. The selection of a drug for therapeutic use involves both these concepts. Drug choice should be made on the basis of specificity of action on the symptom with minimal side effects.

Potency

The potency of a drug is one of the most misunderstood concepts in the area of drug use. *Potency refers only to the amount of drug that must be given to obtain a particular response.* The less the amount needed to get a particular effect, the more potent the drug. Potency has nothing to do with the effectiveness of the drug. Neither is potency related to maximum effect of a drug. These relationships are indicated in Fig. 4-4. If drug A is one-half as potent as drug B, then you can get the same effect by using twice the dose of drug A as of drug B. Potency refers only to relative effective dose; the ED 50 of a potent drug is lower than the ED 50 of a less potent drug. Rarely is it true that two drugs will differ only in their potency.

Time-dependent factors in drug actions

Fig. 4-5 roughly describes one type of relationship between the administration of a drug and its effect over time. Between points A and B there is no observed effect, although the concentration of drug in the blood is increasing. At point B the threshold concentration is reached, and from B to C the observed drug effect increases as drug concentration increases. At point C the maximal effect of the drug is reached but its concentration continues increasing to point D. Although deactivation of the drug probably begins as soon as the drug enters the body, from A to D the rate of absorption is greater than the rate of deactivation. Beginning at point D the deactivation proceeds more rapidly than absorption and the concentration of the drug decreases. When the amount of drug in the body reaches E, the maximal effect is over. The action diminishes from E to F, at which point the level of the drug is below the threshold for effect, although there is still drug in the body up to point G.

It should be clear that if the relationship described in Fig. 4-5 is true for a particular drug, then increasing the dose of the drug will not increase the magnitude of its effect. Aspirin is probably the most misused drug in this respect—if two are good, four should be better, and six will really stop this headache. No way! When the maximum possible therapeutic effect has been reached, increasing the dose may prolong the effect, but such an increase primarily serves to add to the number of side effects. If a high dose is used originally there may be some shortening of the time of onset (the amount of time between taking the drug and the experiencing of effects), but in the case of aspirin there will also be an increase in gastric irritation.

A different type of relationship between a drug and its effect is presented in Fig. 4-6, A. In this case the effect of the drug parallels the concentration of the drug in the body. In Fig. 4-5 the situation was shown where a drug's maximum effect was in some way limited—perhaps all available receptor sites were occupied, or perhaps the system on which the drug was acting had reached its limit for change. Alcohol is one of the drugs where as the concentration in the blood increases, the effects on the central nervous system increase. And with alcohol the drug effect can continue to increase until loss of consciousness or death occurs.

Alcohol is also a good example for the relationship shown in Fig. 4-6, B. This graph shows how drugs can have a cumulative effect so that, with repeated doses of a drug, you get increasing effects. Usually *cumulative*

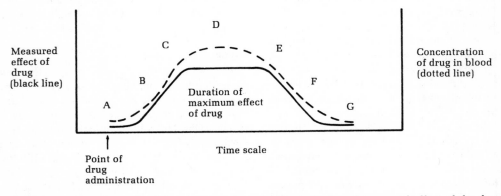

Fig. 4-5. Possible relationship between drug concentration in body and measured effect of the drug.

effects occur when a second dose is given before the first dose has been deactivated. Similar to cumulative effects are those called *additive*, which refer to the fact that different drugs can act on the same system. Even though low doses may be taken of each drug, together the effect may be the same as a high dose of a single drug. Alcohol and the barbiturates are drugs that show additive effects—sometimes their combined depressant effects are lethal.

One of the important changes in manufacturing drugs related to the temporal aspects of drug effectiveness is the development of time-release preparations. These compounds are prepared so that following oral use the active ingredient is released into the body over a 6- to 10-hour period. With a preparation of this type a large amount of the drug is initially made available for absorption and then smaller amounts are released continuously for a long period. The initial amount of the drug is expected to be adequate to obtain the response desired and the gradual release thereafter is designed to maintain the same effective dose of the drug even though the drug is being continually deactivated. In terms of Fig. 4-5, a time-release preparation would aim at eliminating the unnecessarily high drug level at *C-D-E* while lengthening the *C-E* time interval. Unfortunately, up to this time there is no way of manufacturing orally active drug products so that drugs are reliably released over more than 8 to 10 hours.

Another drug phenomenon that is temporally related is tolerance. *Tolerance* refers to a situation in which repeated administration of the same dose of a drug results in gradually diminishing effects. That is, the second dose does not give as great an effect as the first dose, and, if the same dose is repeated a number of times, eventually the drug has no

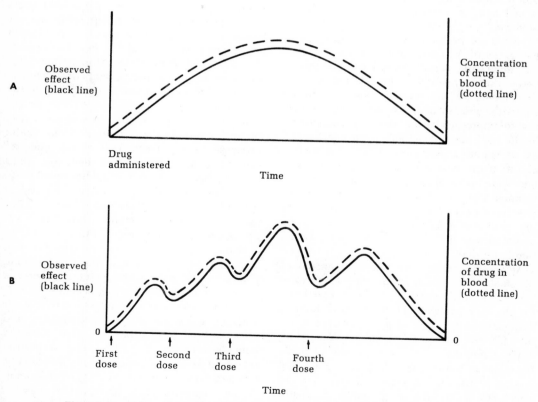

Fig. 4-6. Possible relationships between observed effects and drug concentration.

effect. Some effects of a drug may show tolerance while others do not, since a drug may have multiple effects that may occur by different mechanisms.

With some drugs, LSD for example, tolerance develops relatively rapidly. If LSD is taken once each day for a week, a dose that gave a good effect the first day would probably give little if any effect on the fifth or sixth day. When tolerance develops rapidly it also diminishes rapidly. In the case of LSD, if the user does not ingest any LSD for a week, the full effect of the dose will again be experienced.

Other agents show a slower onset and decrease of tolerance. The barbiturates and the opiates are good examples of the situation where repeated use of a drug gradually requires larger and larger doses of the drug to maintain the level of effect. A rapidly occurring decrease in response to repeated administration of some drugs (within minutes or at the most hours) is given a special name—*tachyphylaxis*.

There are probably a number of ways in which the phenomenon of tolerance develops, but most are poorly understood. In some cases there appears to be an increase in the activity of the enzyme system that deactivates the drug. Another possibility is that tolerance occurs because of an exhaustion of stores of the endogenous agent causing the effect. For most drugs, there is little knowledge of the underlying process. Tachyphylaxis is believed to result from the activation of compensatory mechanisms that prevent the reoccurrence of the initial drug effect or to the persistent occupation of receptors by earlier doses, but again, much more information is needed.

An understanding of the mechanism of physical dependency and the withdrawal symptoms does provide a clue to one basis for the development of tolerance. Tolerance can occur with either stimulant or depressant drugs. When tolerance develops to a compound, it is sometimes accompanied by physical dependence to the drug. Physical dependence is said to have occurred when stopping the administration of the drug results in "withdrawal symptoms." The actual symptoms observed vary from drug to drug but are based on the drug-induced changes in the activity of the cells involved.

The mechanisms underlying physical dependence are not well understood. One simple, and certainly incomplete, explanation is that when a depressant drug is administered it sometimes has its effects by slowing the metabolic processes of cells. To offset this decrease in metabolic activity, the cells initiate processes that return cellular activity to normal even though the drug continues to have a depressant effect on the metabolism. Under this condition, to continue to affect the output of the cells, the amount of drug must be increased, since it now must depress not only the normal activity but also the compensation that homeostatic mechanisms brought into play. This necessary increase in drug dose to obtain the same effect is tolerance.

When administration of the drug is abruptly stopped, its depressant effect on cellular mechanisms disappears over a period of hours as the drug is deactivated. The compensatory mechanisms that were initiated in an attempt to maintain normal cellular functioning continue to act. Without the drug-induced depression to counteract them, the compensatory systems increase the activity of the cells above normal, and this cellular hyperactivity and hypersensitivity are the cause of the withdrawal symptoms. Homeostatic processes again come into action and, as the compensatory systems decrease their activity, the withdrawal symptoms subside.

Still debated is the question of physical dependency to stimulant drugs (see p. 172). When stimulant use stops, overactive compensatory mechanisms may continue to operate and decrease body functions below normal. This may be withdrawal in the case of stimulants. Over time, homeostatic processes return the body to its predrug baseline.

To recapitulate briefly, tolerance can occur with both stimulants and depressants and refers to the observable fact that repeated administration of the same dose of a drug results in fewer and fewer effects. Conversely, when tolerance develops to a drug, the amount of the drug given each time must increase in order to obtain the same effect with repeated administration. Physical dependence refers to the situation where compensatory mechanisms in the body counteract the effect of the drug and continue to act when the drug is no longer given.

Some mention must be made of the phrase *psychological dependence,* which occurs frequently in the literature. It usually refers to the fact that some individuals will be highly motivated to obtain and use a drug because of its pleasurable effects and not just to avoid the occurrence of withdrawal symptoms. Since the same behavior occurs toward other objects and experiences, not just toward drugs, the use of a special term to denote drug-seeking behavior seems unnecessary and suggests incorrectly that this behavior is unique.

CONCLUDING COMMENT

The reader must feel like he's playing all the roles of the blind men trying to describe an elephant. Here, no here, no, no, over there! At some point certain concepts and terms have to be learned. This has been the chapter of earth, air, fire, and water! Hopefully after hopscotching over the field of pharmacology and touching down only at a few places, there is some better appreciation of the kinds of problems and considerations one must take into account in studying social and physiological actions and effects of a drug.

Some of these factors are legal, as in the brand-generic name controversy. Some have to do with the possible changes in the effects of a drug over time: cumulative effects, additive effects, and tolerance. Still other factors deal with the classification of drugs. Whether social or biological, all are important in understanding the world of drugs. Tuning up is over. The next chapter presents the themes necessary for understanding the pharmacodynamics of drugs.

PRECEDING QUOTES

1. Osler, W.: Science **17:**170, 1891.
2. Holmes, O. W., in an address presented before the Massachusetts Medical Society, May, 1860.
3. Dunlop, D.: Abuse of drugs by the public and by doctors, British Medical Bulletin **26**(3):236, 1970.
4. Modell, W.: Hazards of new drugs, Science **139:**1185, 1963.

REFERENCES

1. Deno, R. A., and others: The profession of pharmacy, ed. 2, Philadelphia, 1966, J. B. Lippincott Co., p. 1.
2. Lewin, L.: Phantastica narcotic and stimulating drugs: their use and abuse, New York, 1931, E. P. Dutton & Co.
3. Task Force on Prescription Drugs: Final report, February 7, 1969, Washington, D. C., 1969, U. S. Department of Health, Education and Welfare, pp. 10, 31.
4. Keep them at hand . . . the leading 200 drugs in 1969, Pharmacy Times **36**(4):29-33, 1970.
5. Brice, G. W., and Hammer, H. F.: Therapeutic non-equivalency of oxytetracycline capsules, Drug Information Bulletin 3:112-114, 1969.
6. Murry, W.: Comparative performance of equivalent drugs, presented at the 1968 Scientific Assembly of the Medical Society of the District of Columbia, Washington Hilton Hotel, November 22, 1968, p. 1.
7. Wheatley, D.: Effects of doctors' and patients' attitudes and other factors on response to drugs. In Rickels, K., editor: Non-specific factors in drug therapy, Springfield, Illinois, 1968, Charles C Thomas, Publisher, pp. 73-79.
8. Rickels, K., and Cattell, R. B.: Drug and placebo response as a function of doctor and patient type. In May, P. R. A., and Wittenborn, J. R., editors: Psychotropic drug response, Springfield, Illinois, 1969, Charles C Thomas, Publisher, pp. 126-140.
9. Rickels, K.: Non-specific factors in drug therapy of neurotic patients. In Rickels, K., editor: Non-specific factors in drug therapy, Springfield, Illinois, 1968, Charles C Thomas, Publisher, pp. 3-26.
10. McNair, D. M., Kahn, R. J., Droppleman, L. F., and Fisher, S.: Patient acquiescence and drug effects. In Rickels, K., editor: Non-specific factors in drug therapy, Springfield, Illinois, 1968, Charles C Thomas, Publisher, pp. 59-72.
11. Shapiro, A. K.: Placebo effects in medicine: psychotherapy and psychoanalysis. In Bergin, A. E., and Garfield, S. L., editors: Handbook of psychotherapy and behavior change: an empirical analysis, New York, 1971, Wiley and Sons, pp. 439-473.
12. Cole, J. O., Bonato, R., and Goldberg, S. C.: Non-specific factors in the drug therapy of schizophrenic patients. In Rickels, K., editor: Non-specific factors in drug therapy, Springfield, Illinois, 1968, Charles C Thomas, Publisher, pp. 115-127.
13. Gorodetzky, C. W.: Marihuana, LSD, and amphetamines, Drug Dependence, National Clearinghouse for Mental Health Information, No. 5, October, 1970, pp. 18-23.
14. Vesell, E. S.: Introduction: genetic and environmental factors affecting drug response in man, Federation Proceedings **31**(4), July-August, 1972.

5 The actions of drugs

The physicochemical effects of a drug occur because it increases
or decreases the activity of cells somewhere in the body. Different drugs
have different effects usually because they act on different groups
of cells, and sometimes because their time sequences of events differ. A
drug does not exert a physicochemical effect until it reaches the cells on
which it acts, and the magnitude of the effect depends particularly
on the concentration of the drug at the site of action.

   M. Weatherall, 1970

Drugs affect behavior indirectly as the chemical composition of a drug
interacts with other chemicals, enzymes, or enzyme substrates. The
alteration of the biochemical cell environment produces a change in
cellular, tissue, and organ function. A modification of the behavior state of
the patient results and determines the nature of his interaction with the
environment. Drugs affect various levels of integration, from simple
to complex—from cellular activity to psychosocial interaction.

   B. Bergersen and E. Krug, 1969

As chemicals, drugs cannot affect behavior directly; they can only
interact with other chemicals—with an enzyme, altering its function, or
with important substrates for enzyme activity . . . . Such biochemical
alterations produce changes at the cellular level which, in turn, affect
tissue and organ function. The end result is a modification of the
behavioral and physiologic "state of the individual . . ."

   Samuel Irwin, 1968

The basic fact in understanding the actions of drugs is that the drug molecule must form a physiochemical bond with a cell or a constituent of a cell. This interaction is necessary for a drug to have its effect, and of concern here are those cases where a drug interacts with neurons. Such interaction can occur either on the surface (the membrane) of the cell or inside the cell. Acting at the membrane, a drug may have physiochemical effect in one of three ways. It may combine with a specialized area of the membrane, a receptor; it may act on the membrane structure itself; and, finally, it may act on one of the mechanisms in the membrane that transports material in and out of the cell. The effects a drug has inside a cell are usually on enzymes, those molecules necessary for the production and deactivation of the neurotransmitter. Drugs sometimes act inside cells by affecting neurotransmitter release or reuptake mechanisms.

There are three very important and perhaps very obvious general concepts that will be used repeatedly in talking about drug action. First is that the action of a drug is always mediated by a naturally occurring process of the body. A drug either mimics, facilitates, or antagonizes a normally occurring phenomenon in order to have its effect. Second is that a drug can have only one of three effects on a cell. It can increase or decrease a cell's normal activity or sensitivity, or it can disrupt the cell so that normal activity is sporadic. The third concept is that the magnitude of the effect obtained with a drug depends on the concentration of the drug at the place of action—that is, the place where the drug forms a physiochemical bond with a part of the cell.

One must appreciate that a drug does have very specific biochemical actions, and failure at times to detail these actions indicates a lack of knowledge. Because of the very specific ways in which drugs act, only minute amounts of pharmacologically active agents are needed at the site of action. Some indication of this specificity is suggested by the fact that 0.00001 milligram of the antidiuretic hormone administered to man results in the retention of body fluid by the kidneys. Similarly, the action of a potent phenothiazine drug is obtained with the delivery of only 10^{12} molecules to a rat, which means 10^{-9} grams of the drug in the entire brain is enough to cause observable changes in the behavior of a rat. If these molecules were put in a monomolecular layer the total area would be only 0.1 square centimeter!

The specificity of action of drugs was first suggested by some work of Claude Bernard (1856) on the peripheral nervous system. He was using the drug curare as a tool to study the interaction between the nervous system and the skeletal muscles. Curare is the poison in which South American natives dip their arrow tips. An animal wounded by one of these arrows collapses within seconds since the effect of curare is to paralyze the animal. The question was, how does this poison work?

Bernard used a preparation in which he could isolate nerves that carry impulses to skeletal muscles. In the absence of curare, electrically stimulating the nerve caused the muscle to contract. Following curare, nerve stimulation had no effect on the muscle. If the muscle were *directly* stimulated, it would contract, showing that it could function normally. Similarly, stimulating the nerve and recording at the point where the nerve joined the muscle showed that the nerve functioned properly. The only possibility left was that curare in some way prevents the nerve from activating the muscle. It is now well established that curare is a specific blocker for the skeletal neuro-muscular junction and does so by occupying the acetylcholine receptor. Acetylcholine is the neurotransmitter normally released by the neuron that causes skeletal muscle contraction when it combines with the receptor.

Drugs are, then, quite specific in their actions when they are at the site of action. No matter whether they act on the cell membrane or inside the cell, they either increase or decrease or disrupt the normal functioning of the cell. This means that a drug does not introduce a new quality of nerve action; it only modifies the normal one. First and foremost, though, the drug must be delivered to the cells with which it interacts.

DRUG ACTION
Overview of events prior to drug action

Tracing the path of drug molecules from their entry into the body to their site of action will sketch some of the factors that must then be detailed. Even though oral intake may be the simplest way to "take a drug," absorption from the gastrointestinal tract is the most complicated way to enter the bloodstream. Here the drug must first be taken up (absorbed), either by diffusion or by an active transport system, by cells lining the gastrointestinal tract. To be absorbed, the drug must have certain characteristics. It must be in solution, be lipid soluble, and be in a suitably high concentration. Not all drugs can fulfill these requirements.

Ease of movement of a drug across cell membranes is important in determining its activity. Since cell membranes have a substantial amount of lipid, those drugs that are lipid soluble readily enter cells and move through capillary walls. Lipid solubility can be fairly well predicted from the chemical structure of the compound; one of the crucial factors is the degree of its ionization. As ionization goes up, lipid solubility goes down. Water solubility is increased with ionization and this acts to keep the drug outside of cells. Because of this, ionized, water-soluble drugs, if absorbed at all, will remain extracellular, be *poorly* metabolized, and be readily filtered out by the kidneys and excreted. Physiologically active drugs and hormones that are not lipid soluble need a special transport system to cross cell membranes.

To move into the blood system clearly requires a series of complex steps in most cases. When a drug is delivered by injection directly into a vein, then it is in the circulation. When an intramuscular or subcutaneous injection is used, the drug enters the bloodstream by diffusion from the intercellular space where it was deposited. If taken orally, a drug must diffuse into capillaries from cells lining the stomach and intestines. Such movement occurs for some agents that move from an area of higher concentration into one of lower concentration. Other compounds cannot so easily cross the cell membrane, and an active transport system, which requires energy, is necessary. The active transport systems can move a compound from an area of low concentration to one of high concentration.

The circulatory system is the mode of transportation for drugs from the place where they entered the body to the site of action. As the blood moves through the filtering system in the kidneys, there is the possibility that the drug will be removed from circulation and excreted. In the liver, which is the primary place of deactivation, the compound may be removed from circulation and metabolized (deactivated).

To reach the extracellular fluid space outside the cell, drug molecules have to move from the blood through capillary walls by diffusion. Before the drug can leave the circulatory system, though, it must be separated from the proteins in the blood with which it may have formed a bond. If a drug acts inside a cell, its last barrier to cross is the cell membrane. Neuron membranes are complex structures that are primarily lipid material built on a protein latticework. The membrane contains some pores or openings that permit quite small molecules to enter and leave the cell by diffusion without energy being expended by the cell. Lipid-soluble agents too large to enter via the pores move directly through the cell membrane. Moving a drug into the bloodstream by absorption through the skin is not very effective since the skin poorly absorbs most material applied to it. Suppositories are rarely used but are an effective drug delivery system that makes possible rapid movement of drugs into the body. They are sometimes necessary in the very young and very old. Direct delivery of a drug into the brain is possible with available techniques and is used at times in animal research.

There are only three primary drug delivery methods used with humans: oral, injection, and inhalation. Inhalation is used with volatile anesthetics and is also the drug delivery system used for nicotine in smoking. It is a very efficient way to deliver some drugs. Onset of drug effects is quite rapid because the capillary walls are very accessible in the lungs and the drug thus enters the blood quickly.

Aerosol dispensers have been used to deliver some drugs via the lungs, but there are three considerations that make inhalation of limited value. First, the material must not be irritating to the mucous membranes and lungs. Second, control of dose is more difficult than with the other drug delivery systems. Last, and perhaps the prime advantage for some drugs and disadvantage for others, there is no depot of drug in the body. This means that the drug must be given as long as the effect is desired, and also that when drug administration is stopped, the effect rapidly decreases.

Injection

Chemicals can be delivered with the hypodermic syringe directly into the bloodstream, deposited in a muscle mass, or under the upper layers of skin. With the intravenous (IV) injection, the drug starts in the bloodstream and does not have to be absorbed first, so the onset of action is faster than with any other means of administering drugs. Another advantage is that very irritating material can be injected this way since blood vessel walls are relatively insensitive. A major advantage frequently is that the material injected, the bolus, can deliver a high concentration of the drug to the brain tissues. The major disadvantage to intravenous injections is that the vein wall loses some of its strength and elasticity in the area around the injection site. If there are many injections into a small segment of a vein, as with an addict who must inject where he can see, the wall of that vein eventually collapses and blood no longer moves through it, necessitating the use of another injection site.

Subcutaneous and intramuscular injections have similar characteristics except that absorption is more rapid from intramuscular injection. Muscles have a better blood supply, and thus more area over which absorption can occur, than the underlying layers of the skin. The rate of absorption can be varied in both methods by adding a vasodilator or vasoconstrictor to increase or decrease the area of absorption. When slow absorption is desired, a less soluble salt of the drug is frequently put in a suspension rather than a solution. Since only material in solution can be absorbed, the suspended material has to first go into solution. An additional factor influencing the rate of absorption is that movement into the blood depends on the concentration of the drug. As more drug enters the bloodstream, the concentration outside decreases and so does the rate of absorption. One disadvantage to subcutaneous injection is that if the material injected is extremely irritating to the tissue, the skin around the site of injection may die and be shed. This method of injection is not very common in medical practice but has long been the kind of injection used by beginning narcotic users. Colloquially this is called "skin popping."

There is less chance of irritation if the injection is *intramuscular* because of the better blood supply and faster absorption. Another advantage is that larger volumes of material can be deposited in a muscle than can be injected subcutaneously. Most of the shots given by a physician are intramuscular injections, and anyone who has had a series of tetanus shots may question the fact that this is one of the less irritating ways of injecting a drug.

Oral administration

Most drugs begin their grand adventure in the body by entering through the mouth. Taking biologically active agents orally is unquestionably the oldest route of administration and probably the easiest. It is not necessarily the most effective since a chemical in the digestive tract has to withstand the actions of the acid of the stomach and the digestive enzymes and not be deactivated by food before it is absorbed. As long as the drug remains in the digestive tract it can be considered to be outside the body. The process of drug absorption from the stomach and intestines is a special area in and of itself.

A good example of the dangers in the gut for a drug is that which develops with tetracycline. This antibiotic readily combines with calcium and aluminum ions to form a compound that is poorly absorbed. If tetracycline is taken with milk (calcium ions) or with antacids (aluminum ions), blood levels will never be as high as if it were taken in the absence of these or similar agents.

There are many competing factors in getting the drug through the cells lining the wall of the gastrointestinal tract on into the capillaries in the area. If taken in capsule or tablet form, the drug must first dissolve and, as a liquid, mix in the contents of the stomach and intestines. However, since as concentration goes down so does rate of absorption, the drug will be less rapidly absorbed when it is diluted by other material in the stomach.

Drugs are frequently prepared as salts, and they are weak electrolytes since this ionization increases their water solubility, which is necessary for the compound to spread throughout the stomach. Once distributed, though, absorption is primarily of the non-ionized form of the drug. If organic molecules are too strongly ionized, they will be poorly absorbed and pass through the intestines to be excreted in the feces. Lipid-soluble and very small water-soluble molecules are readily absorbed into capillaries and go into the general circulation. There is very little drug absorption during the first 5 minutes, even on an empty stomach, but by 30 minutes most has been absorbed. After 6 to 8 hours, essentially all of the drug will have been absorbed.

Once in the bloodstream the dangers of entering via the oral route are not over. The veins from the gut go first to the liver. If the drug is the type that is rapidly taken up and metabolized by the liver, very little may get into the general circulation. A drug may thus be ineffective via the oral route but very effective if given by injection.

The brain has a high lipid content and thus is a target organ for drugs with high lipid solubility. Drugs that act on the central nervous system are usually active when given orally because the lipid solubility of these agents increases their absorption from the gastrointestinal tract. Similarly, because of the high lipid solubility and low water solubility, these agents are usually not excreted but are reabsorbed in the kidneys and thus show cumulative effects.

As with all generalizations, there are exceptions. If a lipid-soluble drug is taken with a fatty meal, the drug will to some extent be taken up and remain in the fat. Since fat is only slowly digested and the drug released, the rate of drug absorption is slowed. A slow absorption rate could possibly lower the drug concentration in the blood to an ineffective level.

Transport in blood

When a drug enters the bloodstream, usually its molecules will attach to one of the protein molecules in the blood, albumin being the most common protein involved. The degree to which there is binding of drug molecules to plasma proteins is important in determining drug effects. As long as there is a protein-drug complex, the drug is inactive and also cannot leave the blood. In this condition, the drug is protected from inactivation by enzymes.

There is an equilibrium established between the free (unbound) drug and the protein-bound forms of the drug in the bloodstream. As the unbound drug moves across capillary walls to sites of action, there is a release of protein-bound drug in order to maintain the bound-free equilibrium. Considerable variation exists among drugs in the affinity that the drug molecules have for establishing a bond with plasma proteins. Alcohol has a low affinity and thus exists in the bloodstream primarily as the ethyl alcohol molecule. The salicylate ion has a high affinity, and about 80% is bound to blood proteins. Acetylsalicylic acid, in contrast, has a low affinity. Differences in blood protein binding are reflected in their effects. Acetylsalicylic acid (aspirin) has a more rapid onset of action but a shorter duration than the salicylates.

Since there are differences in the affinity of drugs for the plasma proteins, one might expect that drugs with high affinity would displace those drugs with weak protein bonds. And they do. This fact is important because it forms the basis for one kind of drug interaction. When a high affinity drug is added to a situation where there is a weak affinity drug already largely bound to the plasma proteins, the weak affinity drug is displaced and will exist primarily as the unbound form. The increase in the unbound drug concentration helps move the drug out of the bloodstream to the sites of action faster and may be an important influence on the effect the drug has. At the very least, there will be a shortening of the duration of action.

Taking into consideration that only the free drug can leave the circulatory system, the same rules apply for leaving the bloodstream and entering cells as for leaving the stomach and moving into blood. Small, lipid-soluble, nonionized molecules diffuse through these cell membranes very easily while larger lipid-insoluble, ionized molecules move more slowly, if at all, without an active transport system.

Blood-brain barrier

The brain is very different from the other parts of the body in terms of the ability of drugs to leave the blood and move to sites of action. There is a barrier that acts to keep certain classes of compounds in the blood and away from brain neurons and glial cells. Thus, some drugs act only on neurons outside the central nervous system, that is, those in the peripheral nervous system, while others may affect all neurons.

The blood-brain barrier is not well developed in infants and only reaches complete development after 1 or 2 years of age in humans. Although the nature of this barrier is not well understood, there are several factors known to contribute to the blood-brain barrier. One is the makeup of the capillaries in the brain. They are different from other capillaries in the body since they contain no pores at all. Even very small, water-soluble molecules cannot leave the capillaries in the brain; only lipid-soluble substances can pass the lipid capillary wall.

If a substance can move through the capillary wall, another barrier unique to the brain is met. About 85% of the capillaries are completely covered with glial cells—there is little extracellular space next to the blood vessel walls. With no pores and close contact between capillary walls and glial cells, almost certainly an active transport system is needed to move chemicals in and out of the brain. There are, in fact, known transport systems for some naturally occurring agents.

A final note on the mystery of the blood-brain barrier is that cerebral trauma can disrupt the barrier and permit agents to enter

that normally would be excluded. Concussion or cerebral infections frequently cause enough trauma to impair the effectiveness of this screen, which normally permits only selected chemicals to enter the brain.

Possible mechanisms of drug actions

Many different types of actions will be suggested as ways in which drugs can affect physiochemical processes, neuron functioning, and ultimately thoughts, feelings, and other behaviors. It is possible for drugs to effect all neurons but many exert actions only on certain presynaptic or postsynaptic processes in some neurons or only on presynaptic neurons. Since the action of a drug is usually quite specific—that is, it affects one phase of the information-processing systems—it is unusual to find a drug that has more than one of the actions to be discussed.

Effects on all neurons. Those chemicals that have an effect on all neurons must do it by influencing some characteristic common to all neurons. One general characteristic of all neurons is the cell membrane. It is semipermeable, meaning that some agents can readily move in and out of the cell, but other chemicals are held inside or kept out under normal conditions. The semipermeable characteristic of the cell membrane is essential for the maintenance of an electrical potential across the membrane. It is on this membrane that some drugs seem to act and, by influencing the permeability, alter the electrical characteristics of the neuron. Some drugs do affect the transport systems involved in maintaining the neuron, but usually the effect is a more general one.

The anesthetics, including the barbiturates and alcohol, are chemicals that have their effects on the central nervous system by influencing the cell membrane. Note that the agents that act in this way are depressants and that there are no drugs that increase the cell's activity level by affecting general membrane characteristics.

Postsynaptic effects. Alteration in the information-processing system is usually accomplished by affecting synaptic functioning. A tremendous increase in possible selectivity of action results from action at the synapse because different synapses involve different types of neurohumors. By using a drug that operates only by mimicking or blocking one kind of neurotransmitter, there is a much greater precision of action than when using a compound that acts on all neuron membranes.

Drugs that act postsynaptically can only make contact with the electrical system via the receptor itself or the enzymes that deactivate the neurotransmitters. When a drug acts at the receptor, it can have one of two possible effects. It may mimic the normal transmitter and thus cause either an increase or a decrease in the excitability of the postsynaptic neuron similar to that produced by the normal transmitter. Carbachol, which mimics the action of acetylcholine at many places in the nervous system, is a good example. It activates cholinergic fibers but, unlike acetylcholine, it is not readily deactivated by cholinesterase. As a result, it continues to have its effect on the receptor for a longer period of time than would acetylcholine. Nicotine, at those places where carbachol is ineffective, also mimics the action of acetylcholine but initially activates and then depresses activity of the postsynaptic neuron.

Some drugs act at the postsynaptic receptor by occupying the site but are unable to influence the electrical characteristics of the neuron. These agents are called "blockers," since by occupying the site they prevent the normal neurotransmitters from having an effect postsynaptically. Atropine and scopolamine are well-known compounds that can occupy some cholinergic receptors and thus prevent acetylcholine from having an effect. These drugs act on both the central and peripheral nervous systems, but if a methyl group is added to their chemical structure to form methylatropine and methylscopolamine, the effects are restricted to the peripheral nervous system. The addition of a methyl group prevents the chemical from crossing the blood-brain barrier and provides a valuable tool for research. By comparing the effects of atropine and methylatropine, valuable clues can be obtained to indicate which actions of the drug are mediated by the central and which by the peripheral nervous systems.

In cholinergic systems the enzyme responsible for deactivating acetylcholine is located postsynaptically. Any drug that prevents this deactivating enzyme, cholinesterase, from acting increases the duration of effect that acetylcholine can have. Cholinesterase inhibitors, then, prolong the effect of acetylcholine, which is released under normal physiological stimulation. Some drugs are short-acting, reversible inhibitors (such as eserine) while others (such as diisopropyl fluro-phosphate—DFP) because of the nature of their effect, are called nonreversible and may alter cholinesterase functioning for days.

Thus drugs acting postsynaptically can have major effects on the information-processing system. Emphasis here has been on the cholinergic system, since alteration of function in the adrenergic system is most readily accomplished presynaptically. It is quite difficult to do this with the cholinergic system.

Presynaptic effects. There are several major ways in which drugs affect synaptic processes by acting on the presynaptic neuron. One of these, blocking the release of the neurotransmitter, is of importance only in the peripheral nervous system and will not be discussed. The other ways of altering the effectiveness of the neurotransmitter are concerned with modifications of its synthesis, storage, uptake, and deactivation processes.

Synthesis of the endogenous neurotransmitters can be blocked by inhibiting one or more of the enzyme systems involved in the construction of the transmitter. Preventing or slowing new synthesis results in a depletion of the transmitter under normal functioning and thus a cessation, or at least an impairment, of synaptic transmission. Interestingly, one of the important enzymes involved in the synthesis of noradrenaline plays a similar role in building serotonin, so that inhibition of that enzyme causes a decrease in the level of both these neurotransmitters.

Some drugs effectively decrease the synthesis of the normal transmitters because they are better substrates for the synthesizing enzymes than the endogenous material. The synthesizing enzymes thus act on these drugs rather than on the normal substrate. Because the manufacturing system is not disrupted, complex molecules are built and stored in synaptic vesicles. Since these are not the same as the normal transmitters but are released in the same way as the real transmitters, these synthesized compounds are called "false transmitters." The false transmitters are usually only moderately, if at all, effective in activating the receptor postsynaptically, so information processing is disrupted by their presence.

When a transmitter is manufactured, it must be stored in a vesicle to prevent its deactivation. Some drugs, such as reserpine, prevent the transmitter from being taken up into vesicles. The transmitter is then open to deactivation by the deactivating enzymes but, more importantly, the vesicles are unable to collect and release the transmitter when the neuron fires. Obviously, without transmitter release, the synapse will cease to function normally.

An important distinction must be made between the cholinergic and the adrenergic systems of neurotransmission. The cholinergic system is relatively straightforward. Acetylcholine is synthesized presynaptically, bound in vesicles, released, bound to the postsynaptic receptor site (thereby changing the electrical characteristics of the dendrite), and deactivated postsynaptically. In adrenergic neurons there are a few differences. First, there are two classes of noradrenaline accumulated presynaptically—a functional store, released in neural firing, and a bound (reserve) form of noradrenaline that is not used in synaptic functioning.

A second difference is that after the transmitter molecule has had its effect at the receptor, it is not usually deactivated but instead is released into the synaptic gap, where it is taken up by the presynaptic neuron and stored again in the vesicles of the functional pool of transmitter substance. Some clinically important drugs impair this reuptake, thereby increasing the noradrenaline level at the receptor. Cocaine and imipramine are drugs that have their primary action in this way.

There are two enzymes important in the breakdown of the adrenergic transmitters.

One of these enzymes, monoamine oxidase (MAO) is also important for the deactivation of serotonin, so use of a MAO inhibitor results in an increase in brain levels of both noradrenaline and serotonin. The increase in noradrenaline, however, is not an increase in the transmitter used in neurotransmission (the functional form) but rather an increase in the reserve form. Therefore, there is no increase in the activity of the adrenergic transmitters after administration of a MAO inhibitor.

There are available inhibitors of the second deactivating enzyme, catechol-O-methyltransferase (COMT), but these have not been used clinically because COMT is relatively unimportant in deactivating noradrenaline. This COMT system seems to function both pre- and postsynaptically, although the postsynaptic site seems to be of primary importance.

A final presynaptic mechanism of drug action causes the continuous release of newly synthesized noradrenaline and also increases the amount of noradrenaline released with each electrical impulse. Amphetamine, a stimulant, acts in this way. Both of these actions (along with a third action of amphetamine, blocking noradrenaline reuptake) increase the activity of the adrenergic system and form the biochemical basis for many of amphetamine's behavioral and experienced effects.

Summary of drug actions. Psychoactive drugs have their central effects only by changing the effectiveness and sensitivity of neurons and thus their information-processing characteristics. There are many ways in which this can be accomplished, however, and a brief survey of these methods gives only a hint of the total complexity. Some drugs act on cell membranes. Those compounds are usually nonspecific depressants since they act similarly on all neurons. By interfering with the synthesis, storage, release, or reuptake of a neurotransmitter, or its combination with receptors, the efficiency of the synapse is modified and information transmission changed. By mimicking the transmitter at the receptor or preventing its normal deactivation, the postsynaptic neuron is changed electrically more than under normal conditions, and integrated functioning is also then impaired.

DRUG DEACTIVATION

Before a drug can cease to have an effect one of two things must happen to it. It may be removed unchanged from the body, or it may be chemically changed so that it no longer has the same effect on the body and then excreted from the body. Few drugs are eliminated unchanged from the body, although this is true of the volatile anesthetics. They are eliminated in the same way they enter the body—through the lungs. Alcohol, if taken in large amounts, may be partially eliminated unchanged via the lungs or sweat glands. Some drugs are excreted unchanged in the urine because they are filtered out, but not reabsorbed, in the kidneys. Even drugs that are primarily deactivated biochemically in the body are occasionally found unchanged in the urine.

Most drugs, though, are metabolized in some way in the body and the end products excreted in the urine. Drug metabolism aims primarily at two ends: inactivation of the agent and increasing the water solubility so that it can be excreted via the kidneys. Ionized, nonlipid-soluble substances are filtered out of the blood plasma in the kidneys and, instead of being reabsorbed, pass on to the urine for excretion. In part, the rate of excretion of ionizable substances depends on the pH of the urine, and this reflects to some extent an individual's diet.

Drug metabolism is not an incidental part of the study of drugs and drug actions. Since a drug continues to act until it is changed or excreted, the duration and intensity of a drug's action are determined to a great extent by the speed of its metabolism. Most drug metabolism is accomplished by special detoxification enzymes in the liver. The liver is *the* organ of drug metabolism; anything that interferes with the normal functioning of the liver will impair the drug-metabolizing capability of the body.

The enzymes in the liver that metabolize drugs are quite different from the other enzymes in the body. These liver microsomal enzymes are unique in that they can utilize oxygen directly for metabolism while most enzymes cannot. Another peculiar quality is that they are almost specific for foreign compounds. They do not act on normally occurring chemicals (except steroids), but the reason for this specificity is still not clear. Interestingly, though these microsomal enzymes are specific for foreign chemicals, they are relatively nonspecific within that group of compounds. Therefore, they metabolize a number of very different drugs.

The activity of these microsomal enzymes can be affected by drugs. Over 200 drugs have been shown to increase the activity of these drug-metabolizing enzymes; meprobamate, phenobarbital, and DDT all have this effect in common. When the enzymes are stimulated, drug metabolism speeds up and the duration of action of the drugs in the body is decreased. Some drug interactions may occur so that one drug may inhibit the metabolism of a second and thus increase the second's effects. Alcohol given after meprobamate decreases meprobamate's metabolism, thereby increasing the effects of meprobamate (perhaps sedation).

Some drugs are deactivated at their site of action and, in fact, some are altered in the process of having an action. Furthermore, some drugs are not active in the form in which they are administered but become quite active after they have been altered by the metabolizing process. Marijuana may be one example of this situation where the metabolite is more active than the original compound.

SOME GENERAL RULES
ABOUT DRUGS IN THE BODY

As mentioned in the preceding section, anything that interferes with liver functions will retard the metabolism of drugs. Such retardation will increase the magnitude and the duration of effect following administration of a drug. The most familiar examples of interference with the liver are illness and damage to the liver such as cirrhosis. However, also important is an adequate diet, since near starvation will result in a reduction of the amount of detoxification enzymes.

In the same line, advanced age may be accompanied by reduced blood flow to the liver and thus a decrease in the rate of drug detoxification. Older people frequently have a lower metabolic rate than the young, and this also acts to prolong drug activity. Impaired kidney function for any reason, clearly, would impair excretion of the drug metabolites. In the elderly there is also a higher percentage of body fat than in the young adult. Because of the accumulation of drugs in body fat, this also tends to prolong the duration of a drug's effect.

This last point must be expanded by a further comment on some unique characteristics of fat in the body. Lipid-soluble drugs are slowly taken up by the fat cells. Since fat cells generally have a relatively poor blood supply, they release the drug more slowly than other cells. This slow release may mean that 3 to 4 hours after a drug has been administered there may be higher levels in the system of a fat person than of a lean individual. Since women have more body fat, they may require less of a very lipid-soluble drug after the initial administration because the drug settles in the fat cells and is then released over a longer period of time than is the case with men. As a familiar example, this seems to be the situation with the barbiturates.

SUMMARY AND CONCLUSIONS

To understand how drug taking is related to the experienced effects of a drug, some appreciation is necessary of each of the steps involved in getting the drug to the site of action, the kind of action it has, and the ways in which the action is stopped.

Since a drug must travel via the circulatory system to reach the area where it is to have an effect, some of the time between taking a drug and experiencing its effect is caused by the problem of getting the drug into the bloodstream. Those compounds that are only slightly ionized and quite lipid soluble should have a shorter time to onset of action if everything else is equal.

Usually, though, everything else is not equal.

Some drugs never do get past the combination of factors that are referred to as the blood-brain barrier. If a drug readily enters the brain, it may be that its mechanism of action is by blocking the receptor for a neurotransmitter. The resulting effects may be experienced as depressing or stimulating, but the onset should be fairly rapid since synaptic functioning is impaired as soon as the drug acts. With other agents and other mechanisms of action there may be only a gradual onset of effects, since the impact of decreased synthesis, or decreased storage, of transmitter substances is realized more slowly in synaptic functioning.

Overriding all of this is the rate of metabolism of the drug. As the activity of the microsomal enzymes in the liver increases, so does the rate at which drugs are metabolized and thus deactivated. These enzymes act in a variety of ways to make the drug easier to excrete (that is, less lipid soluble and more water soluble). However, their specific actions need not concern the reader. Suffice it to say that the ability to metabolize drugs is related to the amount of liver microsomes that contains the detoxifying enzymes.

The processes and concepts outlined in this chapter will be used repeatedly in explaining differences in drug actions. Note especially that drugs can only increase or decrease or disrupt the activity of neurons and that the differential effects result from where the drug acts in the nervous system. By incorporating these principles of pharmacology, new dimensions will be added to the understanding of drug effects.

PRECEDING QUOTES

1. Weatherall, M.: Basic pharmacological principles. In Joyce, C. R. B., editor: Psychopharmacology: dimensions and perspectives, Philadelphia, 1968, J. B. Lippincott Co., pp. 1 and 2.
2. Bergersen, B., and Krug, E.: Pharmacology in nursing, ed. 11, St. Louis, 1969, The C. V. Mosby Co., p. 310.
3. Irwin, S.: A rational framework for the development, evaluation, and use of psychoactive drugs, American Journal of Psychiatry 124(8):4, 1968.

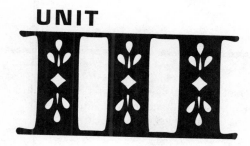

UNIT

The nondrug drugs

6 Alcohol

That poignant liquor, which the zealot calls the mother of sins, is pleasant and sweet to me. Give me wine! wine that shall subdue the strongest, that I may for a time forget the cares and troubles of the world.

Anonymous

Beverage alcohol is fecal matter. Alcohol is not made of grapes or grain or other attractive foods. It is these which are devoured by the ferment germ, and the germ then evacuates alcohol as its waste product. The thought of swallowing the excrement of a living organism is not an aesthetic idea but people will do such things.

Liquor, The Servant of Man

The chief difference between the normal drinker and the abnormal one is that the first man drinks in moderation socially, in order to make reality more pleasurable while the second drinks in order to escape from reality.

Alcohol: One Man's Meat

An alcoholic is someone who drinks too much, and you don't like anyway.

Anonymous

FERMENTATION AND
FERMENTATION PRODUCTS

Many thousands of years before the World Health Organization declared ethyl alcohol a drug intermediate in kind and degree between habit-forming and addicting drugs, Neolithic man had discovered booze. The best evidence now is that beer and berry wine were known and used about 6400 B.C. while grape wine dates from 300 or 400 B.C. Mead, which is made from honey, is possibly the oldest alcoholic beverage, and some authorities suggest it appeared in the Paleolithic Age, about 8000 B.C. Thus, early use of alcohol seems to have been worldwide; beer was drunk by the American Indians whom Columbus met.

Fermentation forms the basis for all alcoholic beverages. Certain yeasts act on sugar in the presence of water, and this chemical action is fermentation. Yeast recombines the carbon, hydrogen, and oxygen of sugar and water into ethyl alcohol and carbon dioxide. Chemically, $C_6H_{12}O_6$ (glucose) + H_2O (water) is transformed to C_2H_6O (ethyl alcohol) + CO_2 (carbon dioxide).

Most fruits, including grapes, contain sugar, and addition of the appropriate yeast (which is pervasive in the air wherever plants grow) to a mixture of crushed grapes and water will begin the fermentation process. The yeast has only a limited tolerance for alcohol; when the concentration is around 15% the yeast dies and fermentation ceases. If white grapes are used, or red grapes with the skins removed, a white wine results. Red wines come from red grapes in which the grape skins are retained in the fermenting mixture. A rosé results if the red grape skins are allowed to remain in the mix for only 1 or 2 days. Champagne is produced by bottling the wine before the fermentation is complete, thus retaining the carbon dioxide.

Cereal grains can also be used to produce alcoholic beverages. However, cereal grains contain starch rather than sugar, and before fermentation can begin the starch must be converted to sugar. This is accomplished by means of enzymes formed during a process called *malting*. In American beer, the primary grain is barley, which is malted by steeping it in water and allowing it to sprout. The sprouted grain is then slowly dried to kill the sprout but preserve the enzymes formed during the growth. This dried, sprouted barley is called *malt*, and when crushed and mixed with water the enzymes convert the starch to sugar. Only yeast is needed then to start fermentation. Usually ground corn is added to the malt to increase the amount of starch available, and all solids are filtered out before the yeast is added for fermentation. Hops (dried blossoms of a special plant) are added with the yeast to give beer its distinctive pungent flavor. In most commercial beers today the alcoholic content is about 4.5%.

Other cultures use other plants as the starting place for fermentation. Cortez, in his expedition to Mexico in 1518, commented on the native alcoholic beverage, pulque, which is made from the agave cactus and has an alcoholic content of about 6%. In home brewing of pulque, a cavity is sometimes made in the body of the cactus and the fermentation carried out there, yielding 5 to 6 quarts of pulque a day until the cactus dies. Mead, made from honey, has an alcoholic content of about 10% and is still available in parts of Great Britain and Denmark. Sake, the traditional rice beer of Japan, is between 12% and 16% alcohol. Apple cider allowed to ferment may develop an alcohol content as great as 14%.

DISTILLED PRODUCTS

To obtain alcohol concentrations above those that can be reached by fermentation, distillation must be used. Distillation is a process in which the solution containing alcohol is heated and the vapors collected and condensed into liquid form again. Since alcohol has a lower boiling point than water, there is a higher percentage of alcohol in the distillate (the condensed liquid) than there was in the original solution.

There is still much debate over who discovered the distillation process and when the discovery was made, but many authorities place it in Arabia around 800 A.D. The term *alcohol* is from an Arabic word meaning "finely divided spirit" and originally referred to that part of the wine collected through distillation—the essence of the wine! Only fermented beverages were used in Europe until the tenth century, when the Italians first distilled wine, thereby introducing "spirits" to the western world. These new products were formally and informally studied and used in the treatment of many illnesses, including senility. The prevalent feeling about their medicinal value is best seen in the name given these condensed vapors by a thirteenth century Professor of Medicine at the French University of Montpellier: "aquae vitae"—the water of life. Around the end of the seventeenth century the more prosaic Dutch called the liquid brandy, meaning burnt wine.

Between the table wines, which are produced by fermentation, and brandies, the distillate of wine, are the fortified wines. These are fermented wines with enough distillate added to bring the alcohol content up to about 20%. Sherry, port, Madeira, and muscatel are familiar examples.

Originally a liqueur was a distilled wine combined with many herbs and used only for medicinal purposes. These cordials have a high sugar content and are usually taken only in very small quantities. Some of the formulations for these beverages, such as Benedictine, are still secret. Some now are distillates of other products. Drambuie, for example, is a distillate of Scotch whisky with the addition of heather, honey, and herbs.

All of the "hard liquors" start from a mash composed of a starchy grain (or other starchy plant such as potatoes) and malted barley to which yeast is added. Unlike the process of making beer, hops are not added and the solid material is not strained out before fermentation is started. This mash is then heated and the distillate condensed.

The name "whiskey" (whisky if it's Scotch, whiskey otherwise) comes from the Irish-Gaelic equivalent of aquae vitae and was already commonplace around 1500. The distillation of whiskey in America started on a large scale toward the end of the eighteenth century and was the basis for the first major political-social drug problem in this country. The chief product of the area just west of the Appalachian Mountains — western Pennsylvania, western Virginia, eastern Kentucky — was grain. It was not profitable for the farmers to ship the grain or flour across the mountains to the markets along the eastern seaboard. Since six barrels of flour could be converted to one barrel of whiskey, which could be profitably shipped East, distillation started on a grand scale.

One of the early distillers who established a good reputation was a Baptist minister living in what was then Bourbon County, Kentucky. In 1789 this minister, Elijah Craig, began storing his whiskey in charred new oak barrels, originating a manufacturing step still used with all American whiskeys (but not with Canadian whiskeys, which are stored in uncharred barrels).

Scotch today is the distillate of fermented malted barley. The distinctive "smokey" flavor of Scotch comes from two sources. The malted barley is dried in kilns in which burning peat provides the heat, and some of the distinctive characteristics of peat are probably picked up by the barley. Also, after distillation the product is stored for at least 3 years in uncharred barrels that were originally used to transport sherry.

A few other distillates will be mentioned briefly. By the seventeenth century distillation techniques made possible the production of relatively pure alcohol. To soften the raw taste of pure alcohol (and possibly to increase its medicinal value) the distillate was filtered through juniper berries and named "jenever" by the Dutch and "genievre" by the French. The British shortened the name first to "geneva" and finally to gin. In its present form, gin is flavored alcohol made primarily from corn to which water is added to give the desired alcohol content. Schnapps is manufactured in the same way but is not so completely distilled and thus still retains some of the flavor of the grain. Pure alcohol diluted with water to the desired alcoholic content is vodka, meaning "little water" in Russian. None of these liquors is aged, instead they are bottled for consumption immediately after distillation.

Rum is the distillate from the fermentation of molasses made from sugar cane. The most profitable and largest industry in New England in colonial days was the manufacture of rum. The same ships were used in a very active trade system that carried rum to Africa to pay for slaves who were then sold in the continental United States to pay for the West Indian molasses that was traded for New England rum which . . . This triangle, and the industry, came to an abrupt halt in 1807 when the importation of slaves was forbidden.

One final note. In the United States the alcoholic content of distilled beverages is indicated by the term *proof*. The percentage of alcohol by volume is one half the proof number, that is, 90 proof whiskey is 45% alcohol. The term "proof" developed from a British Army procedure to gauge the alcohol content of distilled spirits before there were modern techniques. The liquid was poured over gunpowder and ignited. If the alcohol content was high enough the gunpowder would go "pooff" and explode! That was proof that the beverage had an acceptable alcohol content, about 57%.

REGULATION OF ALCOHOL USE

Alcohol is different from most of the recent psychoactive drugs in western civilization in that the problem has never been to prevent its introduction—it has always been everywhere! There have been repeated attempts to control its use and, on occasion, to eliminate its availability. Throughout Europe from the fourteenth through the twentieth century, all of these attempts to suppress alcohol have failed.

Early attempts at regulation of alcohol consumption in England consisted of edicts handed down by religious authorities. Some of these were recorded as early as the sixth century A.D. The first national English legislation to curb intemperance was passed in 1327; it tried to limit the number of establishments that could sell alcoholic beverages. It was rapidly repealed, and a different approach was tried over 150 years later, in 1494. This was the first licensing law and gave justices of the peace the authority to determine where alcoholic drinks could be sold. Nothing succeeded. The consumption of alcohol in one form or another increased regularly. When legal production or sale was prohibited or highly taxed, illegal quantities increased.

In 1688 distillation was opened wide in England; upon paying a small tax, anyone could become a distiller—and almost everyone did! Gin drinking became a national passion, and although laws changed and home distillation was made illegal, consumption increased. The crowding of urban central-city poverty areas with the workers of the industrial revolution, coupled with low-cost, easily available, alcohol, contributed to the increase in alcohol consumption and in public drunkenness.

Parallel with this increased drinking was the negative reaction to it resulting in the formation of temperance groups. In 1825 concern was expressed[1] that "women of the middle and high classes of society entered the small private doors of gin shops to take their drams with the common women." In 1834 one report on drunkenness comments on the ". . . great number of women and sometimes decent women . . ." and of "the young prostitutes from twelve to fourteen years of age who were charged with being drunk and disorderly." One well-enforced act in 1839 started the decline in public drunkenness in England by placing penalties on selling spirits to those under 16 years of age and by establishing closing times for Saturday and Sunday—the days of greatest drunkenness.

Across the Atlantic a new nation was developing and, remembering that one of the reasons the Pilgrims settled for Massachusetts was that "our victuals were much spent, especially our beer," it will be worthwhile to trace some of the high spots in this country's concern over the use of alcohol. The very first law was passed in Maryland in 1642, when drunkenness was punishable by a fine of 100 pounds of tobacco. Shortly thereafter, in 1650, Connecticut passed a law forbidding drinking more than a half hour at a time. Connecticut in 1659 followed with a $5 fine for being drunk in your own home!

Virginia had other problems and in 1664 passed a law prohibiting ministers from drinking to excess. Virginia ministers were a difficult group to change, though, and 100 years later, in 1760, Virginia had to pass another law prohibiting ministers from "drinking to excess and inciting riot." At about the same time, 1755, Georgia indicated what it thought about tavernkeepers by forbidding a liquor license "to any tradesman who was capable of making his livelihood by honest labor"!

When the United States of America was 1 year old, Congress passed the first federal law regarding alcohol. This 1790 law authorized giving every soldier a daily ration of a quarter pint of rum, brandy, or whiskey. This fringe benefit was lost in the army in 1830, but the navy in its wisdom continued to dole out the ration until 1862. (It was over 100 years later that the British sailors lost their grog ration!) The second federal law regarding alcohol was the excise tax that started the Whiskey Rebellion.

Alcohol had played an important role in the development of the United States as early as 1791. In that year the federal government imposed an excise tax on whiskey. West of the Appalachian Mountains where most whiskey was made, the farmers refused to pay and tarred and feathered revenue officers who tried to collect the tax. In 1794 President George Washington called in the militia that occupied counties in western Pennsylvania and sent prisoners to Philadelphia for trial. The militia and the federal government carried the day. The Whiskey Rebellion was an important test for the new government since it established clearly that the federal government had the power to enforce federal laws within a state.

At no time did drinking in the United States reach the epidemic levels it had in England. An expanding frontier, fewer overcrowded slum areas, and a pioneer ideology resulted in almost everyone drinking in the colonial period, but not too much. As society changed in the early part of the nineteenth century, heavy drinking increased, and with each new public drunkard there appeared two or three temperance workers. Temperance movements were everywhere in the early part of the nineteenth century and acquired national status with the formation of the American Temperance Society in 1827, which, it is important to note, advocated temperance, not abstinence. In 1834 Congress provided the plot for a thousand western movies by passing a law forbidding the sale of liquor to Indians.

Around 1840 to 1850 things changed. Up to this time there had not been a great deal of nondistilled alcohol used in the United States. Beer and wine were bulky, so they didn't help win the west. It was only with the advent of artificial refrigeration and the addition of hops, which helped preserve the beer, that there was an increase in the number of breweries.

At first, encouraged by temperance groups who preferred beer consumption to the use of liquor, breweries were constructed everywhere. Surprisingly, it was the great number of breweries that made abstainers out of temperants and brought about the first wave of state prohibition statutes that evolved into national prohibition in 1920. With too many breweries there was an overproduction of beer. To sell their beer many brewers bought taverns or formed partnerships with tavern owners or offered special inducement to bartenders to push the sale of their beer. The brewers also found that it was necessary to supply distilled spirits to the taverns to satisfy the consumers. This alliance worked well, and the consumption of malt beverages increased greatly but did not cause a decrease in the consumption of liquor.

The first state prohibition period began in 1851 when Maine passed its prohibition law. Between 1851 and 1855 thirteen states passed statewide prohibition laws, but by 1868 nine had repealed them. There was a continual battle throughout this period between the "wets" and the "drys." The strength of the feeling is seen in an 1865 Presbyterian Church decision declaring that liquor manufacturers and sellers were not eligible to be members of a Presbyterian church. Another indication of the pervasiveness of temperance beliefs is that our sixteenth President, Abraham Lincoln, was a temperance organization member.

The National Prohibition Party, organized in 1869, and the Woman's Christian Temperance Union, in 1874, provided the impetus for the second wave of state-wide prohibition that developed in the 1880's. From 1880 to 1889 seven states adopted prohibition laws, and by 1896 four had repealed them. In 1895 the American Anti-Saloon League was organized, but it was 12 years later (1907) that the final state prohibition movement began.

Much of the prohibition activity gathered its energy and justification from changes occurring in a bit of Americana.

> The saloon was for centuries an honorable institution. In colonial times, well-meaning legislators made its presence mandatory in certain townships and defined its purpose as the "refreshment of mankind in a reasonable manner," and this same happy regard for a necessity of life was probably close to the American consensus at least until after the Civil War. The saloon of the early nineteenth century was dedicated to the values of fellowship, equality, and euphoria. It was a warm and quiet retreat where men could explore the pleasures of friendship away from the nagging cares of creditor or clerk, wife or clergyman. It was a place where one could lift the burdens of caste, of status, and of the more restrictive social inhibitions, and thus freed, could grasp for the dim image of his own individuality. The saloon was also a glittering release from the drab and gray monotonies of an agrarian reality, a momentary refuge from worry or trouble, humiliation or shame. It offered an honest and felicitous distinction between relief and abandon to a grateful clientele. In a society not yet oppressed by the god of precision—when a man could spell his own name differently every day of the week if he wanted to and when no one measured the trueness of a furrow in millimeters—a reasonably soft cloud of alcoholic haze was a luxury one could hardly afford to be without. Until the agrarian America that produced the saloon no longer existed, the saloon sustained many an honorable man.*

In 1899 a group of educators, lawyers, and clergymen described the saloon as "the workingman's club, in which many of his leisure hours are spent, and in which he finds more of the things that approximate luxury than in his home, almost more than he finds in any other public place in the ward." They went on to say: "It is a centre of learning, books, papers, and lecture hall to them. It is the clearing-house for common intelligence, the place where their philosophy of life is worked

out, and their political and social beliefs take their beginnings."*

Truth lay somewhere between those statements and the sentiments expressed in a sermon:

> The liquor traffic is the most fiendish, corrupt and hell-soaked institution that ever crawled out of the slime of the eternal pit. It is the open sore of this land . . . . It takes the kind, loving husband and father, smothers every spark of love in his bosom, and transforms him into a heartless wretch, and makes him steal the shoes from his starving babe's feet to find the price for a glass of liquor. It takes your sweet innocent daughter, robs her of her virtue and transforms her into a brazen, wanton harlot . . . . The open saloon as an institution has its origin in hell, and it is manufacturing subjects to be sent back to hell . . .†

Prohibition was not just a matter of "wets" versus "drys," or a matter of political conviction or health concerns. Intricately interwoven with these factors was a middle-class, rural, Protestant, evangelical concern that the good and true life was being undermined by ethnic groups with a different religion and a lower standard of living and morality. One way to strike back at these groups was through prohibition. As one Anti-Saloon League leader put it: "There is one thing greater than democracy . . . and that is the will of God."†

If you can serve God's will, protect the virtue of your women, reduce temptation, and decrease your anxiety level by voting prohibition, it is not surprising that between 1907 and 1919 thirty-four states enacted legislation enforcing statewide prohibition while only two states repealed their prohibition laws. By 1917 64% of the population lived in dry territory and in the 1908 to 1917 period over 104,400 licensed bars were closed. The effect on alcohol consumption? A 16% increase in per capita consumption of distilled liquors to a level higher than it had been for over 45 years! Beer consumption on a per capita basis over this same period decreased 3%.

*From Clark, N. H.: The dry years: prohibition and social change in Washington, Seattle, 1965, University of Washington Press, pp. 54-55.

*From Koren, J.: Economic aspects of the liquor problem, New York, 1899, Houghton, Mifflin & Co., pp. 215-217.
†From Clark, N. H.: The dry years: prohibition and social change in Washington, Seattle, 1965, University of Washington Press, pp. 66-67.

It should also be remembered that the fact that there was a state prohibition law did not mean that the residents didn't drink. They did, both legally and illegally. They drank illegally in speakeasies and other private clubs. They drank legally from a variety of the many patent medicines that were freely available. A few of the more interesting ones were Whisko, "a nonintoxicating stimulant" at 55 proof; Golden's Liquid Beef Tonic, "recommended for treatment of alcohol habit" with 53 proof; and Kaufman's Sulfur Bitters, which "contains no alcohol" but was in fact 20% alcohol (40 proof) and contained no sulfur!

1917 was the beginning of the end. In January the United States Supreme Court upheld a law passed by Congress in 1913 forbidding interstate shipment of alcoholic beverages into areas where the manufacture and sale of liquor was "illegal."[1] In March Congress passed an anti–liquor advertising bill,[2] which prohibited the use of the United States mail to advertise "... spirituous, vinous, malted, fermented, or other intoxicating liquors of any kind ..." in an area that locally restricted their advertising. At this time, although only 64% of the population was dry, 90% of the land area was, so this law effectively stopped all but local advertising.

In August of 1917 the Senate adopted the resolution authored by Andrew Volstead, which submitted the national prohibition amendment to the states. The House of Representatives concurred in December and 21 days later on the eighth of January, 1918, Mississippi became the first state to ratify the Eighteenth Amendment. A year later, January 16, 1919, Nebraska was the thirty-sixth state to ratify the amendment and the deed was done!

As stated in the amendment, 1 year after the thirty-sixth state ratified it, national prohibition came into effect: January 16, 1920. The amendment was simple with only two operational parts:

Section 1. After one year from the ratification of this article the manufacture, sale or transportation of intoxicating liquors within, the importation thereof into, or the exportation thereof from the United States and all terri-

tory subject to the jurisdiction thereof for beverage purposes is hereby prohibited.
Section 2. The Congress and the several States shall have concurrent power to enforce this article by appropriate legislation.

The Eighteenth Amendment was repealed by the Twenty-first Amendment proposed in Congress on February 20, 1933, and ratified by thirty-six states by the fifth of December of that year. So ended an era. The Twenty-first Amendment was also short and sweet:

Section 1. The eighteenth article of amendment to the Constitution of the United States is hereby repealed.
Section 2. The transportation or importation into any State, Territory, or possession of the United States for delivery or use therein of intoxicating liquors, in violation of the laws thereof, is hereby prohibited.

How effective was national prohibition? There are many ways of approaching this question, but only one is relevant here: Did it reduce the consumption of alcoholic beverages? In the early years it certainly did, and authoritative estimates place beer consumption in 1920 at about 2 gallons per adult, while in 1917, the last normal consumption year, it was 32 gallons per adult. Distilled spirits dropped from an average of 2.6 gallons per adult in 1917 to 0.5 gallons per adult in 1920. Wine consumption, however, may have even shown a slight increase, going from 0.5 gallons in 1917 to 0.8 gallons per adult in 1920.

By 1930 things were different. Wine consumption had increased to 1.4 gallons, beer to 11.5, and distilled spirits to 2.2 gallons per adult! On a strictly wet-dry basis it would seem that prohibition failed, since 10 years after initiation alcohol consumption was almost as high as it was before enactment.

All other measures of the effectiveness of national prohibition seem to follow the alcohol consumption curve. Deaths resulting from alcoholism in 1920 were only about 20% of the rate in 1917. By 1929, though, the rate was 70% of the 1917 level. Cirrhosis of the liver followed the same dip and rise.

Prohibition did have some effects that lasted beyond 1933. One obvious effect was the elimination of many of the abstinence and temperance groups. With their goal achieved (they believed), their motivation and their membership dwindled to almost nothing in the early twenties. It is doubtful whether these groups could have withstood the urbanization, industrialization, and education that had progressed continually. Of more importance, however, prohibition showed clearly that to attempt to eliminate an already existing pleasure is a mighty hard thing to do. Americans now spend $25 billion a year to purchase alcoholic beverages and consume 19.6 gallons of beer, 1.9 gallons of distilled spirits, and 1.6 gallons of wine per capita.

CHEMISTRY, METABOLISM, AND PERIPHERAL EFFECTS

With alcohol's rich history and its importance as a factor in many social changes, modern science might be expected to know all there is to know about alcohol as a drug. This is hardly the case, but it has been well studied, and this and the next section present the current status of our knowledge of alcohol as a pharmacologically active agent. The discussion here will be limited to ethyl alcohol, C_2H_5OH, and the term "alcohol" refers specifically and only to ethyl alcohol.

Alcohol is unique in that it requires no digestion and can be absorbed unchanged from the stomach and, more rapidly, from the small intestine. In an empty stomach the overall rate of absorption depends on the concentration of alcohol in the stomach and initial part of the small intestine. Even though concentration is the primary factor, the absorption rate can be altered. For example, alcohol taken with or after a meal is absorbed more slowly. This is because the food remains in the stomach for digestive action, and the protein in the food retains the alcohol with it in the stomach.

Plain water, by decreasing the concentration, slows the absorption of alcohol, but soda water speeds it up. The carbon dioxide in the soda acts to move everything quite rapidly through the stomach to the small intestines. It is this emptying of the stomach and the more rapid absorption of alcohol in the intestines that give champagne and sparkling burgundy a faster onset of action than wine. Once absorbed into the bloodstream alcohol passes almost immediately through the liver. Alcohol is acted on in the liver by the enzyme *alcohol dehydrogenase*, which is present primarily in the liver and is *the factor that limits the rate of disappearance of alcohol from the body*. The steps in the metabolism of ethyl alcohol are well known and shown in Fig. 6-1.

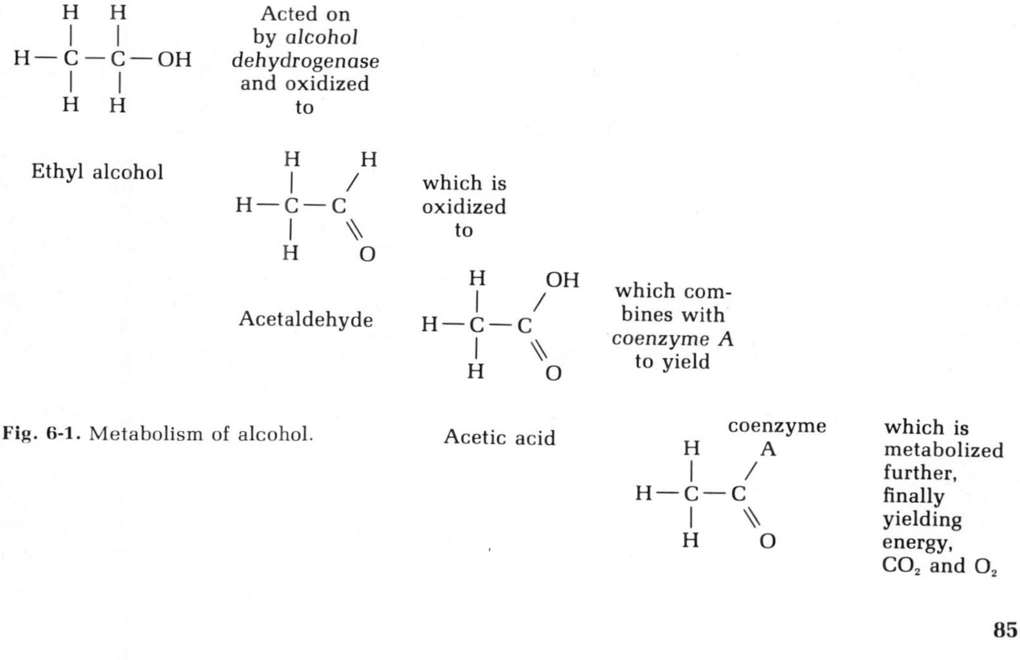

Fig. 6-1. Metabolism of alcohol.

The rate of oxidation of alcohol is not influenced by its level in the blood. The determining factor is the activity of the enzyme alcohol dehydrogenase, and in moderate drinkers the maximum amount of alcohol that can be metabolized is between 0.25 and 0.33 ounce an hour. Since alcohol does not bind itself or form deposits anywhere in the body, when absorbed it must stay in the body fluids until oxidized. If intake is faster than oxidation, blood alcohol concentration increases. There is some evidence that in heavy, habitual alcohol users there is an increase in the rate at which alcohol can be oxidized. Such a relationship suggests that the heavy alcohol consumer can drink more than a moderate user and still have the same blood level of alcohol.[3]

The body excretes very little alcohol under most conditions, perhaps about 2%. With a large intake, up to 10% to 15% may be eliminated unchanged through the kidneys, lungs, and skin. The rest is almost immediately oxidized for its energy content—about 200 calories per ounce. Alcohol is an ideal energy supply since it requires no digestion, is rapidly absorbed, and has a short metabolic pathway. It cannot be stored in the body or converted to any form that can be stored. Therefore the energy produced in the metabolism of alcohol must be used immediately. Since the calories in alcohol are not stored, they do not make a person fat. Alcohol is used, though, to meet the energy requirements of the body, and what sometimes causes a weight gain (even a beer belly!) is the food a person eats in addition to the intake of alcohol. The other foods can be, and are, converted to fat and stored if their energy is not needed for ongoing body needs. Alcohol is not an ideal food since it alone has no nutritional value other than energy production.

A few effects of alcohol intake should be discussed prior to the psychoactive effects. A relatively large and/or prolonged intake of alcohol frequently results in the consumer suffering from a hangover the next day. The complete basis for the symptoms of a hangover is not known, but the symptoms are familiar to a high percentage of even moderate drinkers who occasionally overindulge: upset stomach, fatigue, headache, thirst. It may be that a hangover is a short-term, mild withdrawal illness.

One of the actions of alcohol is to act on the brain to decrease the output of the antidiuretic hormone responsible for retaining fluid in the body. This effect probably means that the body excretes more fluid than is taken in with the alcoholic beverages, but this does not seem to be the primary basis for the thirst experienced the next day. The underlying cause probably lies in the fact that alcohol causes fluid inside cells to move outside the cells, and this cellular dehydration, without a decrease in total body fluid, is known to be related to, and perhaps to be the basis of, an increase in thirst.

The nausea and upset stomach typically experienced can probably be attributed to the fact that alcohol is a gastric irritant. The consumption of even moderate amounts causes local irritation of the mucosa covering the stomach. It has been suggested that the accumulation of acetaldehyde, which is quite toxic even in small quantities, contributes to the nausea and headache, but this now seems unlikely.

The headache may also be partly an allergic reaction to congeners. These are natural products of the fermentation and preparation process and some are quite toxic. Beer, with a 4% alcohol content, has only a 0.01% congener level, while wine has about 0.04% and the distilled spirits between 0.1% and 0.2%. Gin, being almost a mixture of pure alcohol and water, has a congener content about the same as wine, while a truly pure mixture of alcohol and water—vodka—is the same as beer in congener level. Interestingly, aging distilled spirits does not decrease the level of congeners but in fact increases it from about 0.15% to about 0.45%. Congeners make the various beverages different in smell, taste, and color.

Finally, the headache may be a reaction to fatigue and to a low blood sugar level. Fatigue sometimes results from a higher than normal level of activity while drinking. This frequently is a reaction to decreased inhibition, a readily available source of energy, and a high blood sugar level. One of the effects of alcohol intake is to increase the blood sugar level for about an hour after ingestion. This is followed several hours later by a low blood sugar level. That this low blood sugar level is not a complete explanation for any of the hangover symptoms is shown by the fact that taking sugar will not reduce the symptoms but it does return blood levels to normal.

A central nervous system effect of alcohol intake is the dilation of the peripheral blood vessels which increases the heat loss from the body but makes the drinker feel warm. It is this action on the peripheral vessels that argues against the use of alcohol in individuals in shock or extreme cold. Under these conditions blood is needed in the central parts of the body and heat loss must be diminished.

CENTRAL NERVOUS SYSTEM EFFECTS

Alcohol is like any other general anesthetic: *it depresses the central nervous system.* It was used as an anesthetic until the late nineteenth century, when nitrous oxide, ether, and chloroform became more widely used. However, it was not just new compounds that decreased alcohol's use as an anesthetic; it has some major disadvantages. In contrast to the gaseous anesthetics, alcohol is almost completely metabolized in the body and the rate of oxidation is slow. This gives alcohol a long duration of action that cannot be controlled. A second disadvantage is that the dose effective in surgical anesthesia is not much lower than the dose that causes respiratory arrest and death. Finally, alcohol slows the blood-clotting time.

The exact mechanism for the effect of alcohol is not clear, but the best evidence is that alcohol acts directly on neuronal membranes and not at the synapse. It is known that alcohol acts on the neuron's capability to produce electrical impulses and thus process information properly. Furthermore, the effect of alcohol on the central nervous system is directly proportional to the level of alcohol in the blood.

At the lowest effective blood level the reticular system begins to malfunction. This disruption results in the cerebral cortex not being regulated and losing its integrational

and inhibitory ability even before the alcohol blood level reaches the point at which the cerebral cortex is directly affected. The general sequence of behaviors affected is the same with alcohol as with all depressant drugs. Complex, abstract, and poorly learned behaviors are disrupted at the lower alcohol levels and, as the dose increases, better learned and simpler behaviors are also affected. Certain inhibitions may be reduced with the result that performance improves in some areas. Removal of other inhibitions by disruption of the cortex's normal activity may result in the appearance of behaviors not normally seen. Even though there may be an increase in behavior, *alcohol is not a stimulant.* It only seems to be a stimulant when it has depressed inhibitions.

The fact that alcohol impairs functioning of the reticular system, which disrupts cortical functions, resulting in behavioral changes, makes it impossible to predict specific behavioral effects following alcohol intake. Which behaviors are suppressed and which will be released from inhibition depend on the individual's history. Some individuals, after taking a moderately depressant dose of alcohol, turn from passive, nonaggressive comrades into belligerent, hostile combatants. Others become convinced they are modern Don Juans and their eyes, hands, and thoughts become more amorous. This is about all that becomes more amorous. Shakespeare, in speaking of alcohol, phrased it well in *Macbeth*: "Lechery, sir, it provokes, and unprovokes; it provokes the desire, but it takes away the performance." Sometimes permanently![3a]

If the alcohol intake is "just right," most people experience a "high," a happy feeling. Below a certain blood alcohol level there are no mood changes, but at some point we become uninhibited enough to enjoy our own charming selves and uncritical enough to accept the clods around us. This point seems to occur when the alcohol has disrupted social inhibitions and impaired good judgment but has not depressed most behavior. We become witty, clever, true continentals! Fortunately most of those around us at this time will also have impairment of judgment, so they can't say any differently!

Another factor contributing to the feeling of well-being is the reduction in anxieties as a result of the disruption of normal critical thinking. The reduction in concern and judgment may range from not worrying about who'll pay the bar bill (another round, garçon—and be quick about it!) to being sure that you can beat the train to the crossing (watch me scare that engineer!). A final effect of alcohol that may make the older person feel better is the anesthetizing of minor aches and pains.

No blood levels were suggested for the points at which an individual begins to feel good or happy, or becomes amorous, or when his sensory and motor functions are seriously impaired. Blood alcohol levels are reported as the number of milligrams (mg) of alcohol in each 100 milliliters (ml) of blood and are expressed as a percentage. Since 100 grams in 100 milliliters would be 100%, 100 mg of alcohol in 100 ml of blood is reported as 0.10%.

Before suggesting blood alcohol level–behavioral change relationships, two factors must be mentioned. One is that the rate at which the blood alcohol rises is a factor in determining behavioral effects. The more rapid the increase, the greater the behavioral effects. Second, it is well to note that a classic study[4] using a variety of simple visual, motor, and visual-motor tests showed disruption of performance at an average blood level of 0.05% in abstainers, 0.07% in moderate drinkers, and 0.10% in heavy drinkers.

These results show clearly that *behavioral tolerance to alcohol does develop.* They also indicate that the better performance of the heavy drinker compared to the moderate drinker after equal amounts of alcohol is not caused solely (if at all) by the greater rate of alcohol metabolism in heavy drinkers. *A higher blood alcohol level is necessary to impair a heavy drinker's performance than to impair a moderate drinker's performance!*

A partial explanation might be that the heavy drinker is better motivated to conceal the alcohol-induced impairment and probably has had more practice! Performance differences may only reflect the extent to which the two groups have learned to overcome the disruption of nervous system functioning. Another explanation may be that the central nervous system in the heavy drinker develops a tolerance to alcohol that does not exist in the moderate drinker. It is established that neural tissue becomes tolerant to alcohol, and tolerance can apparently develop even when the alcohol intake is well spaced in time.

In any dose-response curve there is considerable variability, and Table 6-1 reports some general relationships between blood alcohol level and behavior. These relationships are approximately correct for moderate drinkers. There are some reports that changes in nervous system function have been obtained at blood levels of as low as 0.03% to 0.04%.

The vomiting reflex may be activated by alcohol at a blood level of about 0.12% or even lower, but only if that level is approached rapidly. With slow, steady drinking the 0.12% level is gradually reached and the vomiting center is depressed. The individual can then continue drinking up to lethal levels if he remains conscious!

The surgical anesthesia level and the minimum lethal level are perhaps the two least precise points in the table. In any case they are quite close, and the safety margin is less than 0.1% blood alcohol. Death resulting from acute alcohol intoxication usually is the result of respiratory failure

Table 6-1. Blood alcohol level and behavioral effects

Blood alcohol level	Behavior
0.05%	Lowered alertness; usually good feeling
0.10%	Slowed reaction times; less caution
0.15%	Large, consistent increases in reaction time
0.20%	Marked depression in sensory and motor capability; decidedly intoxicated
0.25%	Severe motor disturbance, staggering; sensory perceptions greatly impaired; smashed!
0.30%	Semistupor
0.35%	Surgical anesthesia; about the LD 1, minimal level causing death
0.40%	About the LD 50

when the medulla is depressed. With respect to this last point, caffeine is an effective respiratory stimulant in cases of alcohol depression of respiration, but there is no clear evidence that it has any antagonistic actions on the behavioral effects that occur at lower blood alcohol levels. Neither is there a basis for believing that making an intoxicated person move around will help reduce blood alcohol levels. The standard "on your feet, keep walking, drink this black coffee" does not accelerate the sobering-up process.

The blood alcohol level and behavior relationship is similarly but more enjoyably described in the following, which is modified from Bogen.[5]

At less than 0.03% the individual is dull and dignified.

At 0.05%, he is dashing and debonair.

At 0.10%, he may become dangerous and devilish.

At 0.20%, he is likely to be dizzy and disturbing.

At 0.25%, he may be disgusting and disheveled.

At 0.30%, he is delirious and disoriented and surely drunk.

At 0.35%, he is dead drunk.

At 0.60%, the chances are that he is dead.

The relationship between blood alcohol levels and alcohol intake, the oral consumption of an alcoholic beverage, is not simple but is reasonably well understood. Remember, alcohol is not appreciably excreted from or stored anywhere in the body prior to metabolism. When taken into the body, alcohol is distributed throughout the body fluids including the blood. The heavier the person, the more body fluid he has and the lower the concentration of blood alcohol. Sex is also important since women have less fluid than men of the same weight because women have more fat! With less fluid the concentration of alcohol will be higher. It cannot be emphasized too often that central nervous system effects of alcohol are related directly to the blood alcohol concentration.

There is no point in detailing all that is known about the rate of absorption or metabolism of alcohol. It is important to appreciate that the relationships and numbers presented here are only typical and cannot be applied directly to a specific individual. Additional points to remember are that spirits are absorbed more rapidly than wine, which is absorbed more rapidly than beer, and that although eating while drinking will slow the absorption of alcohol and reduce peak blood concentrations, the absorption will continue for a longer period of time.

The relationships among alcohol intake, blood alcohol level, sex, and weight are indicated in Table 6-2.

In the 150-pound person, the average rate of metabolism of alcohol is about 0.30 ounce per hour of absolute alcohol; this lowers the blood alcohol level approximately 0.010% per hour. Thus, if a 150-pound man has six drinks over a 4-hour period his blood alcohol level would roughly be 0.11%. Although not completely studied, the rate of metabolism possibly depends on the size of the liver and thus the size of the body. As a result, the rate of alcohol metabolism may be higher in the heavier person than in the lower weight individual, but this has not yet been shown.

Two rules of thumb are often used to approximate how much an individual can (should) drink. One concerns itself with the amount of the alcoholic beverage a person can metabolize in an hour and is determined by dividing body weight in pounds by five times the percentage of alcohol in the beverage. For the hypothetical 150-pound person this yields about 7.5 ounces of beer. The other guide aims at the 0.15% blood alcohol level (the point at which an individual is legally drunk in every state) and includes a correction for the number of hours that have elapsed since drinking stopped. The formula gives the number of ounces of the beverage that, when ingested, will give a blood alcohol level of 0.15% at any number of postdrinking hours. H is the number of hours since drinking stopped. For 90 proof whiskey the formula is $8 + H$, for wine $36 + 4H$, and for beer $80 + 10H$. Both of these guides are rough approximations and should be taken with a grain of salt (like tequilla).

Blood alcohol level gives a good estimate of the alcohol concentration acting on the

Table 6-2. Relationships among sex, weight, oral alcohol consumption, and blood alcohol level

Absolute alcohol (ounces)	Beverage intake*	Blood alcohol levels (mg/100 ml)					
		Female (100 lbs)	Male (100 lbs)	Female (150 lbs)	Male (150 lbs)	Female (200 lbs)	Male (200 lbs)
1/2	1 oz spirits† 1 glass wine 1 can beer	0.045	0.037	0.03	0.025	0.022	0.019
1	2 oz spirits 2 glasses wine 2 cans beer	0.09	0.075	0.06	0.05	0.045	0.037
2	4 oz spirits 4 glasses wine 4 cans beer	0.18	0.15	0.12	0.10	0.09	0.07
3	6 oz spirits 6 glasses wine 6 cans beer	0.27	0.22	0.18	0.15	0.13	0.11
4	8 oz spirits 8 glasses wine 8 cans beer	0.36	0.30	0.24	0.20	0.18	0.15
5	10 oz spirits 10 glasses wine 10 cans beer	0.45	0.37	0.30	0.25	0.22	0.18

*In 1 hour.
†100 proof spirits.

brain, and the concentration of alcohol in the breath gives a good estimate of the alcohol concentration in the blood. There is a ratio of 1 to 2,100 between the concentration of alcohol in breath (1) and the concentration in blood (2,100). These relationships between breath level/blood level/central nervous system effects/behavioral effects are put to practical use by police. By determining alcohol level in the breath, statements can be made about blood alcohol levels, which form the basis in most states for conviction as a drunken driver.[5a]

DRINKING AND DRIVING

Blood alcohol levels are important because of their relationships to behavior. They assume greater importance if someone decides to mix his drink with driving. Blood alcohol levels as determined via a breath test are sometimes routinely monitored at roadblocks on special occasions such as New Year's Eve. Many states now consider an individual with a blood level of less than 0.05% to be legally sober. A blood level of 0.05% to 0.1% is questionable, while a level over 0.1% usually is sufficient to declare the individual legally drunk. In no state is the necessary level to be declared legally drunk greater than 0.15%. According to FBI statistics 40% of all arrests in the United States are for "drunkenness."

Someone has said that driving after one or two drinks is like driving at night with sunglasses on. There is no question that drinking does impair driving ability. Whether the disruption results from changes in visual sensitivity, motor coordination, speed of response, or judgment cannot be answered; all probably contribute.

The United States Department of Transportation estimates that alcohol is involved in more than 28,000 automobile accident deaths each year and about 800,000 automobile accidents. Most accidents involving alcohol occur in the late afternoon, evening, or night, and the odds are 8 to 1 that a driver killed in a single vehicle crash between 9 and 12 P.M. has been drinking heavily. One California study of single car accidents in which the driver died within 15 minutes of the crash and in which a valid blood test was taken showed that 70% of the males and 40% of the females had blood alcohol levels of 0.1% or more.

The National Safety Council has stated that alcohol is a causal factor in about half of the automobile accidents killing the driver, as well as in a third of the accidents fatal to adult pedestrians. It has also reported that usually these alcohol-associated deaths involve alcoholics, not social drinkers. Other work showed that, compared to no blood alcohol, an auto accident was two and one half times as likely with blood levels between 0.1% and 0.15% and ten times as likely if the level was over 0.15%. Levels this high are apparently not necessary, though, to cause an impairment in driving skills, since another study reported a 25% to 30% deterioration (in skilled drivers) at blood levels of 0.04%.

WHO DRINKS?

Perhaps it is better to ask, who doesn't use alcoholic beverages? Few drugs are more pervasive than alcohol, and most people use it in moderation. It is estimated that 9% of the 95 million drinkers in the United States are alcoholics or at least problem drinkers. Concern over the social cost of alcohol abuse and the increasing emphasis on treatment and rehabilitation was formalized in May of 1971 with the creation of the National Institute on Alcohol Abuse and Alcoholism as part of the National Institute of Mental Health. Much work needs to be done.

Some researchers feel that many individuals who become alcoholics have a faulty biochemical makeup that may be genetically based. There is not much evidence to support this idea, but it must be admitted that some human studies do suggest a genetic basis for alcoholism.[5b-d] The burden of proof is on the biochemists since the personal and cultural factors that predispose an individual to become an abuser of alcohol have been studied frequently with consistent results.

There are clear differences even between primitive tribes that use alcohol only sparingly and those that are referred to as drinking tribes. The more sober tribes live in settled communities with structured social systems that spell out social level and social rights and obligations. The drinking tribes typically have a much looser social structure, with property being held communally and few ties to land. These tribes frequently are nomadic or survive by hunting rather than by growing crops. In brief, in primitive societies if one has to account for his behavior, provide for himself, and receive according to his output, drinking is usually well controlled. If there is no need for self-control, then heavy drinking is not atypical.

Such relationships could be seen in the rural Ireland of the eighteenth and nineteenth centuries. Public drunkenness was widespread and has been related to a very diffuse social organization with little attachment to the land. Also, Ireland at that time suffered from outside rule, which resulted in low respect for authority and little interest in self-control. Some of these general attitudes may be reflected in the finding that the highest alcoholism rate in the United States today is among the Irish-Americans.

Differences between countries in alcohol consumption and in drinking patterns are apparent. Although Italians consume the equivalent of 15 quarts of pure alcohol per year per adult, public intoxication is much less frequent in most of Italy than one might expect. Except in the industrial north, drinking in Italy is associated with meals and family gatherings. It will be interesting to see whether public drunkenness moves south along with the industrialization of Italy.

France is probably the country that has the greatest drinking problem in the world. It has been estimated that adults over 20 in France consume the equivalent of 32 quarts a year of pure alcohol. The French Government estimates that 15% of adult French males are alcoholics and that 30% consume alcohol in amounts dangerous to their health. This high level of consumption is maintained by a variety of factors including nationalism, the relating of wine drinking to virility by the French, and a very strong wine lobby that places ads in the subway such as: "Water is for frogs"!

In the United States there is not such an overt campaign, but over $300 million is spent each year on advertising by the alcoholic beverage industry, and we consume the equivalent of 9 quarts of pure alcohol per adult each year. Much of the advertising content is directed toward associating beer and wine with good times, family gatherings, and virility. Spirits are merchandised more by associating them with cocktail parties, high status, and upper social level behavior. Such advertising must be effective, since in 1972 Americans spent about $25 billion on alcoholic beverages.

Not all Americans drink, but about 80% of urban adults report having used alcoholic beverages, while less than half of the rural adults have indulged. A 1973 survey found that 53% of the adults and 24% of the adolescents had consumed some alcoholic beverage within the week prior to the survey. Generally the higher the economic and education level, the greater percentage of drinkers. Drinking homes beget drinkers, and most abstainers come from nondrinking homes.

In urban areas religious factors also influence drinking patterns, with over 90% of both male and female Jews reporting the use of alcohol. Interestingly, there is a very low percentage of Jews who become alcoholics, and this may develop from the fact that Jews are introduced to alcohol—wine—in the home and in religious ceremonies. About 90% of Catholic and 80% of Protestant males report drinking, while females in these groups report 80% and 70%, respectively.

CHRONIC ALCOHOLISM

To define alcoholism is difficult because the term is used with different meanings by various authorities. Here an alcoholic will be considered to be an individual who uses alcohol to an extent that it interferes with his social and occupational behavior. With this criterion, it has been estimated that there are 5 or 6 million alcoholics in the United States, with a male-female ratio of about 4 to 1. An analysis of the 1950 statistical reports suggested that about 9% of American men were alcoholics and that they drank almost 50% of the alcohol consumed.

California has the highest percentage of alcoholics, followed by New Jersey, New Hampshire, and New York. The highest rate of alcoholism in an identifiable ethnic group is in the Irish-Americans. A better predictor of alcoholism than where a person lives or what his national origins are is the kind of home he comes from. Forty percent of alcoholics come from a broken home and 40% (some overlapping) report problem drinking in at least one parent. Late birth position in a family is associated with alcoholism, but this may be caused, at least partly, by the greater likelihood of a broken home or loss of a parent early in the life of a later-born child.

One study of juvenile drinkers who had been referred to an alcoholism clinic reported that one or both parents were alcoholic. Further, these juveniles expressed much anxiety over drinking but, since drinking made them less anxious, they continued. One motivation for their drinking was to prove that they could drink better than their alcoholic parent. Another basis was suggested by the fact that they typically engaged in group, not solitary, drinking and may have been looking for a substitute for the family ties they were unable to form at home.

Alcoholics have been extensively studied psychologically and a fairly consistent pattern emerges. Unfortunately, you can't tell whether the characteristics existed before, and, in part, led the individual to heavy drinking, or whether the personality traits are the result of heavy drinking and the social stresses resulting from the drinking behavior. At any rate, alcoholics apparently have a very low frustration tolerance and therefore little ability to persevere in a task. Minor difficulties disrupt their performance, and frequently the alcoholic just gives up trying to function adequately. Those traits, coupled with reported tendencies to act impulsively, sometimes with considerable hostility, make it easy to understand why alcoholics also report feelings of isolation. Many studies suggest that one of the basic problems is an intense conflict between wanting to be both dependent and independent, and it may be that alcohol is an attempt to reduce this conflict.

When alcohol intake occurs regularly and in large quantities over a period of years, physical dependence on the drug occurs, and withdrawal from the drug results in a dangerous change in the body physiology. Before the addiction to alcohol reaches this point, physical symptoms sometimes develop, with facial appearance first affected. The capillaries around the conjunctiva of the eyes become enlarged and the skin of the face, forehead, and under the eyes becomes puffy and filled with fluid.

In an individual with a fair complexion, the skin may appear continually flushed and, after prolonged use, a "whiskey nose" may develop. The frequent hoarseness of the alcoholic results from the accumulation of fluid in the mucous membranes of the nose, pharynx, larnyx, and vocal cords. Continual ingestion of alcohol leads to an inflamed stomach associated with nausea and loss of appetite.

The chronic heavy user of alcohol may develop alcoholic polyneuropathy in which there are neurological and motor disturbances suggesting impaired function of peripheral nerves. It has been shown in these individuals that there is a considerable reduction in the speed with which impulses travel in some peripheral neurons.

Two closely related terminal stages of prolonged alcoholism are Wernicke's disease and Korsakoff's psychosis. It seems clear that the Korsakoff disorder is the behavioral manifestation of the brain lesions constituting Wernicke's disease. Wernicke's disease involves hemorrhages and loss of nerve cells in certain parts of the hypothalamus and thalamus, which result in profound disruptions in the ability to learn new material or to recall previously learned material. Individuals with these lesions are usually confused and disoriented as to time and place and are diagnosed as having Korsakoff's psychosis.

As with any central nervous system damage, these neurons do not regenerate. There can be some recovery of function with treatment if alternate neural pathways develop and general health and morale are improved. However, these lesions are not the result of a direct action by alcohol on the brain. Rather, they probably result from a vitamin B_1 (thiamine) deficiency. The same kind of damage in the same areas has been obtained in animals fed a thiamine-deficient diet. The vitamin deficiency in alcoholics results from a reduction in food intake caused by the large number of calories obtained through the use of alcohol. Some estimates are that up to half of the total energy needs in alcoholics may be met by the metabolism of alcohol, which contains none of the other essential foodstuffs.

The evidence is still to come on a final answer to the question of whether alcohol itself has any permanent effect on the brain or other nervous tissue. Recent evidence is convincing, however, that alcohol has a direct damaging effect on the liver. A 1974 report on baboons found that ". . . a nutritious diet will not prevent the development of alcoholic hepatitis and cirrhosis when excessive alcohol is chronically consumed."[5e] Baboons are reasonably close to man physiologically, so future work may yield similar results in humans.

The physical dependence associated with prolonged heavy use of alcohol is best seen when alcohol intake is stopped. *The abstinence syndrome that develops is medically more severe and more likely to cause death than withdrawal from narcotic drugs.* The withdrawal symptoms, which include tremor, convulsions, delirium, and hallucinations, do not appear until blood alcohol levels drop below the intoxication level. These withdrawal symptoms alone may be enough to keep the drinker drinking.

Tremors are one of the most common physical changes associated with alcohol withdrawal and may persist for a long period after alcohol intake has stopped. The classical drunk, bending over to sip his cup, attests to the frequency of tremors. Anxiety, insomnia, feelings of unreality, nausea, vomiting, and many other symptoms are also common.

The withdrawal symptoms do not develop all at the same time or immediately after abstinence begins. The initial signs may develop within a few hours (tremors, anxiety), but the individual is relatively rational. Over the next day or two hallucinations appear and gradually become more terrifying and real to the individual. If no medication is given, delirium tremens develops in some individuals.

In one double-blind, multiple hospital study, 7% of the patients given placebos suffered convulsions during withdrawal while 6% showed delirium tremens (the DT's).[6] In another study convulsions were reported in 12% of the patients, delirium tremens in 5%, and hallucinations in 18%.[7] The symptoms that do develop seem to result from the fact that the cells of the body, and particularly the central nervous system, have been functioning reasonably normally in spite of the depressant action of alcohol. When the alcohol is reduced, the cells become hyperactive. Released from the depression induced by the drug, the cells overreact and became hyperexcitable.

Optimal treatment of the patient seems to be the administration of antianxiety agents such as chlordiazepoxide (see Chapter 10), since in comparing the effectiveness of several compounds in blocking withdrawal symptoms this drug reduced the incidence of convulsions and delirium tremens to less than 1%.[6] This probably is a result of a high degree of cross-tolerance (cross-dependence) between alcohol and chlordiazepoxide, so one drug can be substituted for the other and withdrawal continued at a safer rate. The use of drugs to decrease alcohol withdrawal signs is clearly only symptomatic treatment. To keep the alcoholic from resuming drinking is a difficult task and one that will not be discussed.

CONCLUDING COMMENT

Alcohol is clearly our most popular minor tranquilizer. It is also, without a doubt, a most important drug of abuse. Some authorities believe that if alcohol were discovered today it would not be approved by the Food and Drug Administration even as a prescription drug! The potential for abuse is high, and the physiological damage resulting from misuse is considerable. Alcohol has reached a place where, even though at times it is bad company and its history is less than charming, few

people would want to see it eliminated. Our society's feelings seem to lean toward those of Horace:

> What wonders does not wine! ... eases the anxious mind of its burden ... Whom has not a cheerful glass made eloquent!

even though in 1900 one author felt:

> Experience shows that in all countries where the alcoholic habit reigns, it accounts for from one-half to three-fourths of the crimes, a great share of suicides, of mental disorders, of deaths, of diseases generally, of poverty, of vulgar depravity, of sexual excesses and venereal diseases and of dissolution of families.*

*From Forel, A.: The alcohol question, American Journal of Insanity 57:303, 1900.

PRECEDING QUOTES

1. Anonymous.
2. Smith, W. H., and Helwie, F. C.: Liquor: the servant of man, Boston, 1940, Little, Brown and Co., p. 25.
3. Strecker, E. A., and Chambers, F. T.: Alcohol: one man's meat, New York, 1938, The Macmillan Co., p. 38.
4. Anonymous.

REFERENCES

1. Gordon, L.: The new crusade, Cleveland, 1932, The Crusaders, Inc., pp. 21-24, 150-151.
2. Reed Amendment, P.L. 380, Section 5, March 3, 1917, Sixty-fourth Congress, Session II.
3. Rubin, E., and Lieber, C. S.: Science 172:1097-1102, 1971.
3a. Lemere, F., and Smith, J. W.: American Journal of Psychiatry 130(2):212-213, 1973.
4. Goldberg, L.: Acta Physiologica Scandinavica, vol. 5, Supp. 16, pp. 1-128, 1943.
5. Bogen, E.: The human toxicology of alcohol. In Emerson, H., editor: Alcohol and man, New York, 1932, The Macmillan Co., pp. 126-152.
5a. Lovell, W. S.: Science 178:264-273, 1972.
5b. Vesell, E. S., Page, J. G., and Passananti, G. T.: Clinical Pharmacology and Therapeutics 12(2):192-201, 1971.
5c. Schuckit, M. A., Goodwin, D. A., and Winokur, G.: American Journal of Psychiatry 128(9):122-126, 1972.
5d. Goodwin, D. W., Schulsinger, F., Hermansen, L., Guze, S. B., and Winokur, G.: Archives of General Psychiatry 28:238-243, 1973.
5e. Rubin, E., and Lieber, C. S.: New England Journal of Medicine 290:128-135, 1974.
6. Kaim, S. C., Klett, C. J., and Rothfeld, B.: American Journal of Psychiatry 125:1640-1646, 1969.
7. Victor, M., and Adams, R. D.: Cited by Fraser, H. F.: Annual Review of Medicine 8:427-440, 1957.

🐚 Nicotine

(About 1580) . . . it was more likely than not that . . . the doctor would prescribe tobacco . . . Did the patient suffer from flatulence? The remedy was a tobacco emetic. Toothache? Tobacco dentifrice. A running sore? Cover it with tobacco leaf. A heavy cough? Smoke of tobacco, deeply inhaled. Pains accompanying gestation or labor? Place a leaf of tobacco, very hot, on the navel. If a form of delirium ensued, blow smoke up the nostrils. Headache? Snuff powdered tobacco. A pain in the neck? Lay on the leaf, green.

> *The Mighty Leaf*

Smoke cigarettes? Not on your tut-tut. Drop it . . . You can't suck coffin-nails and be a ring-champion . . . You never heard of a strong arm, a porch-climber, or a bank burglar using a cigarette, did you? They couldn't do it and attend to biz. Why, even drunkards don't use the things. . . . Who smokes 'em? Dudes and college stiffs—fellows who'd be wiped out by a single jab or a quick undercut. It isn't natural to smoke cigarettes. An American ought to smoke cigars, an Englishman a briar, a Harp a clay pipe and a Dutchy a Meerschaum. It's the Dutchmen, Italians, Russians, Turks and Egyptians who smoke cigarettes and they're no good anyhow.

> *John L. Sullivan, 1905*

No research demonstrates that any ingredient as found in cigarette smoke causes cancer or cardiovascular, respiratory, or other illnesses in humans. No research has demonstrated any physiological process through which cigarette smoke results in illness.

> *The Tobacco Institute, 1970*

Cigarette smoking is now as important a cause of death as were the great epidemic diseases such as typhoid, cholera, and tuberculosis . . .

> *Smoking and Health Now, Report of the Royal College of Physicians, January, 1971*

Cigarette smoking is the greatest preventable cause of illness, disability and premature death in this country.

> *Surgeon General, U. S. Public Health Service, 1969*

. . . the control of cigarette smoking could do more to improve health and prolong life . . . than any other single action in the whole field of preventive medicine.

> *Report to the World Health Organization, 1970*

TOBACCO

Tobacco is as American as the ice cream soda. Along with corn, sweet potatoes, ordinary potatoes, chocolate, and the hammock, tobacco is a contribution of the New World to civilization. Not to be outdone, civilization gave the New World mumps, measles, and smallpox! Christopher Columbus records that tobacco leaves were given to him as a gift by the natives of San Salvador on the twelfth of October, 1492. A fitting birthday present.

In 1497 the first report of smoking appeared in print in a book on native customs written by a monk who accompanied Columbus on his second trip. No one "smoked" in the early days of tobacco use; inhaling smoke was called "drinking." The poor fellow who introduced tobacco drinking to Europe was Rodrigo de Jerez. He was the first European to touch Cuba and possibly the first to smoke tobacco. When he continued his habit in Portugal and his friends saw the smoke coming out his mouth and nose, they were convinced the devil had possessed him. The priest agreed, and Rodrigo spent the next several years in jail, only to find upon his release that people were doing the same thing for which he had been jailed!

The word "tobacco" came from one of two sources. "Tobaco" referred to a two-pronged tube used by natives to take snuff, and some early reports confused the issue by applying the name to the plant they incorrectly thought was being used. Another idea is that the word developed its current usage from the province of Tobacos in Mexico, where everyone used the herb. Be that as it may, in 1598 an Italian-English dictionary published in London translated the Italian "nicosiana" as the herb "tobacco" and that spelling and usage gradually became dominant.

The early interest in tobacco was in its medical value. A 1529 report[1] indicated it was used for "abscesses and sores on the head," "cold or catarrh," "persistent headaches." One writer[2] has recorded that fourteen books mentioning the use of tobacco as a medicine were published in Europe between 1537 and 1559. With the medical use of tobacco already well publicized and the importation of the plant from Brazil to Portugal before 1550, everything was set for a French ambassador to Portugal to make a name for himself. And that's just what Jean Nicot did.

Nicot was sent to Lisbon in 1559 to arrange a royal marriage that never took place, but he became enamoured with the medical uses of tobacco. He tried it on enough people to convince himself of its value and sent glowing reports of the herb's effectiveness to the French court. Although tobacco had been introduced earlier to Paris, Nicot received the credit. By 1565 the plant had been called nicotiane, and Linnaeus sanctified it in 1753 by naming the genus Nicotiana. When a pair of French chemists isolated the active ingredient in 1828, they acted as true nationalists and called it nicotine.

To fully appreciate the history of tobacco you must know that there are over sixty species of Nicotiana but only two major ones. *Nicotiana tobacum,* the major species grown today in over 100 countries, is large leafed. Most importantly, *tobacum* was indigenous only to South America, and the Spanish had a monopoly on its production for over 100 years. *Nicotiana rustica* is a small leaf species and was the plant existing in the West Indies and eastern North America when Columbus arrived.

Medical history—short form

Tobacco was formally introduced to Europe as an herb useful for the treatment of almost anything. A conservative (!) statement summarizing the feelings of many physicians about the usefulness of tobacco appeared in a 1591 book: "To seek to tell the virtues and greatness of this holy herb, the ailments which can be cured by it, and have been, the evils from which it has saved thousands, would be to go on to infinity."[3]

Sir Anthony Chute in his 1595 book[4] summarized much of the earlier material and said: "Anything that harms a man inwardly from his girdle upward might be removed by a moderate use of the herb." Others, however, felt differently in this period: "If taken after meals the herb would infect the brain and liver" and: "Tobacco should be avoided by (among others) women with child and husbands who desired to have children."[5]

A few years later, in 1617, Dr. William Vaughn phrased the last thought a little more poetically:

Tobacco that outlandish weede
It spends the braine and spoiles the seede
It dulls the spirite, it dims the sight
It robs a woman of her right.[*]

In the absence of knowledge anything is worth trying and, although the golden age of snuff had not yet arrived, snuff was very popular during the great plague of 1665. It was felt that the regular use of snuff was prophylactic. At the very least, it made it more difficult to smell the stench. Belief in the value of tobacco was fed by reports like that in 1674 by a traveler to the New World:

...it helps the digestion, the gout, the tooth ache, prevents infection by scents, it heats the cold and cools them that sweat, feedeth the hungry, spent spirits restoreth, purgeth the stomach, killeth nits and lice, the juice of the green leaf healeth green wounds, although poison. The syrup for many diseases. The smoke for the Phthisick, cough of the lungs, distillation of rheume, and all diseases of a cold and moist cause, good for all bodies cold and moist taken upon an empty stomach...

But:

...taken upon a full stomach...it moderately drieth the body, inflameth the blood, hurteth the brain, weakens the eyes and sinews.[†]

The slow advance of medical science through the eighteenth and nineteenth centuries gradually removed tobacco from the doctor's black bag. Special note must be made of a series of experiments reported in 1805 by Dr. D. Legare, since his work pushed back the boundaries of ignorance and clearly disproved an old folk remedy. Beyond the shadow of a doubt, Dr. Legare personally proved that, contrary to general opinion, blowing smoke into the intestinal canal did *not* resuscitate

drowned animals or people! Another unsung hero of the men in white coats.

Early history

In the sixteenth century the English had real heroes to love and to copy—men like Sir Walter Raleigh (who wasn't always a pipe tobacco) and Sir Francis Drake (who never was). They sailed the seven seas and, like most sailors of the day, took up pipe smoking. During the Elizabethan era, smoking became a national pleasure for the English, even though few people smoked on the continent.

One thorn in the British side was the Spanish monopoly on tobacco. When the settlers returned to England in 1586 after failing to colonize Virginia, they brought with them seeds of the *rustica* species and planted them in England, but this species never grew well. The English crown again attempted to establish a tobacco colony in 1610 when they sent John Rolfe as leader of a group to Virginia. From 1610 to 1612 Rolfe tried to cultivate *rustica* for sale in London, but it wouldn't sell because the small-leafed plant was weak, poor in flavor, and had a sharp taste.

In 1612 Rolfe's wife died, but, more important, he somehow got hold of some seeds of the Spanish *tobacum* species. This species grew beautifully and sold well in 1613. The colony was saved and every available plot of land was planted with *tobacum*. By 1619, as much Virginia tobacco was sold in London as Spanish tobacco. That was also the year that King James prohibited the cultivation of any tobacco in England and declared the the tobacco trade a royal monopoly.

Tobacco became one of the major exports of the American colonies to England. The Thirty Years' War spread smoking throughout central Europe, and nothing stopped its use. Measures such as one in Bavaria in 1652—which said "tobacco-drinking was strictly forbidden to the peasants and other common people..." and made tobacco available to others only on a doctor's prescription from a druggist[6]—probably slowed tobacco use, but only momentarily.

In 1660 England raised the duty on tobacco, and for the first time tobacco appeared on

---

[*]Quoted in Dunphy, E. B.: Alcohol and tobacco amblyopia: a historical survey, American Journal of Ophthalmology 68(4):573, 1969.

[†]From Stewart, G. G.: A history of the medicinal use of tobacco, 1492-1860, Medical History 11:241, 1967.

the tax books. Gradually increasing costs made adulteration a worthwhile occupation and, in 1716, Parliament passed the Pure Tobacco Act to control adulteration. That this is a never-ending problem is suggested by a 1918 decision of the Mississippi Supreme Court, which said:

> We can imagine no reason why, with ordinary care, human toes could not be left out of chewing tobacco, and if toes are found in chewing tobacco, it seems to us that somebody has been very careless.*

During the eighteenth century smoking gradually diminished, but the use of tobacco did not. Snuff replaced the pipe in England. At the beginning of the eighteenth century the upper class was already committed to snuff. The middle and lower classes only gradually changed over but, by 1770, very few people smoked. The reign of King George III (1760-1820) was the time of the big snuff. His wife Charlotte was so addicted to the powder that she was called "Snuffy Charlotte," although for obvious reasons not to her face. On the continent Napoleon had tried smoking once, gagged horribly, and returned to his 7 pounds of snuff a month.

Middle history

In the colonies trouble developed and, being democratic, the richest man in Virginia (perhaps the richest in the colonies) was made commander-in-chief of the Revolutionary Army. In 1776, in one of his appeals, George Washington said: "...if you can't send money, send tobacco."[7] One hundred and forty-one years later an American commander-in-chief was to echo those words when Pershing said: "You ask me what we need to win this war. I answer tobacco as much as bullets."[8] In the Revolutionary War tobacco played an important role since it was one of the major products for which France would lend the colonies money. Knowing the importance of tobacco to the colonies, one of Cornwallis' major campaign goals in 1780 and 1781 was the destruction of the Virginia tobacco plantations.

*Quoted in Brooks, J. E.: The mighty leaf, Boston, 1952, Little Brown, and Co., p. 303.

After the war, the American man in the street rejoiced and rejected snuff as well as tea and all other things British. The aristocrats who organized the republic were not as emotional, though, and installed a communal snuff box for members of Congress. Only in the mid-1930's did this remembrance of things past disappear. However, to emphasize the fact that snuff was a nonessential, the new Congress put a luxury tax on it in 1794.

> If you don't smoke and you don't snuff,
> how can you possibly get enough?

By chewing, which gradually increased in the United States. Chewing was a suitable activity for a country on the go; it freed the hands, and the wide-open spaces made an adequate spitoon. There were also other considerations; Boston, for example, had passed an ordinance in 1798 forbidding anyone from being in possession of a lighted pipe or "segar" in public streets. The original impetus was a concern for the fire hazard involved in smoking, not the individual's health, and the ordinance was finally repealed in 1880. It is difficult to indicate how much of a chewing country we were in the nineteenth century. In 1860 only seven of 348 tobacco factories in Virginia and North Carolina were for smoking tobacco. The amount of tobacco for smoking did not equal the amount for chewing until 1911 and did not surpass it until the 1920's. Even as cigarettes began developing in Europe, American chewing tobacco was expanding.

The Civil War shut Southern "Bright" (that is, light-colored when cured) tobacco out of northern markets, but Ohio and Kentucky had a different variety of tobacco, "Burley," that was darker and better suited for chewing. Burley had a low sugar content and thus could absorb up to 25% of its weight in licorice, rum, and molasses, while the Bright tobacco from Virginia and North Carolina could only absorb about 4% of its weight. The tobaccos from west of the Appalachian Mountains reached their peak in the 1890 to 1910 period. The 1890's particularly were times of price wars and intense competition. By selling at less than cost, consumption of chewing tobacco increased so that by 1897 one-half of all tobacco in the United States was prepared for chewing. The names of some of the brands are indicative of the savageness of the competition: "Battle Ax," "Scalping Knife," "Crossbow."

Although the writing was on the wall before the turn of the century, it was not until 1945 that the last bow was made to the chewer when cuspidors were removed from all federal buildings. In that same year at the National Tobacco Spitting Contest the winner spat 21 feet, 2 inches. That wasn't as good as Mark Twain, but they're getting there. The 1970 competition established a world's record that still stands: 25 feet, 10 inches!

Recent history

The transition from chewing to cigarettes had a middle point, a combination of both smoking and chewing—cigars. Cigarette smoking was coming, and the cigar manufacturers did their best to keep cigarettes under control. They suggested that cigarettes were drugged with opium so you could not stop using them, that the paper was bleached with arsenic and thus was harmful to you. They had some help from Thomas Edison in 1914:

> The injurious agent in Cigarettes comes principally from the burning paper wrapper. . . . It has a violent action in the nerve centers, producing degeneration of the cells of the brain, which is quite rapid among boys. Unlike most narcotics, this degeneration is permanent and uncontrollable. I employ no person who smokes cigarettes.*

Most cigars had been hand-rolled or at least made by hand-shaping in a mold, but as sales increased machines had to be used. There was an aversion to machine-made cigars, so some advertising was educational in nature. As an example of the high level of advertising before television and Madison Avenue:

> Spit is a horrid word, but it's worse on the end of your cigar. Why run the risk of cigars made by dirty, yellowed fingers and tipped in spit?†

*Quoted in Brooks, J. E.: The mighty leaf, Boston, 1952, Little, Brown and Co., p. 274.
†From Brooks, J. E.: The mighty leaf, Boston, 1952, Little, Brown, and Co., p. 273.

The efforts of the cigar manufacturers worked for a while, and cigar sales reached their highest level in 1920 when 8 billion were sold. As sales increased, though, so did the cost of the product. The whole world knows that "What this country *needs* is a really good five-cent cigar," but how many know that this statement was made by a Vice-President of the United States as an aside in the Senate when one of the members was going on at great length about the needs of the country. If the country got one, it was not enough. The dudes, the effete, were beginning to have their day.

Thin reeds filled with tobacco had been seen by the Spanish in Yucatan in 1518. In 1844 the French were using them, and the Crimean War circulated the cigarette habit throughout Europe. The first British cigarette factory was started in 1856 by a returning veteran (Crimean War), and in the late 1850's an English tobacco merchant, Philip Morris, began producing hand-made cigarettes. On the continent the use of this new dose form must have developed fairly rapidly, since a company in Austria began making double cigarettes in 1865—both ends had a mouth-piece and the consumer cut them in two—and sold 16 million in 1866.

In the United States cigarettes were being produced during this same period—14 million in 1870—but it was in the 1880's that their popularity increased rapidly. The first patent on a cigarette-making machine was given in 1881, and by 1885 over 1 billion cigarettes a year were being sold. Cigarette smoking increased each year. At the turn of the century there was a preference for cigarettes with an aromatic component, that is, Turkish tobacco. A new cigarette in 1913 capitalized on the lure of the Near East while rejecting it in actuality. Three hundred years after John Rolfe saved the Virginia colony with American-grown Spanish tobacco, a true American cigarette was created, Camels. Camels were a blend of Burley's and Bright's with just a hint of Turkish tobacco—you had the camel and pyramid on the package, what more could you want? Besides, eliminating most of the imported tobacco made the price lower, and the Camel cigarette ran away with the market for many, many years.

Chesterfield had been started in 1912, and the name Lucky Strike—which started as a smoking plug after the Civil War—was revived in 1916 as a cigarette. The name didn't have the relevance it had had in the 1860's and 1870's during the gold rushes, but then neither did Old Gold, which appeared first in 1885 and then in 1926 as a cigarette. Those who lived in the 1930's and 1940's will never forget the "Call for Philip Morris!" booming out from the radio after that cigarette was introduced in 1933. Those not so fortunate cannot appreciate it but should remember that their children will never thrill to the throaty: "You . . . can . . . take Salem out of the country, but! . . ."

The first ad showing a woman smoking appeared in 1919. To make the ad easier to accept, the woman was oriental looking and the ad was for Turkish type cigarettes. King-size cigarettes appeared in 1939 in the form of Pall Mall and became the Number 1 seller. Filter cigarettes as filter cigarettes, not cigarettes that happen to have filters along with a mouthpiece, appeared in 1951 with Winston, which is now far and away the best seller (1972: 86 billion cigarettes; number 2 was Marlboro with 70 billion). Total cigarette sales in the United States are over $10 billion a year. Per capita use by persons 18 and older declined from the 1963 all-time high of 4,345 to a low of 3,985 in 1970. Consumption is again increasing and was over 4,100 in 1973.

Tobacco—pro and con

It's clear that throughout the history of tobacco there have been those who oppose its use as well as those who defend it. Some of these thoughts have already been indicated, but others, particularly the more recent ones, are mentioned in this section.

In 1600 pipe smoking was *the* thing to do in England, even though the King opposed it for social, medical, and moral reasons. It was more than a passive opposition, and in 1604 King James (yes, it's *that* King James) wrote and published a very strong antitobacco pamphlet stating that tobacco was "harmfull to the braine, dangerous to the lungs."[9] Never

one to let morality interfere with business, he also supported the growing of tobacco in Virginia in 1610 and, when the crop prospered, he declared the tobacco trade a royal monopoly.

Two hundred and eight years later, in the last two decades of the nineteenth century, pure food and pure body zealots began to prowl the American landscape. As cigarette use increased, so did the antitobacco crusaders. From 1895 to 1907, twelve states banned cigarettes. In 1921 fourteen states had cigarette prohibition laws, and there were over 90 anticigarette bills being considered by the legislative bodies of 28 states. By 1928, however, all the cigarette prohibition laws had been repealed.

Anything was fair play. There were calls to ban the nursery rhyme "Ole King Cole" since he was debauching by calling for his pipe. In 1908 New York City made it illegal for a woman to use tobacco publicly. In the 1920's you hadn't "come a long way, baby," and women were expelled from schools and dismissed from jobs for smoking. The best of the antitobacco statements in that period was by a Dr. Tidswell: ". . . The most common cause of female sterility is the abuse of tobacco by males."

By the 1930's cooler heads prevailed, and the antitobacco people were saying:

Fifty per cent of our insanity is inherited from parents who were users of tobacco; sometimes the victim is a smoker himself, which hastens it on. Thirty-three per cent of insanity cases are caused direct from cigarette smoking and the use of tobacco . . .*

And in 1931:

Judge Gimmill, of the Court of Domestic Relations of Chicago, declared that, without exception, every boy appearing before him that had lost the faculty of blushing was a cigarette fiend. The poison in cigarettes has the same effect upon girls; it perverts the morals and deadens the sense of shame and refinement.
The bathing beaches have become resorts for women smokers, where they go to show off with a cigarette in their mouths. The bathing apparel in the last ten years has been reduced from knee skirts to a thin tight-fitting veil that

---

*From Eaglin, J.: The CC cough-fin brand cigarettes, Cincinnati, 1931, Raisbeck & Co., Printers, p. 97.

scarcely covers two-thirds of their hips. Many of the girl bathers never put their feet in the water, but sit on the shore, show their legs and smoke cigarettes.*

During this period the cigarette industry remained quiet and sales increased. These were the days of "not a cough in a carload" ads. As early as 1939 a major authority on cancer stated: "...the increase in the incidence of pulmonary carcinoma is due largely to the increase in cigarette smoking."[10] There was only a slight disruption in the increasing sales pattern in the early 1950's when scientific reports first linked smoking and lung cancer. In 1951 a long-term study of 30,000 British physicians was started. A report in the British Medical Journal in 1964 summarized the results to date, saying: "...the death rate of cigarette smokers from cancer of the lung has been thirteen times the rate of non-smokers, and that the death rate of heavy cigarette smokers [25 or more cigarettes a day] has been over thirty times the rate of non-smokers..."[11] In that same year, 1964, the whole mess finally hit the fan when an Advisory Committee to the United States Surgeon General declared: "Cigarette smoking is causally related to lung cancer in men; the magnitude of the effects of cigarette smoking far outweighs all other factors."

Regular reports by the Surgeon General since 1967 have detailed and expanded on the relationship between cigarette smoking and disease and premature death in humans. The reports have not been concerned with bathing suits or insanity but have been just as emphatic and more convincing.

... studies from several countries continue to confirm that cigarette smoking is one of the major risk factors contributing to the development of coronary heart disease ... [and] suggest that cigarette smoking is a major risk factor in the development of peripheral vascular disease.
Cigarette smokers have higher death rates from pulmonary emphysema and chronic bronchitis and more frequently have impaired pulmonary function and symptoms of pulmonary disease than nonsmokers.
Cigarette smoking has been clearly identified as the major cause of lung cancer in the United States. For both men and women, the risk of developing lung cancer is directly related to total exposure to cigarette smoke as measured by the number of cigarettes smoked per day, the total lifetime number of cigarettes smoked, the duration of smoking in years, the age at initiation of smoking, the depth of inhalation of tobacco smoke, and the "tar" and nicotine levels in the cigarette smoke.
... recent studies have documented a statistically significant dose-response relationship between the number or amount of cigarettes smoked and late fetal and neonatal mortality ... if a woman gives up smoking by the fourth month of pregnancy, she will have the same risk of incurring a fetal or neonatal loss as a nonsmoker.
... cigarette smoking impairs exercise performance ... involving maximal work capacity. Some of these effects are mediated by reduced oxygen transport and reduced cardiac and pulmonary function.*
The level of carbon monoxide attained in ... rooms filled with tobacco smoke has been shown to equal, and at times to exceed the legal limits for maximum air pollution ... such levels ... may on occasion, depending upon the length of exposure, be sufficient to be harmful to the health of an exposed person. This would be particularly significant for people who are already suffering from chronic bronchopulmonary disease and coronary heart disease.†

Additional comments are needed on the effect of smoking on life expectancy; Table 7-1 makes clear that relationship.[12] Since statistics are usually a little hard to remember, the entire table is approximately summarized in the following verse.

One minute of life for one minute of fun?
Count me in, what harm can be done?
Two hours of life for one pack of the weed?
How can that ever be a dastardly deed?
Forty of them for one morning of me?
That's not a good deal from what I can see.
A day of my life for a carton of such?
You're out of your gourd, I like me too much!

A second comment relates to sex differences. Women haven't been smoking as long or as much as men, but they're doing their best to

*From Eaglin, op. cit., p. 97.

*From U. S. Department of Health, Education and Welfare: The health consequences of smoking, Washington, D. C., 1973, Public Health Service, U. S. Government Printing Office, pp. 23, 35, 67, 135 and 247.
†From U. S. Department of Health, Education and Welfare: The health consequences of smoking, Washington, D. C., 1972, Public Health Service, U. S. Government Printing Office, p. 7.

Table 7-1. Life expectancy (years) at various ages: estimate for United States males*

Age	Never smoked regularly	Cigarette smokers by daily amount			
		1-9	10-19	20-39	40+
25	48.6	44.0	43.1	42.4	40.3
30	43.9	39.3	38.4	37.8	35.8
35	39.2	34.7	33.8	33.2	31.3
40	34.5	30.2	29.3	28.7	26.9
45	30.0	25.9	25.0	24.4	23.0
50	25.6	21.8	21.0	20.5	19.3
55	21.4	17.9	17.4	17.0	16.0
60	17.6	14.5	14.1	13.7	13.2
65	14.1	11.3	11.2	11.0	10.7

*From Hammond, E. C.: World costs of cigarette smoking in disease, disability, and death, World Conference on Smoking and Health, New York, September 11, 1967.

be equal. In 1970, 43% of the adult male population, but only 31% of adult females, were cigarette smokers. Since about 1960 the percentage of teenage males who smoke cigarettes has been decreasing while the percentage of teenage females using cigarettes has regularly increased since 1955. The efforts of women are being rewarded, and since 1960 the increase in lung cancer and heart disease among women smokers has been greater than that in male users![12a]

In 1965 Congress spoke softly and required cigarette packs to be labeled: "Caution: cigarette smoking may be hazardous to your health." In 1970 Congress finally used the big stick and beginning November 1, 1970, required that cigarette packs be labeled: "Warning: the surgeon general has determined that cigarette smoking is dangerous to your health." As of January, 1972, *all* cigarette advertising had to contain this same health warning, as well as the average nicotine and tar content of a cigarette. In mid-1973 the Civil Aeronautics Board required all airlines to provide a no-smoking area for each class of service on every flight. Later that year the Chairman of the Federal Consumer Product Safety Commission said that ". . . cigarettes would rank at or near the top of our consumer product hazard index. . . ." He had earlier suggested that the Commission might set maximum levels for tar and nicotine content of cigarettes and in February, 1974, the Commission began studying a proposal to ban cigarettes with tar levels of 22 milligrams or greater.

In an attempt to decrease the glamour around cigarette use and the appeal to youth, Congress prohibited radio and television cigarette ads beginning January 2, 1971. By 1973 similar bans existed in twenty foreign countries, including Russia! Following the ban on TV and radio ads, cigarette advertising quadrupled in newspapers and doubled in magazines for 1971 compared to 1970.

Perhaps King James was half right, but there were misgivings by some people. A majority of the witnesses testifying at the congressional hearings on the cigarette-labeling bill disagreed with the report of the Surgeon General. None of these dissenting individuals, however, represented the views of any medical or health organization. Concern was expressed over the fact that no one had ever induced lung cancer (similar to the human type of lung cancer) through smoking in any experimental animal. The feeling of those medical authorities who thought the Surgeon General's statements too strong was summarized in 1969 by witnesses at a Congressional Committee hearing: "the evidence incriminating cigarettes as a cause of disease is based on statistical association. The purported pathologic and experimental corroboration is tenuous and contradictory." And again: ". . . on the basis of the evidence available today, no one knows the cause of cancer of the lungs."[13]

The last statement is certainly true! This in no way negates the data in Table 7-1, and it is interesting that the tobacco industry does not deny these facts, only the conclusions. They suggest that smokers are in some way a different breed than nonsmokers and that this is the basic difference between those who develop lung cancer and heart disease and those who don't. There is no question that smokers and nonsmokers do differ on a number of factors, but the final convincing bit of information implicating cigarette smoke as a causative factor in lung cancer and other pathological changes in the respiratory system was the study of the smoking beagles. The charges and counter-charges initiated by this study between the American Cancer Society and The Tobacco Institute are interesting but too involved to relate here. The December, 1970, report of the research sums up the evidence:

> ... the types of histologic changes produced in the lung parenchyma by cigarette smoking were found to be the same in the beagle as in man; in both species there is a dose-response relationship; in both species the degree of damage to the lung parenchyma increases with increasing duration of cigarette smoking ... *findings in this study strongly suggest that smoking cigarettes with an efficient filter will produce less damage to the human lung parenchyma than smoking identical cigarettes without filters.**

The effects of moderate cigarette smoking on the lungs has recently been shown in males and females 15 to 19 years old. Although most of the subjects smoked less than twenty cigarettes daily and had been smoking for only 1 to 5 years: "Cough, phlegm, and short-ness of breath were much more common among smokers than among nonsmokers, with no significant difference between the sexes." Air flow in the lungs was significantly lower in smokers and probably results from partial obstruction of the small airways in the lung.[14]

It is impossible to present here a complete picture of the smoking-health relationships. It is clear that males, and the evidence is also developing for females, who are heavy cigarette smokers are the males (females) who show more lung cancer, more respiratory disease, and more heart disease. When com-

pared to comparable nonsmokers, smokers report more somatic and psychological complaints.[15] That the psychological dis-turbances may lead to, rather than result from, cigarette smoking is suggested by a report showing more rebellion and asocial behavior in those elementary school students (especially males) who later became cigarette smokers than in those who remained nonsmokers. Carrying the study one step farther, it was shown that the adult smokers had more re-bellious attitudes than the nonsmokers.[16] These same people drink more coffee and more alcohol, are more competitive, and show more drive in their everyday life.[17, 18]

Be that as it may, and there obviously are differences between smokers and nonsmokers, one study that began in 1959 started with over 1 million men and women from which about 37,000 pairs of males were selected. The members in a pair were matched for age, race, height, residence, occupation, education, marital status, and alcohol consumption. They differed on one factor: in each matched pair, one smoked cigarettes, one didn't. Briefly, after 3 years over twice as many of the cigarette smokers were dead.[19]

Where do we go from here? What nature has done, man can do better. In late 1973 a British textile company began selling synthetic cigarettes—half tobacco and half cellulose. The United States will not be far behind. When that happens we can only look back with sadness at the passing of an era.

NICOTINE

Nicotine was isolated in 1828 and has been studied irregularly since then. It does not have therapeutic actions, so no drug company has exhaustively looked at its effects, but since it has proved to be a valuable pharma-cological tool for studying synaptic functions as well as being the active ingredient in to-

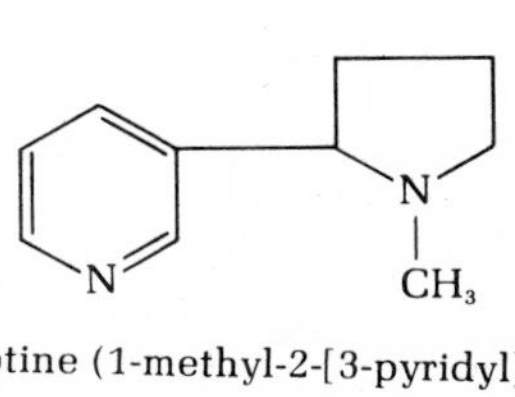

*From Hammond, E. C., and others: Effects of cigarette smoking on dogs, Archives of Environ-mental Health **21:**752, 1970.

Fig. 7-1. Nicotine (1-methyl-2-[3-pyridyl]pyrrolidine).

bacco, there is some relevant information. The structure of nicotine is shown in Fig. 7-1, and it should be noted that there are both d and l forms, but they are equipotent.

Nicotine is a naturally occurring, liquid alkaloid that is colorless and volatile. On oxidation it turns brown and smells much like burning tobacco. Tolerance develops to its effects, along with the dependency that led Mark Twain to remark how easy it was to stop smoking — he'd done it many times!

Acting with almost as much speed as cyanide, nicotine is well established as one of the most toxic drugs known. In man, 60 milligrams is a lethal dose, and death follows intake within a few minutes. A cigar contains enough nicotine for two lethal doses (who needs to take a second one?), but not all of the nicotine is delivered to the smoker or absorbed in a short enough period of time to kill a person.

Nicotine and tar levels in cigarettes usually vary together, with the amount of tar being about ten times greater than that of nicotine. These levels have regularly decreased. In 1954 most cigarettes made in the United States had a tar level between 35 and 53 milligrams, while in 1972 most were between 14 and 29 milligrams. The typical filter cigarette now contains between 1 and 2 milligrams of nicotine. Inhalation is a very effective drug delivery system, with 90% of inhaled nicotine being absorbed. The physiological effects of smoking one cigarette have been mimicked by injecting about 1 milligram of nicotine intravenously.

Nicotine is primarily deactivated in the liver, with between 80% and 90% being modified prior to excretion via the kidneys. This final step in eliminating the deactivated nicotine from the body may be somewhat slowed by nicotine itself, since it acts on the hypothalamus to cause a release of the hormone that acts to reduce the loss of body fluids.

Physiological effects

Outside the central nervous system, nicotine has been well studied, and it has very clear effects on most cholinergic synapses. Nicotine mimics acetylcholine by acting at the cholinergic receptor site and stimulating the dendrite. Nicotine is not rapidly deactivated, and the continued action prevents incoming impulses from having an effect, thereby blocking transmission of information at the synapse. Thus nicotine first stimulates and then blocks the synapse. This blockage of cholinergic synapses is responsible for some of its effects, but others seem to be the result of a second action.

Nicotine also causes a release of adrenaline from the adrenal glands as well as from other sympathetic sites and thus has in part a sympathomimetic action. An additional action that should be identified is that it stimulates and then blocks some sensory receptors such as the chemical receptors found in some large arteries and the thermal and pain receptors found in the skin and tongue.

In acute poisoning, nicotine causes tremors that develop into convulsions, terminated frequently by death. The cause of death is suffocation resulting from paralysis of the muscles used in respiration. This paralysis stems from the blocking effect of nicotine on the cholinergic system that normally activates the muscles. With lower doses there is actually an increase in respiration rate because the nicotine stimulates oxygen-need receptors in the carotid artery. At these lower doses of 6 to 8 milligrams there is also a considerable effect on the cardiovascular system as a result of the release of adrenaline. Such release leads to an increase in coronary blood flow along with vasoconstriction in the skin and increased heart rate and blood pressure.

Within the central nervous system, nicotine seems to act at the level of the cortex to increase somewhat the frequency of the electrical activity, that is, to shift the EEG toward an arousal pattern. In animal studies this alerting pattern following nicotine administration could be increased further by stimulation of the reticular formation so that if the observed cortical arousal is a real effect, it is only a partial basis for the behavioral effect.

Nicotine effects when delivered via smoking

In the smoking individual there are many effects of nicotine that are easily discernible.

The heat releases the nicotine from the tobacco into the smoke. Inhaling while smoking one cigarette has been shown to inhibit hunger contractions of the stomach for up to 1 hour. That finding, along with a very slight increase in blood sugar level and a deadening of the taste buds, may be the basis for a decrease in hunger following smoking.

In line with the last possibility, it has long been an old wives' tale that when a person stops smoking he begins to nibble food and thus gains weight. Some reports suggest that this is not the only reason and that the weight gain is also the result of a lower metabolic rate in the nonsmoking individual. One report showed that when over-a-pack-a-day smokers stopped smoking, there was a three beat per minute decrease in heart rate and a 10% decrease in oxygen consumption. Slowing of the heart rate decreases, to some extent, the energy needs of the body. It seems more probable that the decrease in oxygen consumption resulted from a general decrease in the rate at which food is utilized for energy, so that with the same food intake more will be shifted into fat storage depots.[20]

In a regular smoker, smoking results in a constriction of the blood vessels in the skin along with a decrease in skin temperature and an increase in blood pressure. The blood supply to the skeletal muscles does not change with smoking, but a routine finding in regular smokers is a higher than normal amount of carboxyhemoglobin (up to 10% of all hemoglobin) in the blood. All smoke contains carbon monoxide, with cigarette smoke being about 1% carbon monoxide, pipe smoke 2%, and cigar smoke 6%. The carbon monoxide combines with the hemoglobin in the blood so that it can no longer carry oxygen. It is this effect of smoking, a decrease in oxygen-carrying ability of the blood, that probably explains the "shortness" of breath smokers experience when they have to exert themselves.

Although it has not yet been proved, it may be that the decrease in oxygen carrying ability of the blood is related to the many results showing that pregnant women who smoke greatly endanger their unborn child.

Smoking while pregnant results, on the average, in lighter weight babies, a 200% to 300% increase in number of premature babies, and twice as many aborted and stillborn babies.[21] Some work suggests that 20% of the babies who died prior to or soon after delivery would have lived had the mother not smoked during pregnancy.[22, 23]

It should be noted that intravenous injections and oral administration of nicotine will decrease smoking behavior. However, no one has yet done an adequate study showing a relationship between the amount smoked and the nicotine level of the cigarettes used.[24, 25]

Behavioral effects

The behavioral effects of nicotine will be mentioned only briefly, since there are few studies relating nicotine intake to performance in humans. One electrophysiological study suggests that smoking increases arousal and possibly "selectively enhances the perception of weak stimuli."[25a] These results are at least compatible with research reporting that subjects could maintain their efficiency in a visual reaction time experiment when allowed to smoke, but not if they were prohibited from smoking.[25b]

In rats and mice, low levels of nicotine increase motor activity and performance. At some dose levels, in some tasks, with some strains, there is a facilitation of learning. The data are as yet unclear and the work is mentioned only because it may develop that nicotine can be shown to be effective under some conditions in improving human learning ability.

POSSIBLE BASIS FOR THE USE OF TOBACCO

There are many psychological theories suggesting reasons for the cigarette habit. The most common suggestion is that smoking represents a need for oral stimulation and points to some findings comparing smokers and nonsmokers. Many studies indicate that the smokers have additional oral habits such as greater alcohol and coffee intake and in their early life showed more thumbsucking. Congruent with this idea is the finding that the longer a smoker was breast-fed the less he smoked and the easier it was for him to stop smoking![26]

Some physiological and behavioral studies suggest that a physiological basis for smoking may be a more parsimonious explanation. Most people smoke in a fairly consistent way, averaging one to two puffs per minute, with each puff lasting about 2 seconds with a volume of 25 milliliters. This rate delivers to the individual about 1 to 2 micrograms per kilogram of nicotine with each puff. There must be something optimal or unique about this dose, since smokers could increase the dose by increasing the volume of smoke with each puff or by puffing more often.

A study using cats suggested that this dose rate is optimal in causing a release of acetylcholine from the cortex and an increase in EEG activation. When cats were given 2 micrograms per kilogram of nicotine intravenously every 30 seconds, 70% of the animals showed EEG activation, more than with other tested doses or delivery times. The similarity of this nicotine dose and administration interval to the human self-selected dose and interval was intentional. Thus, it may be that one of the rewards a smoker receives, and which keeps him smoking, is cortical arousal and an alerting of functions.[27, 28] Some studies with humans point in this direction, but gross EEG's do not permit clear separation of the cortical arousal resulting from the pharmacologic effect of nicotine and the arousal that is a result of the smoking behavior.

Other work[29] points in another direction as an explanation for smoking behavior. Heavy smokers compared to nonsmokers show a higher level of cortical activation even in the absence of smoking. On the basis of the frequent finding that nicotine causes an initial stimulation and then a transient depression of synaptic activity, it has been suggested that smokers may be inducing brief periods of tranquilization (that is, a decrease in cortical arousal). This would agree with reports that cigarette smoking increases during periods of stress and tension.

CONCLUDING COMMENT

Nicotine, like most interesting drugs, has multiple effects on the body. Some individuals may use the drug for one effect while others use it for quite a different one. From its rapid spread through western culture it is obvious that nicotine is having some effect that many people want. It also seems clear that cigarette smoking causes serious diseases.

Until recently, when life expectancy increased to its present point, nicotine could be seen only as a very potent drug that either stimulated or calmed an individual when used in moderation. There is no question that the use of nicotine in its present drug delivery system—cigarettes—is a major health problem. It is probable, though, that rather than give up nicotine, a safer method of administration will be developed.

PRECEDING QUOTES

1. Brooks, J. E.: The mighty leaf, Boston, 1952, Little, Brown and Co., pp. 38-39.
2. Quoted in Brooks, J. E.: The mighty leaf, Boston, 1952, Little, Brown and Co., p. 259.
3. The cigarette controversy/eight questions and answers, Washington, D. C., 1970, The Tobacco Institute, p. 10.
4. Smoking and health now, a report of the Royal College of Physicians, London, 1971, Pitman Medical and Scientific Publishing Company Ltd., p. 9.
5. Cited in Diehl, H. S.: Tobacco and your health: the smoking controversy, New York, 1969, McGraw-Hill Book Co., p. 1.
6. Fletcher, C. M., and Horn, D.: Smoking and health, WHO Chronicle 24(8):345-370, 1970.

REFERENCES

1. Stewart, G. G.: A history of the medicinal use of tobacco, 1492-1860, Medical History 11:232, 1967.
2. Ibid., p. 233.
3. Ibid., p. 237.
4. Ibid., p. 238.
5. Ibid., p. 238.
6. Corti, Count: A history of smoking, London, 1931, George G. Harrap & Co., Ltd., pp. 113-114.
7. Heimann, R. K.: Tobacco and Americans, New York, 1960, McGraw-Hill Book Co., p. 73.
8. Ibid., p. 226.
9. Ibid., p. 250.
10. Ochsner, A.: Comment at the International Cancer Congress of 1939, cited in news release of the American Cancer Society, December, 1970.
11. Doll, R., and Hill, A. B.: Mortality in relation to smoking: ten years' observations of British doctors, British Medical Journal 1:1460, 1964.
12. Hammond, E. C.: World costs of cigarette smoking in disease, disability, and death,

World Conference on Smoking and Health, New York, September 11, 1967; Summary of proceedings, American Cancer Society, New York; Hammond, E. C.: Life expectancy of American men in relation to their smoking habits, Journal of the National Cancer Institute **43**:951-961, 1969.

12a. Spain, D. M., Siegel, H., and Bradess, V. A.: Women smokers and sudden death, Journal of the American Medical Association **224**(7):1005-1007, 1973.

13. Committee on Interstate and Foreign Commerce, House of Representatives: Cigarette labeling and advertising—1969, Washington, D. C., 1969, U. S. Government Printing Office, pp. 1214 and 1256.

14. Seely, J. E., Zuskin, E., and Bouhuys, A.: Cigarette smoking: objective evidence for lung damage in teenagers, Science **172**:741-743, 1971.

15. Matarazzo, J. D., and Saslow, G.: Psychological and related characteristics of smokers and nonsmokers, Psychological Bulletin **57**(6):493-513, 1960.

16. Stewart, L., and Livson, N.: Smoking and rebelliousness: a longitudinal study from childhood to maturity, Journal of Consulting Psychology **30**(3):225-229, 1966.

17. Lawton, M. P., and Phillips, R. W.: The relationship between excessive cigarette smoking and psychological tension, American Journal of the Medical Sciences **232**:397-402, 1956.

18. Jenkins, C. D., Rosenman, R. H., and Zyzanski, S. J.: Cigarette smoking: its relationship to coronary heart disease and related risk factors in the Western Collaborative Group Study, Circulation **38**(6):1140-1155, 1968.

19. Hammond, E. C.: Smoking in relation to mortality and morbidity, Journal of the National Cancer Institute **32**(5):1161-1187, 1964.

20. Glauser, S. C., and others: Metabolic changes associated with the cessation of cigarette smoking, Archives of Environmental Health **20**:377-381, 1970.

21. The health consequences of smoking, Public Health Service Publication No. 1696, Washington, D. C., 1967, U. S. Government Printing Office.

22. Russell, C. S., Taylor, R., and Law, C. E.: Smoking in pregnancy, maternal blood pressure, pregnancy outcome, baby weight and growth, and other related factors, British Journal of Preventive Social Medicine **22**:119, 1968.

23. Mulcahy, R., and Knaggs, J. F.: Effect of age, parity, and cigarette smoking on outcome of pregnancy, American Journal of Obstetrics and Gynecology **101**:844, 1968.

24. Jarvik, M. E., Glick, S. D., and Nakamura, R. K.: Inhibition of cigarette smoking by orally administered nicotine, Clinical Pharmacology and Therapeutics **11**(4):574-576, 1970.

25. Glick, S. D., Jarvik, M. E., and Nakamura, R. K.: Inhibition by drugs of smoking behaviour in monkeys, Nature **227**:969-971, 1970.

25a. Hall, R. A., Rappaport, M., Hopkins, H. K., and Griffin, R.: Tobacco and evoked potential, Science **180**:212-214, 1973.

25b. Frankenhaeuser, M., Myrsten, A., Post, B., and Johansson, G.: Behavioral and physiological effects of cigarette smoking in a monotonous situation, Psychopharmacologia (Berl.) **22**:1-7, 1971.

26. McArthur, C., Waldron, E., and Dickinson, J.: The psychology of smoking, Journal of Abnormal Social Psychology **56**(2):267-275, 1958.

27. Armitage, A. K., Hall, G. H., and Morrison, C. F.: Pharmacological basis for the tobacco smoking habit, Nature **217**:331-334, 1968.

28. Hall, G. H.: Effects of nicotine and tobacco smoke on the electrical activity of the cerebral cortex and olfactory bulb, British Journal of Pharmacology **38**:271-286, 1970.

29. Brown, B. B.: Some characteristic EEG differences between heavy smoker and non-smoker subjects, Neuropsychologia **6**:381-388, 1968.

8 Caffeine

Certainly our Countrymens pallates are become as *Fanatical* as their Brains; how else is't possible they should *Apostatize* from the good old primitive way of Ale-drinking, to run a *Whoreing* after such variety of distructive *Foreign* Liquors, to trifle away their *time*, scald their *Chops*, and spend their *Money*, all for a little *base, black, thick, nasty bitter stinking, nauseous* Puddle water: Yet (as all Witches have their Charms) so this ugly *Turkish* Enchantress by certain *Invisible Wyres* attracts both Rich & Poor . . .

> *The Women's Petition Against Coffee, 1674*

But why must innocent COFFEE be the object of your Spleen? That harmeless and healing Liquor, which Indulgent Providence first sent amongst us, at a time when Brimmers of Rebellion, and Fanatick Zeal had intoxicated the Nation, and we wanted to drink at once to make us Sober and Merry: Tis not this incomparable fettle Brain than shortens Natures standard, or makes us less Active in the Sports of Venus, and we wonder you should take these Exceptions . . .

> *The Men's Answer To The Women's Petition Against Coffee, 1674*

Tea and coffee arouse the dull, calm the excitable, prevent headaches, and fit the brain for work. They preserve the teeth, keep them in their place, strengthen the vocal chords, and prevent sore throat. To stigmatize these invaluable articles of diet as "nerve stimulants" is an erroneous expression, for they undoubtedly have a right to rank as nerve nutrients.

> *Dr. Jonathan Hutchinson, 1911*

COFFEE

The absolute coercion which is imposed on the Americans of the United States by the Prohibition Act with respect to alcohol has necessarily had the result of greatly increasing the use of other excitants and also narcotics. ...The consumption of coffee has also developed in an undreamt-of manner. In 1919 929.2 million pounds were consumed and in 1920 as many as 1,360 million pounds. The consumption therefore increased from 9 to 12.9 pounds per head per year, and is approaching the threshold of abuse.*

The repeal of prohibition must have pushed Americans over the threshold because in 1935 per capita consumption of coffee reached 13.7 pounds, and by 1946 it was at an all-time high of over 20 pounds per person. Although it might be reassuring to Dr. Lewin, the coffee industry is not at all pleased with the fact that consumption in 1972 was at 13.8 pounds per person and has been declining until recently.

That decline seems to be occurring even though there have been no pamphlets such as one appearing in England more than two centuries ago by a Woman's Liberation group: "The Women's Petition Against Coffee, representing to public consideration the grand inconveniences accruing to their sex from the excessive use of the drying and enfeebling Liquor." It was the men who used coffee excessively, and the petition claimed it made them as "unfruitful as those *Desarts* whence that unhappy *Berry* is said to be brought." Perhaps women had a right to complain! No fear, the evidence gradually accumulated that there was no truth to the idea that coffee diminishes sexual excitability and results in sterility.

The origin of coffee falls midway between the unknown beginnings of alcohol and the well-authenticated history of tobacco. There are many legends from which to choose, but the best is that of Kaldi, the shepherd in Arabia, who couldn't understand why his goats were bouncing around the hillside like a bunch of kids. He followed them up the mountain one day and ate some of the red berries the goats were munching on. "The results

*From Lewin, L.: Phantastica narcotic and stimulating drugs, New York, 1931, E. P. Dutton & Co., Inc., p. 253.

were amazing. Kaldi became a happy goatherd. Whenever his goats danced he danced and whirled and leaped and rolled about on the ground." Kaldi took the first coffee trip! A holy man took in the scene and "that night he danced with Kaldi and the goats." A veritable orgy. The legend has it that Mohammed then told the holy man how to boil the berries in water and have the brothers in the monastery drink the liquid to keep awake so they could continue their prayers.[1]

Coffee drinking in Arabia became very popular, and the drink was called Qahwah, which also was the word for wine. About 900 A.D. the use of coffee is mentioned in an Arabian medical book as good for almost everything, including curing measles and reducing lust. The use of coffee spread throughout the Islamic world, and in Mecca people spent so much time in the coffeehouses that the use of coffee was outlawed and supplies of the coffee bean were burned. Speakeasies developed and wiser heads prevailed, so the prohibition was withdrawn.

As with most new drugs, coffee entered Europe in the doctor's black bag as a medicine. It didn't stay there long. Around the middle of the seventeenth century coffeehouses existed in both England (1650) and France (1671) and a new era appeared. Coffeehouses were all things to all people—a place to relax, a place to learn the news of the day, a place to seal bargains, a place to plot. In England, Charles II was so disturbed by the coffeehouses acting as "hot-beds of seditious talk and slanderous attacks upon persons in high stations" that they were outlawed. Eleven days, that's how long it was before the ruling was withdrawn, and the coffeehouses developed into the "penny universities" of the early eighteenth century. A penny a cup and you could listen to and learn from some of the great literary and political figures of the times. Lloyds of London, the insurance house, started in Edward Lloyd's coffeehouse around 1700.

The French were slower to embrace the hearty cup. Cheap wine made the need for another social drink less essential in France than in England. French coffeehouses did make one major contribution to western culture, the cancan! This must have almost emptied the cafes, but French ingenuity came through. One cafe owner was able to convince his cancan girls to perform without bloomers! Coffee consumption increased in spite of the competition, and in 1972 France consumed over 11 pounds of coffee per person.

In the English colonies across the Atlantic, coffee drinking increased, but tea was the colonists' drink. Cheaper, and more available than coffee, tea had everything—including, beginning in 1765, a tax on its importation! The British act, taxing the colonists' tea helped fan the fire that lit the musket that fired the shot heard round the world! That story is better told in connection with tea, but the final outcome was that to be a tea drinker was to be a Tory.

Coffee became the new nation's national drink. With increasing demand for coffee worldwide, the Dutch had spread coffee cultivation to the East Indies in 1696. Prior to the rise of Brazil as the giant, most American coffee came from Java, and this term rapidly became a synonym for coffee (actually the island was Sumatra).

Today 65% of America's coffee comes from the Western Hemisphere, with Brazil supplying about 30%. This coffee is the *Arabica* species, which has a caffeine content ranging from 0.5% to 1.5% and averaging 1.0%. The African species, *Robusta*, has a slightly higher caffeine level of about 2%.

Although the practice of roasting coffee is over 600 years old, the first commercial roasting was done in 1790 in New York City. Prior to that time each home or business roasted its own green coffee beans with mixed results. Roasting is an important part of preparing coffee for use, since heating the bean to about 400° F. and then rapidly cooling it with water develops the characteristic flavor and aroma of the beverage. About 85% of the caffeine is dissolved by brewing and ends up in the cup.

It wasn't always as easy to "make a pot of coffee" as it is today, and preparation has come a long way from mixing ground coffee in water. Although the percolator was invented in 1827, it was not widely sold in the United States until about 1876. The vacuum method was originally developed in 1840 but took its present form in 1900, 3 years before expresso coffee appeared in Italy. The real convenience in coffee making began in 1860 when ground coffee was first packaged and sold in paper bags. The vacuum pack appeared in 1900 and helped preserve freshness from the roaster to the consumer. Although instant coffee was developed before 1900, its widespread use began in the 1950's, and in 1972 it accounted for 28% of all coffee sold in the United States. (In Great Britain 85% of the coffee consumed is instant coffee.)

Coffee is America's national nonalcoholic drink. Americans spent over $1.4 billion in 1972 for 2.8 billion pounds of coffee made from 9,800 billion coffee beans to be able to make over 150 billion cups of coffee. Sixty-four percent of Americans over age 10 drink coffee daily, while only 51% drink milk, 47% soft drinks, and 27% tea as of winter 1973. In 1972 on a total population basis (all ages) Americans consumed about 36 gallons of coffee, 7 gallons of tea, and 30 gallons of soft drinks.

TEA

Perhaps the major differences between tea and coffee are summed up in the legends surrounding their origins. The wild shepherd of Arabia suggests that coffee is a boistrous, everyday drink. Tea is a very different story. According to one legend, Daruma, the founder of Zen-Buddhism, fell asleep one day while meditating. Resolving that it would never happen again he cut off both eyelids. From the spot where his eyelids touched the earth grew a new plant. From its leaves a brew could be made that would keep a person awake.

The first report of tea that seems reliable is in a Chinese manuscript around 350 A.D. Its use must have spread slowly since it was seen primarily as a medicinal plant. The nonmedical use of tea is suggested by a 780 A.D. book on the cultivation of tea, but the real proof that it was in wide use in China is the fact that a tax was levied on it in the same year. Before this time the cultivation and use of tea had spread to Japan through Buddhist monks.

Europe had to wait eight centuries to savor

the herb that was "...good for tumors or abscesses that come from the head, or for ailments of the bladder... it quenches thirst. It lessens the desire for sleep. It gladdens and cheers the heart." The first European record of tea in 1559 says: "One or two cups of this decoction taken on an empty stomach removes fever, headache, stomach-ache, pain in the side or in the joints...." It was 50 years later, in 1610, that the Dutch delivered the first tea to the continent of Europe.

In 1600 an event occurred that had tremendous impact on the history of the world and on present patterns of drug use. In that year the British East India Company was formed, and Queen Elizabeth gave the company a virtual monopoly on everything from the east coast of Africa across the Indian and Pacific oceans to the west coast of South America! This was a period in which the primary imports from the Far East were spices. The company prospered, but a major conflict developed between the Dutch and English trade interests over who belonged where in the East. A resolution was reached in 1623 that "gave" the Dutch East India Company the islands (the Dutch East Indies) while the English East India Company had to be content with India and other countries on the continent!

The British East India Company concentrated on importing spices, and the first tea was brought to England by the Dutch. As the market for tea increased, the English East India Company expanded its imports of tea from China. Profit from the China tea trade colonized India, brought about the Opium Wars between China and Britain, and made England switch from coffee to tea. In the last half of the eighteenth century the East India Company carried out a "Drink Tea" campaign unlike anything ever seen to that time. Advertising, low cost on tea, and high taxes on alcohol made the British tea drinkers.

Coffee had arrived first, so most tea and chocolate were sold in coffeehouses rather than in tea- or chocolatehouses. Even as tea's use as a popular social drink expanded in Europe, there were some prophets of doom. A 1635 publication by a physician claimed, at the very least, that using tea would speed the death of those over 40 years old, but increasing use was not slowed. By 1657 tea was being sold to the public in England. This was no more than 10 years after the English had developed the present word for it—tea. Although spelled "tea," it was pronounced "tāy" until the nineteenth century. Prior to this period the Chinese name "ch'a" had been used, Anglicized to either "chia" or "chaw."

With the patrons of taverns off at coffeehouses living it up with tea, coffee, and chocolate, tax revenues from alcoholic beverages declined. To offset this loss, coffeehouses were licensed, and a tax of 8¢ was levied on each gallon of tea and chocolate sold. To keep the profits resulting from the expanding tea trade at home, Britain banned Dutch imports of tea in 1669, thereby giving the English East India Company a monopoly.

Almost 100 years later it was the same profit motive that led to the American Revolution. Because it had given the East India Company a monopoly on importing tea to England and then to the American colonies, the British government imposed high duties on tea when it was taken from warehouses and offered for sale. But, as frequently happens, when taxes went up, consumption did not go down but smuggling increased. It developed in Britain to the point where more smuggled tea than legal tea was being consumed. The American colonies were becoming big tea drinkers and helping the King and the East India Company stay solvent. The Stamp Act of 1765 and the Trade and Revenue Act of 1767 (Townshend Act) imposed many import taxes on the colonies. Under political and economic pressures Parliament did repeal almost all of these revenue measures but, as a symbol of its authority, did not eliminate the import tax on tea.

These measures made the colonists very unhappy over paying taxes they hadn't helped formulate and in 1767 resulted in a general boycott on consumption of English tea. Coffee use increased, but the primary increase was in the smuggling of tea. The drop in legal tea sales filled the tea warehouses of the East India Company and put the company in financial trouble. In 1773, to save the company, Parliament gave the East India Company the right to sell tea to the American colonists without paying the tea taxes. The company was also allowed to sell the tea through its own agents and thus eliminate the profits of the merchants in the colonies.

Several boatloads of this tea, which would be sold cheaper than any before, sailed toward different ports in the colonies. The American merchants would not have made any profit on this tea, and they were the primary ones who rebelled at the cheap tea. Some ships were just turned away from port, but the beginning of the end came with the 342 chests of tea that turned the Boston harbor into a teapot on the night of December 16, 1773.

The revolution in America and the colonists' rejection of tea helped tea sales in Great Britain, since to be a tea drinker was to be loyal to the Crown. Many factors contributed to change the English from coffee to tea drinkers, and whatever the crucial reason the preference for tea persists today. Although the use of coffee increases yearly and that of tea declines, the English are still tea drinkers. In 1972 the per capita consumption in the United Kingdom was 8 1/2 pounds of tea and only 5 pounds of coffee. In that same year Americans averaged about 3/4 pound of tea (enough for 150 cups) and twenty times that amount of coffee.

Although the coffee bean is picked only once or twice a year, tea is plucked every 7 to 10 days during warm weather. Only new leaves are picked so replacements grow fairly rapidly. An experienced plucker may collect enough in a day to make 10 pounds of tea leaves. The leaves are dried, rolled to crush the cells in the leaf, and then kept in a damp area for oxygen to be absorbed. This oxidation turns the green leaves a copper color and makes "black tea" from "green tea." In the United States black tea is used almost exclusively, but some Oolong tea, partially oxidized tea leaves, and green tea are sold.

1904 is the magic year for tea drinkers. Two major innovations occurred. At the fair in St. Louis iced tea was sold for the first time! It now accounts for 70% of all the tea consumed in this country. Fifteen hundred miles to the east in New York City, a tea merchant mailed samples of his tea to many potential purchasers. Back came the orders—send us tea and send it in those same little bags you used to send out the samples! From the hand-sewn silk sample bags used in 1904, there has evolved the modern teabag machinery that cuts the filter paper, weighs the tea, and attaches the tab. Convenience has taken two additional major steps since 1950: instant tea in the 1950's and instant tea mixes (with flavoring and sweetening added) in the 1960's.

CHOCOLATE

Long before Columbus landed on San Salvador, Quetzalcoatl, Aztec god of the air, gave man a gift from Paradise—the chocolate tree. Linnaeus was to remember this legend when he named the cocoa tree *Theobroma*, food of the gods. The Aztecs treated it as such, and the cacao bean was an important part of their economy with the cacao bush being cultivated widely. Montezuma II, the emperor of Mexico in the early sixteenth century, is said to have consumed nothing other than fifty goblets of chocolatl every day. The chocolatl (from the Mayan words "choco" [warm] and "latl" [beverage]) was flavored with vanilla but was far from the chocolate of today. It was a thick liquid about like honey that was sometimes frothy and had to be eaten with a spoon. The major difference, though, was that it was bitter; the Aztecs didn't know about sugar cane and had no sweetening material.

Cortez introduced sugar cane plantations to Mexico in the early 1520's and supported the continued cultivation of the *Theobroma cacao* bush. When he returned to Spain in 1528, Cortez carried with him cakes of processed cocoa. The cakes were eaten as well as being ground up and mixed with water for a drink. For almost a century the Spanish kept the method of preparing chocolate from the cacao bean a secret, but it eventually spread, as did the use of chocolate.

During the seventeenth century chocolate drinking reached all parts of Europe, primarily among the wealthy. Maria Theresa, wife of France's Louis XIV, had a thing about chocolate, and this furthered its use among the wealthy and fashionable. Gradually it became more of a social drink, and by the 1650's chocolatehouses were open in England although, primarily, the sale of chocolate was added to that of coffee and tea in the established coffeehouses.

In the early eighteenth century there were health warnings against the use of chocolate in England, but its use expanded. Its use and importance are well reflected in a 1783 proposal in Congress that the United States raise revenue by taxing chocolate as well as coffee, tea, liquor, sugar, molasses, and pepper.

Although the cultivation of chocolate never became a matter to fight over, it too has spread around the world. The New World plantations were almost destroyed by disease at the beginning of the eighteenth century, but cultivation had already begun in Asia, and today a large part of the crop comes from Africa.

Until 1828 all of the chocolate sold was a relatively undigestible substance obtained by grinding the cacao kernels after processing. The preparation had become more refined over the years, but it still followed the Aztec procedure of letting the pods dry in the sun, then roasting them prior to removing the husks to get to the kernel of the plant. The result of grinding the kernels is a thick liquid called chocolate liquor. In 1828 a Dutch patent was issued for the manufacture of "chocolate powder" by removing about two-thirds of the fat from the chocolate liquor. The chocolate powder was the forerunner of today's breakfast cocoa.

The fat removed, cocoa butter, became important when someone found that if you mixed it with sugar and some of the chocolate powder you could easily form it into slabs or bars. In 1847 the first chocolate bars appeared, but it was not until 1876 that the Swiss made their contribution to the chocolate industry by inventing milk chocolate. By FDA standards, milk chocolate today must contain at least 12% milk solids, but better grades contain almost twice that amount.

The active ingredient in chocolate is theobromine. It has physiological actions that closely parallel those of caffeine, but it is much less potent in its effects on the central nervous system. The average cup of cocoa contains less than 5 milligrams of

caffeine but approximately 100 milligrams of theobromine.

COCA-COLA

...it is clear that the only question arising under section 7 is whether the caffeine in the Coca-Cola is an "added poisonous or other added deleterious ingredient which may render such article injurious to health"...*

In 1886 Dr. J. C. Pemberton of Atlanta, Georgia, formulated a green nerve tonic containing caramel, fruit flavoring, phosphoric acid, caffeine, and a secret mixture called Merchandise No. 5. A friend, F. M. Robinson, suggested the name by which it is still known: Coca-Cola. The unique character of Coca-Cola and its later imitators is a blend of fruit flavors that makes it impossible to identify any of its parts.

An early ad for Coca-Cola suggested its varied uses:

This "INTELLECTUAL BEVERAGE" and TEMPERANCE DRINK contains the valuable TONIC and NERVE STIMULANT properties of the Coca plant and Cola (or Kola) nuts, and makes not only a delicious, exhilarating, refreshing and invigorating Beverage (dispensed from the soda water fountain or in other carbonated beverages), but a valuable Brain Tonic, and a cure for all nervous affections—SICK HEAD-ACHE, NEURALGIA, HYSTERIA, MELANCHOLY, &c.†

Business did not boom, and Asa Candler bought the formula, name, and rights and incorporated Coca-Cola in 1892. Candler changed the advertising for the company and sold Coke only as a beverage. Although the spread of Coca-Cola across the country and around the world is an amazing story, it is not this aspect that is of interest here.

Our story begins with an 1892 letterhead of Candler's that describes Coca-Cola as: "The new and popular fountain drink, containing the tonic properties of the wonderful coca plant and the famous cola nut." In 1903 the company admitted to the presence of a small amount of cocaine, but none was found in a 1906 government analysis.

*Sixth Circuit Court of Appeals, 1914: 215 Federal Reporter 539, June 13, 1914.
†From Huisking, C. L.: Herbs to hormones, Essex, Connecticut, 1968, Pequot Press, Inc., p. 138.

There is little question but that the name Coca-Cola was originally conceived to indicate the nature of two of its ingredients. This suggestion of the use of the coca leaves and the cola (kola) nuts was supported by the use as late as 1916 of a pictorial representation of the leaves and nuts on each bottle. In 1909 the FDA seized a supply of Coca-Cola syrup and made two charges against the company. One was that it was misbranded because it contained "no coca and little if any cola" and secondly that it contained an added poisonous ingredient—caffeine.

Prior to the 1911 trial in Chattanooga, Tennessee, the company paid for some research into the physiological effect of caffeine. When all the information was in, the company won—and the government appealed the decision. In 1916 the Supreme Court of the United States upheld the lower court by rejecting the charge of misbranding, stating that the company has repeatedly said that "certain extracts from the leaves of the coca shrub and the nut kernels of the cola tree were used for the purpose of obtaining a flavor" and that "the ingredients containing these extracts" with the cocaine eliminated is called Merchandise No. 5.

The question of whether caffeine was an "added poisonous ingredient" was not so readily resolved. Caffeine was added, but it was an essential part of the Coca-Cola formula. In that respect it was not added above and beyond the essential ingredients— it was one of them. The Supreme Court said that the lower courts should decide if the caffeine made the drink injurious to health.[2] At that time the company materially reduced the amount of caffeine in its syrup, and the government never felt it had a case worth pursuing beyond that point. At present the Food and Drug Administration requires that a "cola" must contain some caffeine but no more than about 5 milligrams per ounce.

A 1931 report indicated that Merchandise No. 5 contained an extract of three parts coca leaves and one part cola nuts, but to this day it remains the secret special formula that makes Coca-Cola what it is, "the real thing," the Number 1 soft drink in the world with over 110 million 6-ounce servings being consumed each day!

The latest reports suggest that Coca-Cola contains less than 4 milligrams of caffeine per ounce. If a new consumer protection group has its way, all of the cola manufacturers will have to indicate on their labels the amount of caffeine their beverages contain. It will be interesting to see whether this labeling requirement can be extended to coffee, tea, and chocolate, where the caffeine is not added but is part of the natural product. In tea and coffee the caffeine level is also higher than the Food and Drug Administration allows in colas.

CAFFEINE

The clinical literature on psychological and physiological reactions to caffeine and caffeine-containing beverages is extensive and confusing. Perhaps more contradictions can be cited than in the literature on any other pharmacologically active agent.*

The xanthines are the oldest stimulants known to man. Xanthine is a Greek word meaning yellow, which is the color of the residue left if the xanthines are heated with nitric acid until dry. The three xanthines of primary importance are caffeine, theophylline, and theobromine. Theophylline, meaning "divine leaf," is found in the "tiny little tea leaves" of *Thea chinensis*; theobromine, "divine food," is the primary active agent in the fruit of the chocolate tree, *Theobroma cacao*; and caffeine is responsible for the activity in coffee *(Coffea arabica)*, cola *(Cola acuminata)*, and tea. Caffeine levels for these beverages are indicated in Table 8-1.

These three chemicals are methylated xanthines and are closely related alkaloids, as can be seen in Fig. 8-1. Most alkaloids are insoluble in water but these are unique since they are slightly water soluble. The cured coffee bean contains about 1.0% caffeine, dry tea leaf about 5%, and cocoa has very little caffeine but about 1.8% theobromine.

These xanthines have similar effects on the body, with caffeine having the greatest

*From Colton, T., Gosselin, R. E., and Smith, R. P.: The tolerance of coffee drinkers to caffeine, Clinical Pharmacology and Therapeutics 9(1):31-39, 1968.

and theobromine almost no stimulant effect on the central nervous system and the skeletal muscles. Theophylline is the most potent agent on the cardiovascular system. Caffeine, so named because it was isolated from coffee in 1820, has been the most extensively studied and unless otherwise indicated is the drug under discussion here.

In man absorption of caffeine is rapid after oral intake, and peak blood levels are reached 30 to 60 minutes after ingestion. Although maximal central nervous system effects are not reached for about 2 hours, the onset of effects may begin within half an hour after intake. The half-life of caffeine in man is 3 to 5 hours, and no more than 10% is excreted unchanged.

Cross tolerance exists between the methyl-

ated xanthines, and loss of tolerance may take more than 2 months of abstinence. The tolerance, however, is low grade and, by increasing the dose two to four times, an effect can be obtained even in the tolerant individual. There is less tolerance to the central nervous system stimulation effect of caffeine than to most of its other effects. The direct action on the kidneys to increase urine output and the increase of salivary flow do show tolerance.

Dependence on caffeine is real, and one withdrawal symptom that has been well substantiated is the headache, which generally develops in habitual users (five cups or more of coffee per day) after about 18 hours of abstinence. Some reports suggest that nausea and lethargy may precede the actual headache, but the only clear symptom is the headache. It has been produced experimentally by giving caffeine chronically to noncaffeine users and then substituting a placebo, as well as by withholding coffee from habitual users.[3, 4]

Table 8-1. Amount of caffeine in beverages

Beverage	Amount of caffeine (milligrams)	Amount of beverage (ounces)
Regular coffee	90 to 125	5
Instant coffee	60 to 80	5
Decaffeinated coffee	30 to 75 (typical; some are quite low)	5
Tea	30 to 70	5
Cocoa	Less than 5 (about 100 mg theobromine)	5
Coca-Cola	45	12
Pepsi-Cola	30	12
Chocolate bar	22	1-ounce bar

Toxicology

Caffeine is not very toxic, but high doses result in convulsions, while still higher doses cause death from respiratory failure. One death in man has been reported following the intravenous injection of 3.2 grams; the oral dose that would be fatal has been estimated at about 10 grams. The toxic effects of caffeine result from 1 gram. The central stimulation and toxic effects can be blocked by central nervous system depressants.[5]

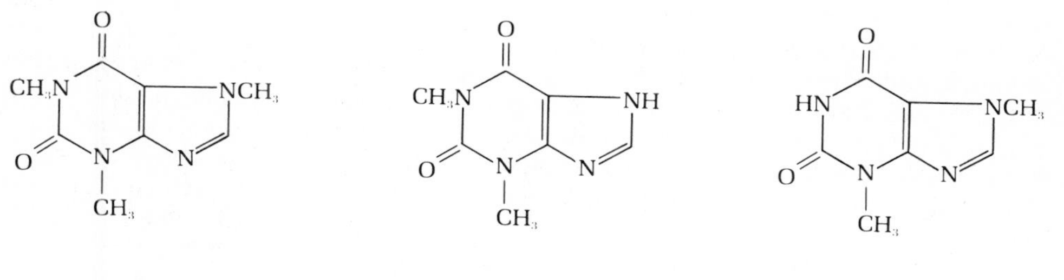

Caffeine
(1, 3, 7-trimethyl-2, 6-dioxopurine)

Theophylline
(1, 3-dimethyl-2, 6-dioxopurine)

Theobromine
(3, 7-dimethyl-2, 6-dioxopurine)

Fig. 8-1. Methylated xanthines.

Physiological effects

The pharmacological effects on the central nervous system are probably the basis for the wide use of caffeine-containing beverages. At a dose level of 150 to 250 milligrams (about two cups of coffee) the cortex is activated and the electroencephalogram (EEG) shows an arousal pattern. Some data suggest that this effect results from a direct action on the cortical neurons. In the absence of tolerance this dose level will increase the time it takes to fall asleep and also cause disturbances in the sleep. There is a good relationship between the mood-elevating effect of caffeine and the extent to which it will keep the individual awake.

In noncaffeine users this 150- to 250-milligram dose level also causes a significant reduction in heart rate (four beats per minute) within 30 minutes. Although this reduction does not occur in habitual users, one report suggests that they have generally higher blood pressure and lower heart rates than nonusers. Habitual users have also been reported to have slightly higher basal metabolic rates than nonusers.

Higher dose levels (about 500 milligrams) are needed to affect the autonomic centers of the brain, and heart rate and respiration may be increased at this dose. The direct effect on the cardiovascular system is in opposition to the effects mediated by the autonomic centers. Caffeine acts directly on the vascular muscles to cause a dilation, while stimulation of the autonomic centers results in a constriction of blood vessels. Usually dilation occurs, but in the brain the blood vessels are constricted, and this constriction may be the basis for caffeine's ability to reduce hypertensive headaches.

There are several reports that caffeine increases the blood level of lipids and glucose. Elevated fat levels in the blood in conjunction with the actions on the cardiovascular system may tie in with reports that heavy coffee (but not tea) users have a higher incidence of angina and myocardial infarction than moderate users or abstainers. It must be mentioned, though, that coffee users seem to have a better chance of surviving a myocardial infarction than do abstainers![6, 6a, 6b]

An interesting sidelight is that caffeine, in the dose range in man of about eight cups of coffee a day, results in an increase in the synthesis of microsomal enzymes in the liver. The stimulation of drug metabolism has thus far only been shown to be true in the rat, but it may be that heavy coffee or tea users will also have increased liver microsomal activity.[7]

Behavioral effects

A nice double-blind study is a good way to summarize the experienced effects of caffeine. In this study abstainers given 150 or 300 milligrams of caffeine reported upset stomachs and jittery and nervous feelings. In the heavy coffee user it was just the opposite; he felt irritable and sleepy when given a placebo in lieu of caffeine. When caffeine was given to heavy users they reported increased alertness and a feeling of contentedness.[8]

Considering the differences in effects experienced by users and nonusers, coupled with the normal variation seen in any drug effects, it is remarkable that any general statements can be made about caffeine effects on performance. Speaking conservatively, a therapeutic dose of caffeine, 200 to 300 milligrams, will partially offset fatigue-induced decrement in the performance of motor tasks, and this effect may in part be caused by a direct action of the agent on muscle. Like the amphetamines, but to a much smaller degree, caffeine prolongs the amount of time an individual can perform physically exhausting work. In addition to effects on physical work, caffeine seems to slow the onset of boredom and to increase attention. The cortical stimulation that reduces drowsiness and increases alertness and reactivity may also cause irritability and excitability so that complex behavior may be disrupted.

Many investigators feel that caffeine does little more than restore performance to pre-fatigue or control levels, but there are reports of increases in the ability to produce verbal association to words after a 200- to 300-milligram dose, as well as an increase in the ability of the individual to process sensory information. The best simple summary is that 150 to 300 milligrams of caffeine offsets fatigue-induced performance decrement in both physical and mental tasks, slows the development of boredom, and may, in a rested, interested individual, increase his motor and mental efficiency above control levels.[9]

CONCLUDING COMMENT

If one were to attempt to indicate the drugs that have had the most impact on the world, caffeine and nicotine would certainly be among the top contenders. Caffeine has remained a popular drug, whether in coffee, tea, or cola, because it's easy to adjust the dose level and the few adverse side effects are far removed from the use of the drug. As a mild stimulant it has few peers.

PRECEDING QUOTES

1 and 2. Meyer, H.: Old English coffee houses, Emmaus, Pennsylvania, 1954, The Rodale Press.
3. Ukers, W. H.: All about coffee, New York, 1935, The Tea & Coffee Trade Journal Co., p. 314.

REFERENCES

1. Uribe Compuzano, A.: Brown gold, New York, 1954, Random House, Inc., pp. 4-5.
2. United States v. Forty Barrels, 36 Supreme Court Reporter 573-581, October Term, 1915.
3. Goldstein, A., and Kaizer, S.: Psychotropic effects of caffeine in man. III. A questionnaire survey of coffee drinking and its effects in a group of housewives, Clinical Pharmacology and Therapeutics 10(4):477-488, 1969.
4. Goldstein, A.: Wakefulness caused by caffeine, Naunyn-Schmiedebergs Archivfur Experimentelle Pathologie und Pharmakologie 248:269-278, 1964.
5. Peters, J. M.: Factors affecting caffeine toxicity, The Journal of Clinical Pharmacology 7:131-141, 1967.
6. Paul, O.: Stimulants and coronaries, Postgraduate Medicine 44:196-199, 1968.

6a. Coffee drinking and acute myocardial infarction, Lancet 1:1278-1281, 1972.
6b. Maugh, T. H., II: Coffee and heart disease: Is there a link? Science 181:534-535, 1973.
7. Mitoma, C., and others: Nature of the effect of caffeine on the drug-metabolizing enzymes, Archives of Biochemistry and Biophysics 134:434-441, 1969.
8. Goldstein, A., Kaiser, S., and Warren, R.: Psychotropic effects of caffeine in man. I. Individual differences in sensitivity to caffeine-induced wakefulness, Journal of Pharmacology and Experimental Therapeutics 149(1):156-159, 1965; Psychotropic effects of caffeine in man. II. Alertness, psychomotor coordination, and mood, Journal of Pharmacology and Experimental Therapeutics 150(1):146-151, 1965.
9. Weiss, B., and Laites, V.: Enhancement of human performance by caffeine and the amphetamines, Pharmacological Review 14(1):1-36, 1962.

GENERAL REFERENCES

Annual Coffee Statistics, No. 36, Pan-American Coffee Bureau, New York, 1972.
Chatt, E. M.: Cocoa, New York, 1953, Interscience Publishers, Inc.
Cheney, R. H.: Coffee: a monograph of the economic species of the genus Coffea L, New York, 1925, New York University Press.
Cummings, W. F.: The Nielsen Report to the tea industry, presented to the 25th Annual Meeting of the Tea Association, November 3, 1970.
Thurber, F. B.: Coffee: from plantation to cup, ed. 5, New York, 1884, American Grocer Publishing Association.
Ukers, W.: The romance of tea, New York, 1936, Alfred A. Knopf, Inc.
Wellman, F. L.: Coffee: botany, cultivation, and utilization, New York, 1961, Interscience Publishers, Inc.
World Coffee and Tea, Vol. II, No. 4, August, 1970.

Over-the-counter drugs

... self-medication is an integral part of health care today. People like to medicate themselves ...

> *George Griffenhagen, 1969*
> *American Pharmaceutical Association*

He who has himself for a doctor, has a fool for a physician.

> *Anonymous*

Home medication is usually employed to improve personal hygiene and to relieve those conditions that can be effectively and safely self-diagnosed and treated by a layman.... those that tend to be self-limited in duration or subject to gradual or spontaneous remissions.... Treatment is directed towards providing symptomatic relief rather than cure of disease or substitutive therapy.

> *Chester S. Keefer, 1969*
> *Boston University School of Medicine*

Why does a woman want to keep supplies of safe and reliable home remedies on hand? The reason is a personal one: to make and to keep her family healthy and comfortable.

> *Mrs. William H. Hasebroock, 1965*
> *Federation of Women's Club*

Self-medication is being practiced today with a degree of sophistication that belongs to the Dark Ages.

> *William S. Apple, 1969*
> *American Pharmaceutical Association*

There is no way in which a drug can be made completely safe, and it certainly cannot be made so by law. Through legislation, a drug can be surrounded by safeguards, but it can never be made completely safe.... in certain dosages, any drug can be toxic.

> *Commission on Drug Safety, 1964*

Self-diagnosis of ailments and prescribing of drugs is as old as mankind, but there's been considerable change from the garlic hung around the neck to the $4 billion industry today that manufactures, packages, and sells the proprietary, that is, over-the-counter (OTC), drugs. Only a few of the over 100,000 OTC products that are manufactured by about 2,000 companies can be mentioned and, in fact, only two general classes of these drugs will be considered in any detail at all.

OTC drugs are chemicals considered to be safe for use by the general public when they are taken according to the directions on the package. A Food and Drug Administration brochure states: "People are capable of treating some of their illnesses ... Mature persons are familiar with the signs and symptoms of the common, minor, everyday ailments which can be self-treated successfully."[1]

These everyday ailments are fairly common. It has been estimated that of every 1,000 people 750 will have the symptoms of an illness each month. Of these about 250 will go to a physician, and the other 500 frequently find OTC drugs are the answer. These estimates may seem high, but for comparison it can be noted that the National Center for Health Statistics reports that one out of every five individuals under 17 has a chronic medical condition. Further, adults average two and children four colds each year.

Since OTC drugs are self-selected, it is imperative that there be adequate information supplied for the use of each compound. Interestingly, very little drug information is now required on the container of a prescription drug. An OTC package, though, must list at least the common or generic names and quantities of its active ingredients, as well as the amount of alcohol, if any, it contains. OTC drug labels also include instructions for using the drug, simple, direct warnings, and limitations on its use, such as: "Discontinue use if pain persists and consult a physician."

These drugs are a consumer product and as such must be sold in a competitive marketplace. The cough and cold remedy market is now $500 million a year. Battling for consumers means one thing is sure—advertising will be heavy!

And so it is. Advertising costs are well over $100 million a year for headache remedies (and Americans responded by spending over $500 million for aspirin and combination analgesics). It isn't the amount of advertising that is of major interest here, but the quality. There are two issues: one is misrepresentation; second is the underlying, general orientation of the ads. Neither issue is settled.

In 1961 the FTC wondered if Bufferin, Excedrin, Bayer Aspirin, and Anacin could all *really* be "faster" or "more effective." It is relatively easy to show that even a placebo is "faster" and "more effective," so there was no trouble for each of the *three* manufacturers involved to support their claims for their products. (Faster and more effective than what? Quiet, don't ask!) Unable to really press its case in court, the FTC withdrew.

In the late 1960's and early 1970's advertising was changed and a new spector arose. In the present phase of these OTC commercials, the ads begin with the causes of the headache and imply that the remedy for the headache also removes the tensions and anxieties of the day, not just the result of the tensions.

In 1972 the FTC accused the Bufferin, Excedrin, Bayer Aspirin, and Anacin manufacturers of deceptive advertising and cited an FDA report that nonprescription analgesics were equally effective when the products contain equivalent quantities of analgesics. The FTC also claimed that it was deceptive advertising to suggest that analgesics were effective in reducing stress and tension. It may be years before the courts finally settle the legal issues, but the scientific issues have long been resolved.

This problem of drugs being suggested as panaceas for the problems of living has been repeatedly considered. A particularly clear statement about the possible connection between the expanding illegal use of drugs and television commercials for OTC compounds was made by New York City's Mayor John Lindsay in early 1970:

In a sense, the impulses driving our children to this (drug addiction) are beyond our effective control. How can any institution, for example, compare with the force of television on the mind of a child? We are told that the average family watches television 5 1/2 hours

119

a day. Thus if a city child begins serious watching when he is 2, then by the time he comes into your schools, he has seen some 8,000 hours of TV.

And what has he been taught? He has been taught to relax minor tensions with a pill; to take off weight with a pill; to win status and sophistication with a cigaret; to wake up, slow down, be happy, relieve tension with pills— that is, with drugs.*

Ever alert, the FTC in mid-1970 initiated a study of the possible relationship between OTC advertising and illegal drug use. The FTC action was in part a response to Congressional prodding. The Chairman of the Senate's Consumer Subcommittee stated lyrically:

It is advertising . . . which mounts so graphically the message that pills turn rain to sunshine, gloom to joy, depression to euphoria and solve problems and dispel doubts.†

The National Association of Broadcasters Code Authority, staying one step ahead of governmental regulations, issued guidelines in 1970 governing TV ads for OTC "stimulants, calmatives, or sleeping aids." In September, 1973, additional guidelines became effective that covered all OTC products. Ads for these products must not be attention-getting to the young or imply a casual attitude toward drug use. They must also avoid suggesting either very pleasurable effects or "immediate relief." In addition, no pill taking is to be shown, and it must be made clear that the drugs are only for occasional use.

Before leaving the question of TV commercials, several points are worthy of comment. As of 1974 there are no studies that show a relationship between these commercials and drug abuse. Since one of every eight commercials is for OTC products, it may be that they are too pervasive.[1a] It's interesting that no one has yet raised the issue of whether OTC commercials contribute to misuse of these OTC drugs themselves. The comparison with cigarettes is not direct, but it is worth considering whether cigarettes could have presented themselves as an OTC drug "for calming that jittery feeling before the big date"

*Quoted in Goddard: tax drugs to fight abuse, American Druggist, March 9, 1970, p. 34.
†From Advertising: the darkening drug mood, Time, August 10, 1970, p. 60.

and included on the package warnings about excessive use.

Another issue is that hard-sell ads such as "this brand is best" may well contribute to the symptomatic relief experienced by users of that brand. Many of the symptoms and indications for OTC compounds are the type that should be particularly susceptible to nonspecific (placebo) effects.

Better times may be coming, at least for the consumer. In January, 1972, the FDA announced a program to determine the safety and effectiveness of OTC products. The procedure will follow that established with the National Academy of Science-National Research Council (NAS-NRC) panels that evaluated prescription drugs (see p. 31). The FDA has established twenty-six OTC product categories and assigned each category to a panel of experts. The panels will review the safety and effectiveness of the drugs involved as well as the labeling of products in each category. Finally they will recommend the conditions under which the drugs are safe and effective and the products not mislabeled. Note well that individual OTC products (there may be as many as half a million, no one knows for sure) will not be evaluated by the panels. This poses no major problem since only about 200 active drugs are involved in the thousands of items marketed as OTC products. The FDA will take legal action against specific products that can be judged to be unsafe, ineffective, or mislabeled.

One early study by NAS-NRC reviewed 420 specific OTC products that were representative of the entire OTC market. Only 25% of these products were found to be effective. This panel found, for example, that of all the toothpaste introduced between 1938 and 1962 only stannous fluoride products were considered "effective as an aid in reducing the incidence of dental caries."

One other set of NAS-NRC results will be mentioned since it may eliminate a whole OTC category when implemented: mouthwashes. The NAS-NRC panel found that mouthwashes have "no therapeutic advantage over . . . water." The supportable claims for many mouthwashes are that they are aromatic, cause the mouth to feel clean, and are a refreshing mouth rinse. No longer will young girls cry in commercials because they weren't kissed on their first date.

PRELUDE

There are many ways to group OTC compounds and only two classes of compounds will be discussed in detail. Brief comment is necessary on two groups of misused OTC preparations. Over $200 million was spent in 1967 on vitamins. Vitamins are organic chemicals that act as essential enzymes in the body but cannot be manufactured by the organism. "A vitamin, if a drug at all, is not one in the ordinary sense, although vitamins may have independent pharmacologic reactions, and all may be poisons if given long enough at excessive levels."[2] The sentiments of most authorities about the large OTC sales of vitamins were phrased nicely by a British physician:

> ... the wholesale consumption of vitamin concentrates by healthy people in this fortunate "welfare state" is a waste of money. There is no scientific evidence that in healthy people vitamins prevent infections, stimulate appetite, help to assuage neuritic pains or aid positive health in any way. Indeed the era of vitamin D deficiency ... has been succeeded by one characterized more by hypercalcaemia due to an excessive intake of concentrates of vitamin D superimposed on the consumption of food-stuffs fortified by it.*

Over $200 million a year is also spent for the 700 OTC laxatives. There is no question that laxatives are much overused and if taken regularly for long periods they impair the capability of the body to maintain "regularity"! "Constipation is probably the most commonly encountered complaint of civilized man and preoccupation with bowel function a phenomenon explicable only by reference to Freudian hypotheses."[3] To conclude this section on these drugs, a remark by Sir Derrick Dunlop is appropriate: "It is now more generally realized that moderate constipation constitutes a far smaller menace to health than over-enthusiastic efforts to treat it ... the abuse of laxatives by the public is still common...."†

*From Dunlop, D.: Abuse of drugs by the public and by doctors, British Medical Bulletin 26(3): 236-239, 1970.
†Ibid.

The $50 million-a-year trade in antiacne preparations and the expanding market for drugs to help people contract and lose weight, as well as dozens of other interesting types of compounds, will have to be ignored. The remaining sections of this chapter deal with two groups of agents, internal analgesics and cough and cold remedies. Prior to each of these topics, some comment is necessary about the physiological changes underlying the symptom(s) from which relief is sought.

PAIN, PLACEBO, AND PEOPLE

Pain is such a little word for such a big experience.

There are some reports of individuals who are normal in other respects but who cannot experience pain. Most people, however, have experienced pain of varying intensities. Two classes of drugs are used to reduce pain or the awareness of pain. Anesthetics (meaning "without sensibility") have this effect by reducing awareness or by blocking consciousness completely. The barbiturates and the volatile anesthetics such as ether are the primary examples of this type of agent. Analgesics (meaning "without pain") are compounds that reduce pain without causing insensibility. The narcotics are a group of drugs in this class, but in this chapter only the OTC internal analgesics such as aspirin and phenacetin will be discussed.

One classification divides pain into two types, depending on its place of origin. Visceral pain arises from the nonskeletal portions of the body, such as intestinal cramps; the narcotics are quite effective in reducing pain of this type. Somatic pain, arising from muscle or bone and typified by sprains, headaches, and arthritis, is reduced by the salicylates (aspirin).

Another system of categorizing pain relates the type of neuron that carries the signal we call pain to the kind of pain experienced. Bright, sharp pain is mediated by large, fast neurons and seems to activate the individual, while dull, aching pain, which depresses the person and causes anxiety, is mediated by small, slow neurons. (To differentiate these two, hit your thumb with a hammer. The initial sensation that causes you to verbalize doubts about the hammer's ancestors is bright pain, while the throbbing experience that soon follows is dull pain.) A third pain experience is labeled burning pain. Neurons intermediate in size and speed produce this. Narcotics attenuate the bright pain and the salicylates the dull.

Pain is unlike other sensations in many ways, having mostly to do with the influence of nonspecific factors. The experience of pain is increased with fatigue, anxiety, fear, boredom, and anticipation of more pain. These are clearly nonspecific factors to be remembered throughout the discussion of analgesics. When pain is experimentally induced in a laboratory, it has been found that redheads report pain at lower stimulus intensities than blondes, who in turn are more sensitive than brunettes. When personality tests were used to select introverts and extroverts, introverts were generally found to have lower pain thresholds.[4] It is certain, at least from experiences in combat zones during war, that a high level of arousal and/or intense concentration on a task crucial for survival can completely block the experience of pain. During combat severe wounds would be unknowingly incurred, and only after the attack ended would the soldier be aware of his then very painful wound.

With a symptom as susceptible to nonspecific factors as pain seems to be, a brief comment on the effectiveness of a placebo in reducing pain seems required. Classic studies have been done by Beecher, who has also summarized reports of many investigators on the effectiveness of placebos in the reduction of pain.[5] These were real situations with a variety of clinical causes ranging from postoperative pain to the aches associated with the common cold. About 35% of the patients in these studies had their pain "satisfactorily relieved" by placebos. That is, when individuals in pain were given an inactive substance along with the suggestions that it would reduce the pain, 35% of the cases obtained relief.

This 35% proportion is quite high when it is appreciated that morphine provides satisfactory relief of pain in only about 75% of patients. It was also found that placebos were most effective in reducing the pain in stressful situations while morphine had its smallest effect in these stressful situations. As might be expected from the last statement, placebos are more effective in pathological (that is, real-life) pain than in experimental pain. The internal analgesics mentioned in the next section have been repeatedly shown to be more effective at therapeutic doses than placebos for certain kinds of pain.

INTERNAL ANALGESICS
Aspirin

The most widely used class of internal analgesics is the *salicylates*. The word itself suggests their long heritage, coming from the Latin "salix" meaning willow. Over 2,400 years ago the Greeks used extracts of willow and poplar bark in the treatment of pain, gout, and other illnesses. Aristotle commented on some of the clinical effects of similar preparations, and Galen also made good use of these formulations.

These remedies fell into disrepute, however, when St. Augustine declared that all diseases of Christians were the work of demons and thus a punishment from God. (See other effects of this edict in Chapter 10.) The American Indian, unhampered by this enlightened attitude, used a tea brewed from willow bark to reduce fever. The salicylates were not rediscovered in Europe until about 200 years ago when an Englishman, Edward Stone, combined two bits of the best information then available and put the result to clinical test. The two pieces of data he combined were: listen to old wives, sometimes they're not just jawboning; and plants acquire the characteristics of the place where they grow. The old wives kept saying willow bark is good for pain and whatever else ails you! Stone phrased the second attitude nicely.

> As this tree delights in a moist or wet soil where aches chiefly abound, the general maxim that many natural maladies carry their cures along with them, or that their remedies lie not far from their causes, was so very apposite to this particular case that I could not help applying it. That this might be the intention of Providence had some little weight with me.*

*From Smith, L. H., Jr., Chairman, Medical Staff Conference: The clinical pharmacology of salicylates, California Medicine 110(5):411, 413, 1969.

Stone prepared an extract of the bark and gave the same dose to fifty patients with varying illnesses and found the results to be "uniformly excellent."

In the nineteenth century the active ingredient in these preparations was isolated and identified as salicylic acid. In 1838 salicylic acid was synthesized, but not until 1859 were procedures developed that made bulk production feasible. Salicylic acid and sodium salicylate were then used for many ills, especially arthritis.

In the giant Bayer Laboratories in Germany in the 1890's there worked a chemist named Hoffmann. His father had a severe case of rheumatoid arthritis and only salicylic acid seemed to help. The major difficulty then, as today, was that the drug caused great gastric discomfort. So great was the stomach upset and nausea that Hoffmann's father frequently preferred the pain of the arthritis. Hoffmann undertook the examination of the salicylates to see if he could find one with the same therapeutic effect as salicylic acid, but without the side effects.

In 1898 he synthesized acetylsalicylic acid and tried it on his father, who reported relief from pain without stomach upset. It should be noted that the same compound had been synthesized in 1853 but was apparently never tested clinically. There are conflicting stories about what happened when Hoffmann took the compound to the head of pharmacology[6, 7] but the compound was tested, patented, and released for sale in 1899 as Aspirin. Aspirin was a trademarked name derived from acetyl and spiralic acid (the old name for salicylic acid).

Aspirin was marketed with an advertising campaign to physicians unique for the chemical industry at that time. The drug, sold as a white powder in individual dosage packets, was then available only on prescription. It was immediately popular worldwide, and the United States market became large enough that it was very soon manufactured in this country. In 1915 the 5-grain (300-milligram) white tablet stamped Bayer first appeared and, also for the first time, aspirin became a nonprescription item. The Bayer Company was on its way. It had an effective drug that could be sold to the public and was known by one name—Aspirin. And they had the name trademarked!

Before February, 1917, when the patent on Aspirin was to expire, Bayer started an advertising campaign to make it clear that there was only one Aspirin and its first name was Bayer. Several companies started manufacturing and selling Aspirin as aspirin, and Bayer sued. World War I intervened and the Germany-based American Bayer Company was seized as alien property and sold to an American-based American company. The question of whether aspirin was a brand or a generic name was solved in 1921 by the famous Judge Learned Hand in Solomon-like fashion! Companies other than Bayer could not use the word aspirin in their price lists, but they could use it to describe their product in advertising to the public. What? This distinction is no longer made, aspirin is aspirin—or is it?

Willow bark has come a long way! There are five major manufacturers of aspirin in the United States, and they sell bulk aspirin to many packaging companies. There are over 300 aspirin-containing products on the American market. Each day Americans gobble down about 44 million aspirin tablets! Twenty-one tons of acetylsalicylic acid a day. Unbelievable, but true. It is the most widely used drug in the world next to alcohol, or, perhaps to better phrase it, following alcohol.

Therapeutic use. Aspirin is truly a magnificent drug. It is the drug against which all others in its class must be compared.[7a] It has three primary effects for which it is usually taken. It is an analgesic that effectively blocks somatic pain in the moderate to severe range. Aspirin also has an antipyretic effect and will reduce body temperature caused by fever. Last, but for many purposes most importantly, aspirin is an anti-inflammatory agent. It reduces the inflammation and soreness in an injured area. No other single drug has this span of effects coupled with a relatively low toxicity.

There is a whole family of compounds stemming from the basic chemical structure of salicylic acid. Aspirin is the drug of choice of all these compounds for general use. Whenever necessary, distinction will be made between the actions of aspirin and the other salicylates, but primary emphasis is on aspirin throughout even though the more general term salicylates will be used at times to indicate the characteristics of the family.

Before discussing the three major effects in detail, quick mention should be made of other actions of aspirin when taken at the usual therapeutic dose level of about 600 milligrams (10 grains, two of the regular aspirin tablets). In a way not yet fully understood aspirin increases fluid retention in the body and increases blood volume, which sometimes results in a slight weight gain. Oxygen consumption is increased, and blood sugar levels increase in normal individuals but decrease in diabetic persons. The mechanisms underlying these actions are understood in part and involve an action of aspirin on the mitochondria of cells. The mitochondria are the energy-producing units of cells, and aspirin interferes in some way with their normal functioning.

Even a 3 year old should know by now that "At the first sign of a cold...turn off your TV. Go to bed, drink plenty of liquids, and take aspirin!" The aspirin has two effects that are relevant here; the fever-reducing action will be discussed first.

The antipyretic (fever-reducing) action of aspirin seems to work via a central mechanism. Aspirin does not lower temperature in an individual with normal body temperature. It has this effect only if the person has a fever. The mechanism by which the salicylates decrease body temperature is fairly well understood. They act on the temperature-regulating area of the hypothalamus to increase heat loss through peripheral mechanisms. Heat loss is primarily increased by vasodilation of peripheral blood vessels and by increased perspiration. Heat production is not changed, but heat loss is facilitated so that body temperature may go down.

Research into the mechanism of action underlying aspirin's analgesic effect is moving rapidly. As recently as 1968[8] a review article could state with reference to the salicylates that: "It is generally assumed that they act on the hypothalamus to cause analgesia...(but) ...recent studies point to a peripheral site of action." A year and a half later another paper reported[9]: "...salicylates appear to work chemically in the area of the peripheral neuron." An older article[10] suggests that salicylates had their analgesic action at the periphery, phenacetin (an analgesic to be discussed) at the thalamus, and narcotics at the cortex. It is doubtful (although it would be nice) that such a clear separation of sites of action is true.

At therapeutic doses, 600 to 1,000 milligrams of aspirin does have analgesic actions that are fairly specific. First, and in marked contrast to narcotic analgesics, aspirin does not affect the impact of the anticipation of pain. It seems probable also that aspirin has its primary effect on the ability to withstand continuing pain and not on the threshold at which pain is identified.[11] This no doubt is the basis for much of the self-medication with aspirin, since moderate, protracted pain is more common than pain near the threshold level.

Other work suggests that aspirin is most effective as an analgesic against the middle range of pain. At low pain levels, it is difficult to show the effectiveness of any compound because of the extreme variability of patients' responses. At the level of "unbearable" pain, in experimental situations, aspirin does not increase the amount of time an individual can tolerate the high pain levels.[12]

The salicylates do not block all types of pain. They are especially effective against headache, musculoskeletal aches and pains, less effective for toothache and sore throat, and almost valueless in visceral pain as well as in traumatic (acute) pain. It has been difficult to develop experimental pain conditions that demonstrate the effectiveness of aspirin and other similar agents in the laboratory, but recent work suggests that some breakthroughs may have been made.[11-13]

More aspirin is probably used for its third major therapeutic use than for either of the other two. The anti-inflammatory action of the salicylates is the major basis for its use in rheumatoid arthritis. One report[7] states that 25% of all patients with rheumatoid arthritis use only aspirin, and over 50% use aspirin in addition to other compounds. These patients consume large amounts of aspirin, perhaps 3,000 milligrams (10 tablets) every day.

Even though the effectiveness of the salicylates in the treatment of rheumatoid arthritis has been known since the 1870's, "the basic mechanism of action . . . remains unsolved."[14] Several tentative hypotheses are still viable, one being that aspirin decreases the permeability of the capillaries, thereby preventing the collection of fluid (which causes pressure and thus pain) in the inflamed area. Another line of thought proposes that aspirin strengthens, intracellularly, the sacs containing the enzymes that cause inflammation of tissue when released. Be that as it may, aspirin is a highly effective anti-inflammatory agent, but higher dose levels are needed for this action than for its analgesic effect.

Recent studies[15-17] suggest that the specific mechanism has been identified whereby aspirin reduces fever and inflammation. Aspirin inhibits the synthesis of some forms of prostaglandins, which are hormone-like substances that have only recently been studied. It is known that some of them are potent inducers of fever. More work may result in the development of new compounds that are more effective than aspirin in reducing fever and inflammation.

More research is needed, but the anticoagulant action of aspirin, in low doses, may decrease the possibility of a heart attack.[17a]

The term "therapeutic dose" has been used repeatedly and 600 to 1,000 milligrams suggested as the dose range. Most reports suggest that 300 milligrams is usually more effective than a placebo, while 600 milligrams is clearly even more effective. Many studies indicate that increasing the dose above that level does not increase aspirin's analgesic action. A 1968[18] double-blind study of patients with postoperative pain indicates that 1,200 milligrams of aspirin may provide greater relief than 600 milligrams, but additional work will be needed to substantiate this. This report also confirmed what has long been a clinical fact: that older patients need less aspirin to obtain the same block of pain. Surprisingly this study found that there was no relationship between analgesic effectiveness, dose, and body weight.

Since the action of a drug depends on its concentration at the cellular site of action, much work has been done to see how aspirin gets there, how fast it gets there, and how long it stays. Aspirin is readily absorbed from the stomach but even faster from the intestine. Thus anything that delays movement of the aspirin from the stomach should affect absorption time. The evidence is mixed[18] on whether taking aspirin with a meal, which delays emptying of the stomach, increases the time to onset of action. It is clear, however, that a water solution of aspirin is more rapidly absorbed than the tablet form and thus gives higher and earlier effective blood levels of the drug.[19] This is a partial basis for the more rapid onset of action of the effervescent aspirins, but excessive use of these drugs disrupts the body's normal acid-base balance and creates other problems.

It is interesting that two famous compounds that the Bayer laboratories in Germany were instrumental in introducing to the world are rapidly transformed to their original form after absorption. Both heroin and aspirin were first synthesized in the Bayer Laboratories. Heroin is more active than morphine because it gets into the brain faster. Once there, it is converted to morphine and has morphine-like actions. Aspirin, either in the gastrointestinal tract or in the bloodstream, is converted to salicylic acid.

Taken orally, aspirin is a more potent analgesic than salicylic acid, since aspirin irritates the stomach less and is thus absorbed more rapidly. Studies of blood levels differentiate the two. In one study,[20] following ingestion of a 650-milligram tablet of aspirin, headache and postpartum pain were not reduced significantly from placebo until 45 minutes had elapsed, and maximum relief was obtained after 60 minutes. Four hours after intake, pain levels were equivalent in the drug and placebo groups. These reports fit well the salicylate blood levels measured in the same patients. At 45 minutes and at 4 hours the levels were the same. Thus, it may be that a salicylate blood level of 30 micrograms per milliliter is the threshold for analgesic effect, with maximum relief at a level of 40 micrograms per milliliter.

From the point of view of an occasional user there are three other important points. Much work has been aimed at developing a sustained-release capsule for aspirin to eliminate the need for taking medicine every 4 hours (or at night) and to maintain more constant blood levels. Usually the capsules are enteric coated (protected with a chemical that will not be acted on by stomach juices but will dissolve in intestinal fluids) and contain coated spheres of the drug that release it into the system slowly to maintain appropriate blood levels for 8 hours. A recent double-blind study[21] suggests that time-release capsules can be made that give the same pain relief as half as much regular aspirin given twice as often. These capsules also provide the additional relief of causing fewer and less intense gastrointestinal disturbances than regular aspirin. Many clinicians, however, feel that the enteric, slow-release form is too erratic in its effects for regular use.

Another factor to be considered when buying aspirin is that most tablets, including aspirin, develop a harder external shell the longer they sit. This hardening effect does not change the amount of the active ingredient but does make the active ingredient less effective because disintegration time is increased by the hard exterior coating. In the same line, moisture and heat speed the decomposition of acetylsalicylic acid into two other compounds: salicylic acid, which causes gastric distress, and acetic acid, vinegar. When the smell of vinegar in your aspirin bottle is strong, discard the aspirin! A colleague[22] phrased it well: when you can smell the vinegar you should either apply a large dose to the commode or continue to use the tablets if you have a corn in your stomach which you want to treat! (Salicylic acid is now used primarily to remove corns!)

And finally: does buffering speed absorption of the aspirin? It can in adequate levels, but:

> . . . several well-controlled clinical trials, comparing ordinary aspirin tablets . . . have shown that buffered aspirin produces effects which are indistinguishable from plain aspirin.*

*From Modell, W., editor: Drugs of choice, 1970-1971, St. Louis, 1970, The C. V. Mosby Co., p. 195.

Going one step further, a report on medical testimony before a Senate subcommittee said:

> Over and over in detailed testimony before a Senate subcommittee this week, the message was the same: No matter how it is dressed up, inexpensive aspirin is the most effective ingredient in costly over-the-counter medicines.*

Adverse effects and misuses

Many studies have shown that the majority of healthy persons who ingest aspirin-containing compounds in therapeutic doses will bleed in varying amounts. Although the amount lost into the gut is usually less than 6 ml. per day, some persons have lost more than 100 ml. In general, the bleeding occurred whether the aspirin is in tablet, soluble or "buffered" form.†

There is some evidence that indicates the blood loss is the same whether the aspirin is taken during or between meals.[23] The bleeding effect is probably the result of a direct action of the aspirin on the gastric mucosa.[24, 25] Preparations that release the aspirin in the intestines reduce but do not stop the blood loss.

It is important to appreciate that the *blood loss has been demonstrated primarily when chronic therapeutic doses (2,000 milligrams and more a day) are used for several days.* The use of two aspirin for headache relief does not cause observable blood loss even if followed in 4 hours by two more aspirin, except in rare cases. There are, however, many people who do consume great amounts of aspirin regularly for a general malaise.[26]

Gastric bleeding is not the only serious effect that can result from overdosage. Referring to OTC analgesics in general, one observer noted:

> . . . the recommended daily dose can be doubled, trebled or even quadrupled for a few days without producing serious toxic effects, but . . . continued use of high doses will invariably lead to intoxication and death.‡

*From United Press International, November 27, 1970.
†From Babb, R. R., and Wilbur, R. S.: Aspirin and gastrointestinal bleeding, California Medicine **110**(5):440, 1969.
‡From Boyd, E. M.: Analgesic abuse: maximal tolerated daily doses of acetylsalicylic acid, Canadian Medical Association Journal **99**:790, 1968.

If you think about it awhile it will become more reasonable, but at first reading it is difficult to believe that:

> ...the incidence of analgesic abuse to doses producing severe toxicity may be calculated to be about the same as the incidence of narcotic addiction in Canada, namely, about 1 in 10,000.*

Concern is being voiced in high places about some of these negative side effects. The 1970 presidential address to the American Academy of Allergy raised the question of whether aspirin should be returned to the list of prescription drugs. Although admitting that the drug was used effectively and safely by millions, the President of the Academy was concerned over the number of actions of aspirin we don't understand, as well as the previously noted adverse side effects to chronic use and overuse.[27]

One other problem that comes from the casual attitude most people have about aspirin is that:

> ...there may be as many as half a million aspirin ingestion accidents a year in children under 5 years of age.... In 1966 there were 225 fatalities due to aspirin and salicylates, with 92 deaths in children under 5 years.... Childhood poisonings, or potential poisonings, are not accidental. The child willfully eats the aspirin.†

Not only does aspirin poisoning occur in young children, but it is increasing. Nor are all aspirin deaths caused by the child eating aspirin he wasn't supposed to. Frequently the overdose of the drug is unknowingly given by the parent.[28, 29] Aspirin is consistently involved in more poisonings in the under-5 age group than the next four or five classes of compounds, such as soaps and bleach, combined.[30]

Usually (10 to 1) the poisoning agent is "baby aspirin." To decrease the seriousness of overingestion, all the major manufacturers of baby aspirin in this country have limited the bottles to 36 1¼-grain tablets, and some have developed a safety lid to make it difficult for children to open the bottle. A far better plan is to use strip packaging where each tablet can be obtained only by ripping open

*Ibid.
†From Crotty, J. J.: The epidemiology of salicylate poisoning, Clinical Toxicology **1**(4):381, 382, 384, 1968.

a foil type container. This would decrease convenience and increase cost to the consumer, and manufacturers are resisting the move on that basis.

A fitting summary and closing comment on this wonder drug is this:

> The assurance with which these preparations are advertised and offered for sale and the casualness with which they are sold from retail establishments of so many types and by vending machines in every conceivable place must contribute to a widespread impression that, in the recommended doses, aspirin preparations are harmless. On the other hand, the frequency with which salicylate preparations are taken for suicidal purposes does indicate that the toxicity of higher doses is realised by at least some sections of the public.*

Phenacetin

Only brief comment can be made about a second OTC internal analgesic, phenacetin. Phenacetin is the P in the APC tablets (A is for aspirin and C is for caffeine). Soldiers know well that at sickcall in the army the APC tablets represent the Army's Perfect Cure—for everything! Phenacetin has two of aspirin's three major properties with analgesic and antipyretic effects. There is some evidence that phenacetin itself has these actions, but it is converted rapidly to acetaminophen, which most authorities feel is the active chemical at the cellular level. It is true that when acetaminophen is given, peak blood levels are reached in about half the 1 to 2 hours required for phenacetin.

Phenacetin has been around since 1887 but has not been studied nearly so extensively as aspirin. Its mechanism of action is thought to be the same as aspirin and the rationale for combining the two is that this prolongs the analgesic effect, because phenacetin is absorbed slower; however, there seems to be no basis for this belief. Phenacetin may cause some depression of mood and energy, and this may be the post hoc justification for the addition of caffeine (a stimulant) to compounds containing phenacetin. Caffeine, in one report,[4] caused a decrease in pain threshold, so its value here is questionable.

*From Blacow, N. W.: Is aspirin safe? Journal of the Indiana State Medical Association **52**(1):41-45, 1969.

Until 1964, compounds containing phenacetin could be marketed as any other OTC compound could. In 1964, the FDA considered the evidence linking prolonged, high-dose usage of OTC analgesics with kidney lesions and dysfunction. Australia reports the greatest misuse of analgesic drugs containing phenacetin. One estimate is that at least 4% of the population may have significant kidney damage as a result.[31] The FDA then required that a warning be placed on all labels of drugs containing phenacetin. The warning reads:

> This medication may damage the kidneys when used in large amounts or for a long period of time. Do not take more than the recommended dosage, nor take regularly for longer than 10 days without consulting your physician.

Thus the United States, Sweden, Denmark, Canada, Switzerland, and Australia now partially restrict its use. When the FDA ruling went into effect, Anacin dropped phenacetin from its formulation rather than include the warning, so it now contains only aspirin and caffeine. All of this occurred in spite of the fact that the evidence is clear that the evidence is not clear.

> Disagreement continues on the importance of excessive use of analgesics as a cause of clinical renal disease. Evidence from animal experiments must be considered inconclusive and the toxic effects and actions of individual analgesics and of their combinations on the kidney are not fully known; therefore it may be considered premature to incriminate a single drug.*
>
> It is suggested that analgesic nephritis is caused by the abuse of several drugs and not by phenacetin alone.†

THE ALL-TOO-COMMON COMMON COLD

No matter how you cut it, they all say the same thing:

> ...the common cold is a syndrome characterized by a catarrhal inflammation of the upper respiratory tract, namely the nose,

pharynx, accessory nasal sinuses and the larynx.*

A cold may be defined as a contagious minor illness with running nose, stuffiness, scratchy throat, cough and little or no fever. †

I am at this moment
Deaf in the ears,
Hoarse in the throat,
Red in the nose,
Green in the gills,
Damp in the eyes,
Twitchy in the joints, and
Fractious in the temper
From a most intolerable and
Oppressive cold.

Charles Dickens‡

You have to feel better, though, realizing that the same man who brought us the original Tiny Tim could be so poetic about something that is "... the most frequent acute illness of man, and ... account(s) for more time lost from work and school than any other cause."[32]

The common cold is caused by a strain of viruses called the rhinoviruses. Over 100 types have been identified, and they are clearly distinct from the viruses that cause influenza, measles, and pneumonia. Success in developing vaccines against poliomyelitis and measles has made some experts optimistic about a cold vaccine being just over the next hill,[33, 34] but others are very pessimistic because of the great variety of viruses. Another problem is that the rhinoviruses can change their immunologic reactivity very readily, so that vaccine good against a rhinovirus in October may be of no value in February.

Americans can hardly wait for a cure. Over 250 million acute cold-like illnesses occur each year in the United States. Colds outnumber other ailments 25 to 1.[35] Occasionally a new virus appears to which no one has developed antibodies, and this can make some viral outbreaks quite dangerous. Influenza is a

---

*From Gault, M. H., Rudwal, T. C., and Redmond, N. I.: Analgesic habits of 500 veterans: incidence and complications of abuse, Canadian Medical Association Journal 98(13):624, 1968.
†From Prescott, L. F.: Renal effects of acetylsalicylic acid, phenacetin, acetaminophen, and caffeine, Current Researches 45(3):309, 1966.

*From Regnier, E.: The administration of large doses of ascorbic acid in the prevention and treatment of the common cold, Review of Allergy 22:835, 1968.
†From Adams, J. M.: Viruses and colds, the modern plague, New York, 1967, American Elsevier Publishing Co., Inc., pp. 151-152.
‡From Dickens, C.: The collected letters of Charles Dickens, 1880, Chapman & Hall Ltd., pp. 92, 93.

viral infection but it is not "just a bad common cold." The 1957-1958 epidemic of the Asian flu was responsible for the death of 78,000 people in the United States. Influenza outbreaks have been recorded as early as the year 1173, but the one that many people still remember occurred in 1918-1919. That post–World War I epidemic was responsible worldwide for 20 million deaths!

Viruses damage or kill the cells they attack. The rhinoviruses zero in on the upper respiratory tract and at first cause irritation that may lead to reflex coughing and sneezing. Increased irritation inflames the tissue and is followed by soreness and swelling of the mucous membranes. As a defense against the infection the mucous membranes release considerable fluid, which causes the "stuffed-up feeling."

Although the incubation period may be a week in some cases, the more common interval between infection and respiratory tract symptoms is 2 to 4 days. Prior to the onset of respiratory symptoms the individual may just "feel badly" and develop joint aches and headaches. When fever does occur it almost always develops early in the cold.

In everyday living, colds are passed via airborne particles—jet-propelled usually through unobstructed sneezing. This may be the reason why some of the old wives' procedures for preventing colds worked. If you wore a necklace of onions everyone was sure to stay away and thus minimize the chance of your being infected! One of the advances of modern science, though, was to show clearly that the "I was in a draft" and "my clothes were soaking wet" type of explanation will no longer do as a basis for a cold. Only man and some of the higher apes are susceptible to colds, and until recently the ability to grow cold viruses in the laboratory was very poor.[36]

The experimental animal-of-choice for studying colds had to be man. In many studies with human volunteers three types of findings seem to recur. First, not all who are directly exposed to the cold virus develop cold symptoms. In fact, only about 50% do. Second, in individuals with already existing antibodies to the virus, there may be only preliminary signs of a developing cold. These signs may last for a brief period (12 to 24 hours) and then disappear. The last finding crosses swords with the old wives so it is best to quote.

> Chilling experiments with volunteers did not show any particular influence on susceptibility to colds. Some volunteers were given an inoculation followed by a hot bath and made to stand in a draft in wet bathing suits. Some took walks in the rain and sat around in wet clothes. Other subjects were given the same chilling treatments with inoculations which contained no virus. No significant differences were found in these various well-controlled groups, and it even turned out in a few experiments that virus inoculation plus chilling sometimes caused fewer colds than chilling alone.[*]

The incidence of colds increases during the winter months, and there may be an early peak in November and then another one in February. The incidence curves are similarly shaped whether for southern or northern United States, and it is suggested that:

> ...the exact temperature and climate in different areas do not control the frequency of colds, but that a change of climate towards a cooler, and possibly damper type might increase the incidence of this disease.[†]

The rhinoviruses discussed here seem to be the causative agent for the common cold in older children and adults. In infants and young children, however, other viruses cause most of their acute respiratory illnesses. A final comment: a cold is only a nuisance but it can, and frequently does, develop into a serious illness. An untreated cold, if there is no new infection, will last 3 to 14 days. With proper treatment, a cold shouldn't last more than 2 weeks.

Prevention and treatment

There are two sure-fire ways to decrease or eliminate the chance of "catching a cold." One is to not be a primate, but for most of us that would be difficult. Everyone, though, is engaging in at least one good health habit that does decrease the chances of getting a cold.

*From Adams, J. M.: Viruses and colds, the modern plague, New York, 1967, American Elsevier Publishing Co., Inc., pp. 73-74.
†From Tyrrell, D. A. J.: Common colds and related diseases, Baltimore, 1965, The Williams & Wilkins Co., p. 30.

Getting older would appear to be the best protection against many of the common cold viruses which attack us.*

Evidence, as of 1974, suggests that high doses of vitamin C will reduce the severity of a cold but not change the incidence of colds.[36a]

It should also be made very clear that there are now no treatments available that reduce the duration or severity of the common cold infection. All treatment discussed here is symptomatic suppression. To deal meaningfully with the available aids to reduce the misery of a cold, quick note will be made of the basis for the major symptoms of an upper respiratory illness or head cold: runny nose and tickly throat.

We will start at the top and run down. The mucous membranes in the nose are wondrous. Under normal conditions the mucus that the membranes secrete is carried by moving cilia toward the back of the nasal cavity at a rate that replaces the mucus at least every hour and usually much more often. The mucus humidifies the air we breathe and traps small particles of dust. In a cold, the blood vessels dilate and they and the mucous membrane release more fluid in the area of the infection. Both the capillary dilation and the mucus contribute to the nasal congestion.

The release of fluid is probably caused by histamine, which is a naturally occurring substance normally released from injured cells. Histamine has many effects, and one is to increase the permeability of capillary walls, thus causing an increase in the amount of fluid in the injured area. This has some protective advantage for the damaged cells, but in the nose it stuffs things up.

A cough is a protective reflex that keeps the lower respiratory tract clear of foreign matter. The mucous membranes in the area contain nerve endings that, if adequately stimulated, send signals to certain autonomic centers in the base of the brain. This "cough control center," when activated, does three things in sequence: causes a rapid intake of air and closing of the epiglottis, increases contraction of chest and abdominal muscles

while constricting the bronchial tubes, thereby putting pressure on the epiglottis, and releases the epiglottis and expels the air at over 75 m.p.h.!

The stimulus for a cough in a cold may be an irritation resulting from a postnasal drip or from an accumulation of mucus within the bronchial tubes as a result of histamine release. Elimination of excessive mucus facilitates the passage of air, which is usually felt to be a good thing in land animals.

There are two pharmacological approaches to reducing swollen membranes. One approach is to use an agent that causes vasoconstriction, since this not only reduces the size of the blood vessels but also decreases their fluid loss. The other approach is to block the action of histamine. Sympathomimetic agents, such as amphetamine in the Benzedrine inhaler (see Chapter 11), are potent vasoconstrictors and thus shrink swollen membranes. The most common sympathomimetic agent used in nasal drops is probably phenylephrine hydrochloride. When these drugs are used and the blood supply to the area reduced, there may be a decrease in the capability of the area to fight the infection and to resist new infection. Another problem is that the duration of the effect decreases each time, and a condition of chronic congestion can result. It is possible that if sympathomimetic nose drops are used excessively, some nervousness and sweating could develop. These effects are for the most part avoided if the directions for use are followed. Although some authorities do not sanction the oral use of sympathomimetic agents for relief of nasal congestion, they do appear in some OTC compounds, the most commonly used being phenylephrine.

Since only $63 million was spent on nasal drops and sprays in 1969, while $200 million were spent on cold and allergy tablets, the oral medication seems preferred. Antihistamines are the major drugs used in these preparations. Their use in the treatment of colds goes back to World War II. At that time, the antihistamines were touted as preventing and curing the common cold, not just as suppressing the symptoms. Before the FDA could step in, all of America believed that

*Adams, op. cit., p. 74.

antihistaminic drugs were "cold cures." Today antihistamines (usually pheniramines) are one of many drugs in cold capsules. A 1972 FDA review doubts that antihistamines reduce cold symptoms but supports their use against coldlike symptoms from allergies.

The antihistamines have one universal side effect, sedation. The pheniramines are selected for use in antiallergy and cold tablets because they have satisfactory antihistamine actions and cause only minor sedation. Often agents in this group of drugs have greater sedating effects. This has been capitalized on by making them part of the formulation used in most OTC sedatives and sleep aids. The antihistaminic agent used in these compounds is typically methapyrilene.

Antihistamines also have some anticholinergic effects (causing dry mouth, at least), and these actions are frequently augmented by the addition of anticholinergic substances such as scopolamine and/or belladonna alkaloids. To briefly summarize this excursion, it should be emphasized that the sympathomimetic agents act by causing vasoconstriction and reducing the fluid loss from the capillaries. The antihistaminic drugs block histamine's effect on capillary walls, which is to increase movement of fluid from blood into tissue, and, via an anticholinergic mechanism, help prevent vasodilation of the capillaries. All of this should decrease congestion in the nasal cavity, and it usually does for most people suffering from an allergy.

Dropping down to the lower respiratory tract and the problem of coughing, the situation is not so clear since coughing is a natural response that occurs to keep the air passages open. Should it be suppressed? How can it be? Coughing caused by a cold can be reduced by making the cough control center less sensitive, reducing the sensory impulses to the center, or improving the situation in the bronchial tubes, that is, reducing the congestion. Of the three, the last is preferable since it should facilitate the passage of air, while the other two methods could even impair it. Codeine is an effective narcotic depressant of the cough control center and acts at doses low enough to permit its inclusion in nonprescription cough remedies. Codeine is also

a mild depressant of the entire central nervous system, and at higher doses than necessary to suppress coughing may reduce the rate of respiration.

The commonly-used drug in OTC cough suppressant preparations is nonnarcotic and named dextromethorphan. In addition to depressing the cough center, this agent may also depress the central nervous system, but usually not at levels that can be safely reached by using OTC preparations.

To conclude this section on the treatment of coughs and colds, it is valuable to summarize and paraphrase from a brochure given to college students for the self-treatment of colds.

1. For your feeling of tiredness, headache, malaise, chilliness, and feverishness:
Two aspirin tablets (a total of ten grains) every three to four hours—you may chew these for slightly faster action.
2. For your uncomfortable throat and cough:
   a. Hot (about as hot as you can tolerate) salt water gargle at least four times a day.
   b. Analgesic throat lozenges. Suck them slowly and use as needed to reduce throat irritation. Actually, any hard candy will provide more-or-less similar relief.
3. For your running and/or stuffy nose:
Phenylephrine hydrochloride nasal drops (0.25% concentration)—Use approximately five drops in each nostril no more than four times a day.

Several principles to be kept in mind when selecting medication for your cold are: do not use antibiotics in any form; nasal drops and sprays should be water based; your cough, although annoying, if productive of sputum may be helping you by reducing or eliminating secretion collection in your trachea and lower respiratory tract so such a cough should not be suppressed too much, if at all.*

The misuse of these cough and cold remedies to produce alterations in consciousness is not uncommon. Chapter 13 gives some idea of the kinds of effects obtained when high doses of sympathomimetic or anticholinergic drugs are taken. Dextromethorphan in high doses can result in sensations that some may interpret as positive feelings. Frequently these OTC compounds have a relatively high

*From Thompson, D. S.: Education for self-care of the common cold, Journal of the American College Health Association 14:181, 1966.

alcohol content and, even without the addition of other psychoactive agents, can cause a high.

CONCLUDING COMMENT

The world of OTC drugs is vast. Perhaps here more than anywhere else in the drug area do the consumer, the manufacturer, the advertiser, and the government need increased interaction. The people who use OTC compounds are not sophisticated in drug use and need to be led by the hand into the land of safe, symptomatic self-treatment. This will require restraints on advertising and on the proliferation of new, but no better, compounds.

With the expanding demands for better medical care and an ever-increasing patient-physician ratio, it seems likely that self-medication will increase along with the potency of the drugs available and in use. It seems essential that some action must soon be taken to plan for the systematic education of everyone in the analysis of his symptoms and the selection of a safe but effective drug.

PRECEDING QUOTES

1. Griffenhagen, G. B., editor: Handbook of non-prescription drugs, Washington, D. C., 1969, American Pharmaceutical Association.
2. Anonymous.
3. Keefer, C. S.: Summary and conclusions, Annals of the New York Academy of Sciences 120(2): 1005, 1965.
4. Hasebroock, Mrs. W. H.: Home remedies in household management, Annals of the New York Academy of Sciences 120:996, 1965.
5. Apple, W. S. Cited in Griffenhagen, G. B., editor: Handbook of non-prescription drugs, Washington, D. C., 1969, American Pharmaceutical Association.
6. Report of the Commission on Drug Safety, 1964, Subcommittee on Responsibilities of the Public on Drug Safety, Federation of American Societies for Experimental Biology, Washington, D. C., pp. 176 and 179.

REFERENCES

1. Food and Drug Administration: The use and misuse of drugs, Publication No. 46, U. S. Department of Health, Education and Welfare, Washington, D. C., 1968, U. S. Government Printing Office.
1a. Final report, hearings on drug advertising: Drug Advertising Project, National Council of Churches, March 1, 1973.
2. Modell, W., editor: Drugs of choice, 1970-1971,
   St. Louis, 1970, The C. V. Mosby Co., pp. 101, 195.
3. Grollman, A.: The efficacy and therapeutic utility of home remedies, Annals of N. Y. Academy of Sciences 120:911-930, 1965.
4. Haslam, D. R.: Individual differences in pain threshold and level of arousal, British Journal of Psychology 58(1):139-142, 1967.
5. Beecher, H. K.: Placebo effects of situations, attitudes and drugs: a quantitative study of suggestibility. In Rickels, K., editor: Nonspecific factors in drug therapy, Springfield, Illinois, 1968, Charles C Thomas, Publisher, pp. 27-39.
6. Stevenson, J. M.: Aspirin, Journal of the Indiana State Medical Association 61:1462-1464, 1968.
7. Salicylates, Chemical and Engineering News 46:50, 1968.
7a. Moertel, C. G., Ahmann, D. L., Taylor, W. F., and Schwartau, N.: A comparative evaluation of marketed analgesic drugs, New England Journal of Medicine 286(15):813-815,1972.
8. Prescott, L.: Analgesics, The Practitioner 200: 84-92, 1968.
9. Smith, L. H. Jr.: The clinical pharmacology of salicylates, California Medicine 110(5):410-422, 1969.
10. Grotto, M., Dikstein, S., and Sulman, F. G.: Additive and augmentative synergism between analgesic drugs, Archives Internationales de Pharmacodynamie et de Therapie 155(2):371, 1965.
11. Wolff, B. B., and others: Response of experimental pain to analgesic drugs: III. Codeine, aspirin, secobarbital, and placebo, Clinical Pharmacology and Therapeutics 10(2):217-228, 1969.
12. Smith, G. M., and Beecher, H. K.: Experimental production of pain in man: sensitivity of a new method to 600 mg. of aspirin, Clinical Pharmacology and Therapeutics 10(2):213-216, 1969.
13. Burn, G. P.: A device for measuring the threshold of pain in man, British Journal of Pharmacology 34:251-258, 1968.
14. Woodbury, D. M.: Analgesic—antipyretics, anti-inflammatory agents, and inhibitors of uric acid synthesis. In Goodman, L., and Gilman, A., editors: The pharmacological basis of therapeutics, ed. 4, New York, 1970, The Macmillan Co., p. 321.
15. Vane, J. R.: Inhibition of prostaglandin synthesis as a mechanism of action for aspirin-like drugs, Nature New Biology 231:232-235, 1971.
16. Smith, J. B., and Willis, A. L.: Aspirin selectively inhibits prostaglandin production in human platelets, Nature New Biology 231:235-237, 1971.
17. Ferreira, S. H., Moncada, S., and Vane, J. R.: Indomethacin and aspirin abolish prostaglandin release from the spleen, Nature New Biology 231:237-239, 1971.
17a. Aspirin revisited: it may lessen risk of thromboembolism, Medical World News, April 5, 1974, pp. 15-17.

18. Parkhouse, J., and others: The clinical dose response to aspirin, British Journal of Anaesthesiology **40**:440, 1968.

19. Levy, G.: Aspirin: absorption rate and analgesic effect, Current Researches **44**(6):837, 1965.

20. Wiseman, E. H., and Federici, N. J.: Development of a sustained-release aspirin tablet, Journal of Pharmaceutical Sciences **57**(9):1535-1539, 1968.

21. Fosdick, W. M., and Shepard, W. L.: Enteric-coated microspherules: a clinical appraisal of two forms of aspirin, The Journal of Clinical Pharmacology **9**:128, 1969.

22. Lewis, C.: Personal communication.

23. Stephens, F. O., and others: The effect of food on aspirin induced gastro-intestinal blood loss, Digestion **1**:275, 1968.

24. Goddard: tax drugs to fight abuse, American Druggist, March 9, 1970, p. 34.

25. Dunlop, D.: Abuse of drugs by the public and by doctors. British Medical Bulletin **26**(3):236-239, 1970.

26. Boyd, E. M.: Analgesic abuse: maximal tolerated daily doses of acetylsalicylic acid, Canadian Medical Association Journal **99**:790, 1968.

27. Should aspirin be put on Rx-only status? American Druggist **161**(6):40, 1970.

28. Crotty, J. J.: The epidemiology of salicylate poisoning, Clinical Toxicology **1**(4):381-386, 1968.

29. Craig, J. O., Ferguson, I. C., and Syme, J.: Infants, toddlers, and aspirin, British Medical Journal **1**:757, 1966.

30. Verhulst, H. L., and Crotty, J. J.: Survey of products most frequently named in ingestion accidents in 1965, The Journal of Clinical Pharmacology **7**:10, 1967.

31. Purnell, J., and Burry, A. F.: Analgesic consumption in a country town, Medical Journal of Australia **2**:389-391, 1967.

32. Douglas, R. G.: Pathogenesis of rhinovirus common colds in human volunteers, Annals of Otology **79**:563-571, 1970.

33. Herman, E., and Stenebring, W., editors: Second Conference on Antiviral Substances, Annals of New York Academy of Science. In press.

34. Vaccines up the nose, British Medical Journal **1**:63-64, 1970.

35. Cold remedies around the world, American Association of Industrial Nurses Journal **13**:29, 1965.

36. Tyrrell, D. A. J.: Hunting common cold viruses by some new methods, The Journal of Infectious Diseases **121**(5):561-571, 1970.

36a. Johnson, O. G.: The food fad boom, FDA Consumer, pp. 5-12, December 1973-January 1974.

133

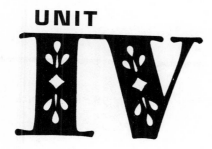

Psychotherapeutic drugs — their use and misuse

10 Tranquilizers and mood modifiers

Doctors pour drugs of which they know little, to cure diseases of which they know less, into human beings of whom they know nothing.

Voltaire

There is a great pleasure in combatting with success a violent bodily disease, but what is this pleasure compared with that of restoring a fellow creature from the anguish and folly of madness and of reviving in him the knowledge of himself, his family, his friends and his Gods!

Benjamin Rush, M.D. 1810

To Pinel's principles for the treatment of psychotics twentieth century psychiatry can add little, except to convert them into modern terminological dress . . .

Joint Commission on Mental Illness and Health, 1961

Fifteen years after the introduction of modern drug therapy to psychiatry, it has become a most valuable form of treatment, widely used although still not completely accepted.

. . . much more effort is needed. . . . although we have many patients who get better, we still have too few who get well.

Drug Treatment in Psychiatry, 1970

The drugs described in this chapter are in part very unlike those previously described. The effects of caffeine, nicotine, and alcohol have been repeatedly experienced, through choice, by a majority of adults in this country. In the case of the over-the-counter agents, a symptom or group of symptoms has to be identified by an individual, and he then prescribes and treats himself and monitors the decline in symptoms. Previously discussed drugs, then, are self-prescribed and self-administered and their effects personally evaluated. The antipsychosis, antianxiety, antidepression, and antimania drugs outlined here are available only by prescription and are used in the treatment of major illnesses.

The illnesses on which these drugs have an effect are different from other illnesses treated with drugs. Psychosis, neurosis, depression, and mania are diagnosed only on the basis of behavioral changes and changes in feeling and thinking. There are no laboratory tests that can identify components of blood or urine that are unique to any of these illnesses. Autopsy never reliably indicates lesions of the nervous system. All of these classes of behavioral and feeling disruptions are called *functional disorders,* in contrast to the *organic disorders* that have a known physiological basis. The causes of these functional disorders are unknown; the only known fact is that there is some disruption of the normal functioning of the nervous system. There is no evidence at this time of any impairment in the organic substrate of the brain, although there are many theories suggesting a biochemical or genetic basis for these illnesses.

HISTORY

A brief history is helpful to appreciate the use of drugs in the treatment of these illnesses and to understand the impact of these psychoactive agents on the field of psychiatry. It is meaningful to divide the history of the treatment of the mentally ill into four eras: pre-Pinel, Pinel to custodial hospitals, custodial hospitals to 1950, and 1950 to present.

Pre-Pinel treatment

Before Pinel's influence began in the last decade of the eighteenth century, there were many different beliefs about the causes of mental illness and they all shared the premise that the mentally ill could not be cured or helped in any way. The ancient belief that the mentally ill were possessed by demons and evil spirits was reaffirmed as late as 1489 in the publication of *Malleus maleficarum* (Witch Hammer), which described many symptoms of mental illness and attributed that behavior to witchcraft. This book was widely used in various inquisitions and witch hunts for almost 300 years.

The attitude of society about what should be done with the mentally ill changed gradually in the western world from one of ignoring them, in the hope that they would go away, to a concern for public safety. This concern initially resulted in the mentally ill being chained in dungeons, but it gradually moved to an enlightened management policy that paralleled the growth of asylums. The asylums were very clearly custodial and the mentally ill, the mentally retarded, and the paupers were all carefully isolated from the sane, normal, moral members of the community.

The famous Bethlehem Hospital (Bedlam) was started in London in 1553 by Henry VIII. The treatment offered the "patients" in asylums and the loss of personal identity reflected the state of the art of medicine as well as society's attitude toward these individuals. A good idea of the general approach to the treatment of the mentally ill is given by the following description.

> About the last of May or the first of June, depending on the weather, they were all bled. Following this, they were given weekly vomits, and after that they were purged. The violent were confined in chains, or caged, or encased in muffs, leggins, or straight-jackets. They snapped and snarled, and tore and tugged at their chains like wild beasts. In the seventeenth century a man might take his entire family on a holiday outing through this chamber of horrors for a sixpence. . .*

Pinel to custodial hospitals

All reforms move slowly in historical perspective and, when the history is long enough, it can be seen that changes occur only through

---

*From Marshall, H. E.: Dorothea Dix—forgotten Samaritan, Chapel Hill, 1937, The University of North Carolina Press, p. 66.

a series of advances and setbacks. Philippe Pinel was trained as a physician in Paris and studied methods of treatment of the insane at the Gheel colony in Belgium. The Gheel community was very much like some of the most modern treatment centers in Europe today. The entire village was devoted to the care of the mentally ill, and most of the patients lived in the villagers' homes and worked at jobs on farms. Only a few were held in the hospital. Treatment consisted of the proper diet, some work, love, and kindness. No restraints or punishments were used.

Pinel published his essay on the diseases of the mind in 1791 and was placed in charge of Paris's Saltpetriere Hospital for Men in 1792. He quite literally cast off the chains of the inmates. He liberated them, and the newspapers of the day were quick to point out the common basis between the French Revolution and the removal of restraints from the mentally ill (that is, the liberation of the individual). In 1793 restraints were considerably reduced in the women's hospital for the mentally ill in Paris, but little was accomplished outside the capital city for 50 years.

Word of Pinel's reforms as well as those instituted by others spread to many medical centers, and at the turn of the century the mode of treatment was "Moral Treatment." Moral Treatment was primarily respect for the individual, concern for his problems, work for his hands, and a calm environment. This treatment increased discharge rates to levels that have only recently been reattained. Wherever Moral Treatment was tried it seemed to be effective. Within 80 to 100 years of its formulation, however, such treatment vanished. Its use decreased partly because of changes in the attitude of the medical scientists and partly because of the effectiveness of the pioneers in the field of mental health such as Dorothea Dix.

In the United States there were no great medical centers. The asylums in this country contained a varied collection of mentally ill individuals without professional treatment or supervision. One of the pioneers in the treatment of the mentally ill in the United States was Dr. Benjamin Rush. He had good credentials; in addition to medical training in this country and in Europe, he was a signer of the Declaration of Independence, director of the Philadelphia Mint, and physician-general of the mid-Atlantic portion of the Continental Army. Later he was Professor of Medicine at the University of Pennsylvania, then the leading medical school in the country.

As an influential physician in this new country he was effective in instituting some reforms in the treatment of the mentally ill. Unfortunately, Rush strongly believed in the influence of physical factors on the functioning of the psyche, and his treatment procedures frequently involved inducing great pain, fear of death, and the letting of 20 to 40 ounces of blood, which he found "wonderful for calming mad people"! Because of Rush's prestige, these treatment methods prevailed and prevented the concepts of Moral Treatment from being widely applied in the United States.

In addition to Rush's influence, treatment of the mentally ill was, in part, determined by the still-persisting common feeling that it was a disgrace to be mentally ill. Many disturbed family members were in fact skeletons-in-the-closet when guests came. With most people abhorring the mentally ill, one could not expect that much would be done to assist them. As a result they were at various times assigned to poorhouses, jails, and county homes. Not only the attitudes of society toward the mentally ill but also attitudes toward hospitals kept hospitals from being built. Medical hospitals were dangerous places in those days—Lister, germ theory, and aseptic conditions were still in the future. If hospitals were bad, and they also cost money, it seemed silly to construct them for people you didn't really care about!

In 1840 the United States government for the first time counted the number of "insane" in the census. A total was reported of 17,434 out of a population of over 23 million, a little less than one in a thousand. By this date there was institutional care for the mentally ill only in eleven of the twenty-six states, and a total of fourteen hospitals for mental disease with a capacity of less than 2,500 beds. Conditions were appalling—the mentally ill, the poor, the criminal, the mentally retarded were all housed indiscriminately wherever they could be placed. Usually poorhouses and prisons were used and filled two to three times normal capacity. Once institutionalized these people were forgotten—out of sight, out of mind.

Onto this scene came Dorothea Dix. Her career is an interesting story and a milestone in mental health history, but unfortunately we must emphasize here only a negative outcome of her efforts. Miss Dix devoted her life to the separation of the mentally ill from the retarded, the poor, and the criminal, and was responsible for the construction of hospitals in many parts of the country for the treatment of the mentally ill. Dorothea Dix concentrated on getting the states to assume responsibility from the local communities. She was responsible for moving the mentally ill out of other institutions into mental hospitals and for dispelling some of the negative attitudes people had about the illness so that family members were hospitalized instead of hidden. However, the construction of hospitals and the commitment of more people to them operated to assure the general neglect of the mentally ill.

The hospitals gradually grew larger and larger, to the point where no treatment could be given because there were not enough professional and other personnel. The hospitals were built away from crowded cities, and the patients became more isolated from the community. The isolation and overcrowding made the hospital role more and more custodial, and discharge rates went down. The few private hospitals that had been able to earlier implement Moral Treatment had to relinquish it for a custodial role.

Not all of the blame for the failure of Moral Treatment to triumph as a treatment for the mentally ill can be attributed to Dorothea Dix. One factor was the developing attitude in the late nineteenth century in some influential scientists that mental illness was a brain disorder and as such should be treated by physical and physiological methods. The fact that the physiological methods available did not work was unimportant; clearly, Moral Treatment was not consistent with this attitude. A second factor, which appealed more to another group of physicians, was culmi-

nating in the work of Freud in Vienna. The psychoanalytic emphasis on the unconscious dynamics underlying symptoms was not easily translated into treatment methods for large numbers of patients. Neither of these important developments can be traced here, but, combined with overcrowded and understaffed hospitals, they seemed to provide adequate justification for "locking up the loonies" and waiting for an effective treatment to appear.

Custodial hospitals to 1950

There is no clear line dividing this period from the preceding one. In 1860, though, mental hospital discharge rates began to decrease. The trend toward lower discharge rates, and thus longer periods of hospitalization, continued from 1860 to 1920. There was no increase in the patient discharge rate, and decrease in duration of hospitalization, until the mid-1950's.

The effective use of malaria-induced fever for the treatment of general paresis in 1917 renewed hope for a physical treatment of the mentally ill. The 1920's had their narcosis therapy, which consisted of long periods of almost continuous drug-induced sleep, up to a week or 10 days in some cases. The first of the old modern physical therapies was developed by Manfred Sakel in Vienna in the late 1920's. Sakel, in 1933, induced coma in schizophrenics by the administration of insulin. The resulting drop in blood glucose level caused the brain neurons to first increase their activity and cause convulsions and then to decrease their activity and leave the patient in a coma. Thirty to fifty of these treatments over a 2- to 3-month period was said to be highly effective, and discharge rates of 90% were reported in the early years of use.

In 1954 a standard text in psychiatry could describe insulin shock therapy as ". . . the only effective method of treating early schizophrenia." A 1957 survey of the literature found, however, that even when initial treatment was reported to be effective, relapse rate was high, and recovery following insulin shock treatment was actually no higher than the rate of spontaneous remission.[1]

Ladislas von Meduna believed strongly that epilepsy and schizophrenia were mutually exclusive illnesses. He had observed, incorrectly, that no epileptic was schizophrenic and no schizophrenic ever had epilepsy. Reasoning that the epileptic convulsions prevented the development of schizophrenia, he felt that inducing convulsions might have therapeutic value for these patients. His first convulsant drug was camphor, but it had disadvantages, the major one being a time lag of hours between injection and the convulsions. In 1934 he started injecting Metrazol (pentylenetetrazol), which induced convulsions in less than 30 seconds, and reported improvement rates in schizophrenics of 50% to 60%.

The use of a drug was not ideal for inducing convulsions since the 30-second interval between injection and loss of consciousness (with the convulsion) produced much anguish in the patient. Ugo Cerletti developed the use of electric shock to induce convulsions. This method has the advantage of inducing loss of consciousness and convulsion at the moment the electric shock is applied. Although originally using mouth and rectum electrodes, he changed to brain electrode placement in 1938 and found it safer and more effective.

Electroconvulsive therapy (ECT) is only rarely used now with schizophrenics. Although early studies in 1943 suggested that almost 70% of the treated schizophrenics showed marked improvement, more recent reports in 1957 are in the neighborhood of 50%. Electroconvulsive therapy, however, is still used with depressed patients with good effect.[1]

Throughout the early part of this history of treatment methods, reference was made only to the mentally ill, the insane, the psychotics. In discussing the last three treatments, use of the specific term schizophrenia was introduced. Before moving on to a consideration of the modern drug treatments, an excursion is necessary into the present categorization of the mentally ill.

CLASSIFICATION OF THE MENTALLY ILL

Only some broad guidelines can be laid down here, but these will be adequate for present purposes. As already noted only functional disorders are relevant—those for which there is no known organic base. There are two major groupings, the psychoses and the neuroses. The psychoses are clearly the more severe disorder since the illness affects the psyche (the mind). The neuroses are less disruptive to the individual, as reflected in the name, which suggests that only the neurons of the nervous system are impaired. Present use of these terms is only because of tradition and does not imply any basis for these illnesses. Particularly remember that there is no neural malfunctioning underlying neurotic behavior. As will be elaborated, the psychoses are a disorder of thinking coupled with a blunting of affect. The neuroses are best viewed as life-adjustment problems.

Within the psychoses there are two dimensions of behavior that must be considered in diagnosis. One dimension refers to the degree of disorganization of thought processes, while the second dimension is concerned with disturbances of mood. Most psychotics differ from nonpsychotics on both these dimensions, and their actual classification is still a problem. In the United States, if a patient has some disorganization of thought he is usually classed as a schizophrenic, even if there is a mood disruption. In Great Britain the emphasis is on the mood, and the same patient would most likely be classified as a depressive.[2]

The first significant attempt to classify the large, heterogeneous group of psychotics was made only a little over 70 years ago by the great German psychiatrist Emil Kraepelin. However, of more importance here is the 1924 work of a Swiss psychiatrist, Eugen Bleuler, who termed one large group of psychotics as schizophrenics and emphasized the splitting of thinking from reality as basic in their illness. The major relevance of Bleuler is that he was the first to separate fundamental symptoms, those existing in every schizophrenic, from accessory symptoms, which were of far less importance and occurred with greater variability.

The fundamental symptoms were primarily disordered associations in thinking and a blunting or loss of affect or feeling. The blunting and loss of affect are reflected well in the apathy and low level of responsiveness of the schizophrenic. The disordered thinking process is indicated by the following type of logic in a schizophrenic patient.

"I'm going to be a good president of the
    United States."
Why?

Because I've had a heart attack!
What does that mean?
President Eisenhower was a good president
and he had a heart attack. I've had a heart
attack so I'll be a good president.

The accessory symptoms are usually the more
dramatic ones. Hallucinations, delusions, and
ideas of persecution are examples. These
symptoms sometimes come and go in the same
patient and certainly do not appear in all
patients.

Although the distinction between fundamental and accessory symptoms is still used,
as is the diagnosis of schizophrenia, few
authorities believe that this group of patients
is really a single entity. Some people, including
Bleuler, even talk of the schizophrenias. Many
schizophrenics also differ from normal on the
mood disturbance dimension. So common is
this that many schizophrenics are labeled
schizoaffective, or schizophrenic with affective disorder.

There are a number of psychotic patients
(and many neurotic patients) who suffer severe
disruptions in their mood. At one end of the
continuum the general characteristics of the
depressed patients have been well described
as: ". . . a phasic, temporary, severe lack of
present or anticipated satisfaction associated
with the conviction that one cannot perform
adequately."[3] The depressed patient may be
further classed as a retarded depressive in
whom there is a slowing and a deterioration
of behavior and thought. This is the type of
patient one usually thinks of as a depressed
patient. The agitated depressive has the
general characteristics mentioned previously,
but the manifestation may be through hyperactivity.

As might be expected, at the other end of
the mood continuum is the manic individual.

The hallmark of the manic episode is psychomotor acceleration, coupled with an ease of
enjoyment and an unrealistically optimistic
attitude toward achievement and the possibility of future enjoyment.*

The group of emotionally disturbed individuals classed as neurotics are not as severely

disrupted in their interactions with the world
as the psychotics. Rarely are neurotics hospitalized for prolonged periods. Their general
characteristics are much anxiety (which may
be directly experienced or partially expressed
in various symptoms), dissatisfaction, and unhappiness. There is no gross deficit in reality
testing, but neurosis is always accompanied
by some decrease in efficiency and effectiveness. This decrease occurs typically without
a major deficit in thinking and has led one
writer to comment: "Neurosis consists of
stupid behavior by an unstupid person."

Neurotic behavior can perhaps best be
understood as maladaptive solutions to life-
adjustment problems. Neurotic symptoms are
behavior that provide short-term relief from
anxiety, feelings of inferiority, and other
similar negative feelings. They become self-
defeating when used frequently, and at that
point the symptoms cause more problems than
they solve. Inability to solve these self-caused
problems results in frustration, increased feelings of inadequacy, and anxiety. When the
discomfort becomes unbearable the individual
seeks help in solving his problems in living.

These, then, are the four large classes of
emotionally disturbed individuals for which
psychotherapeutic agents have been sought
and found: the schizophrenics, the depressives,
the manics, the neurotics. The next section
returns to treatment methods and will trace
some of the interactions between drug therapy,
patient population, and society.

TREATMENT OF SCHIZOPHRENIA

From 1945 to 1955 there was an average
increase each year of 13,000 patients residing
in state mental hospitals. This was a continuation of a long-term trend and the result of a
dedicated effort to move mentally ill individuals into hospitals so that treatment could
be provided and the community protected.
Because of these increases, although the population of the United States doubled from 1903
to 1952, the population of state mental hospitals
quadrupled from 133,000 to over half a million.

The year 1955 was the high water mark of
residents in mental hospitals. If the 1945 to
1955 rate of increase had continued, there
would have been about 750,000 patients in
state mental hospitals by 1971. Instead, though,

*From Klein, D. F., and Davis, J. M.: Diagnosis and
drug treatment of psychiatric disorders, Baltimore,
1969, The Williams & Wilkins Co.

141

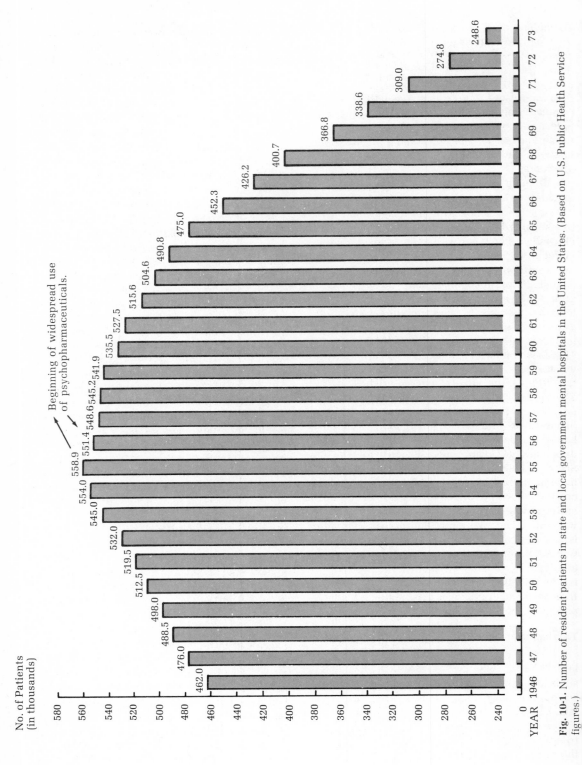

Fig. 10-1. Number of resident patients in state and local government mental hospitals in the United States. (Based on U.S. Public Health Service figures.)

the number has decreased each year since 1955 so that in 1973 there were about 300,000 fewer patients in those hospitals than in 1955. The 1946 to 1973 mental hospital population changes are clearly seen in Fig. 10-1. This decline in the resident population has occurred in spite of a large increase in the number of admissions to state hospitals. In 1955 there were 178,000 patients admitted to state mental hospitals, while in 1966 there were over 330,000. The crucial factor is that the average period of hospitalization in 1955 was 6 months while in 1966 it was about 2 months. Parallel with this increasing discharge rate from hospitals has been an increase in aftercare facilities. In 1970 there were 185 operating community mental health centers and almost 200 more approved and/or under construction.

Many authorities feel that the primary factor underlying the decline in mental hospital population in the United States can be identified as the introduction of new psychoactive agents into treatment programs in 1954 and 1955. There are three basic questions to be answered when considering any class of drugs used in the treatment of a behavioral disturbance. The first is, as a result of the drug treatment, is there a decrease in the frequency of the behaviors that brought the individual to, and keeps him in, the hospital? That is, are the drugs effective? Do they reduce symptoms? Second, are there adverse side effects that inevitably occur when the individual is receiving a therapeutic dose? Phrased differently, how safe is the drug? Can it be used without harm to the patient? The last question is, if an individual is released from the hospital while still under medication, can he function adequately in the community? To what extent is the medicated psychotic patient who is free of major symptoms different from nonpsychotic, nonmedicated individuals?

Treatment and effect

Of the individuals in mental hospitals the largest group, about 50%, are diagnosed as schizophrenic. It is estimated that signs of schizophrenia are shown by 2% of the population at some time in their life.[3]

The only class of drugs to be considered in treatment of schizophrenia is the phenothiazines. Two other classes of drugs have been used minimally: reserpine and similar drugs, which were used briefly in the early 1950's, and the butyrophenones, which have only recently been introduced into this country.

Although a phenothiazine was first synthesized in 1883 and one was tried as an insecticide in 1934, the present story will be brief and begins in 1950 in France with promethazine. Promethazine was used to potentiate surgical anesthesia and was successful enough to start a search for other phenothiazines. In 1950 chlorpromazine was synthesized and by 1952 its use to potentiate anesthesia had been described. In addition, reports were that, by itself, chlorpromazine did not induce a loss of consciousness although it did decrease the interest of the patient in what was going on around him.

As a result of this last characteristic chlorpromazine was tried in France in the treatment of the mentally ill. The very first report of this work, in 1952, mentioned that not only was anxiety reduced but also that the drug acted on the psychotic process itself. Chlorpromazine was first used in the United States in 1954 for the treatment of psychomotor excitement and manic states. The use of chlorpromazine and other phenothiazines with similar actions has expanded dramatically. One estimate is that between 1953 and 1963 over 50 million patients received chlorpromazine, and no one attempts to estimate the number to the present time. In 1967 about 85% of all patients in state mental hospitals were receiving some phenothiazine medication, usually in tablet form.

The chemical structure of some of the phenothiazines is indicated in Fig. 10-2. These agents differ in their potency, as indicated, but at therapeutic doses have essentially the same effect on the schizophrenic symptoms. Side effects do vary from one compound to another, and frequently the therapeutic use of a specific agent is determined by how well the patient tolerates a particular side effect.

In one of the early reports (1955) dealing with the effects of chlorpromazine on a large number of hospitalized psychotic patients it was stated that:

> In patients who show a great deal of initial excitement, particularly those with manic and schizoaffective disorders, the medicament is

Phenothiazine
nucleus

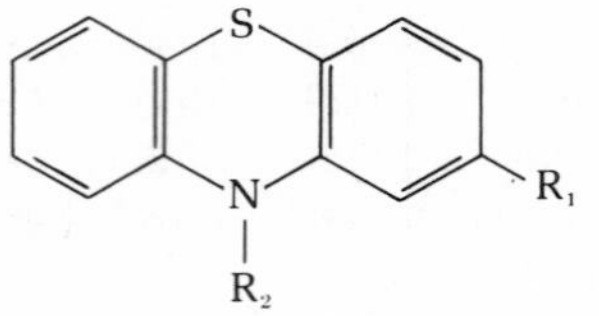

Generic name	Brand name	Clinical potency	R_1	R_2
Chlorpromazine*	Thorazine	7	— Cl	$-CH_2-CH_2-CH_2-N\begin{smallmatrix}CH_3\\CH_3\end{smallmatrix}$
Triflupromazine	Vesprin	5	— CF$_3$	Same as above
Prochlorperazine	Compazine	4	— Cl	$-CH_2-CH_2-CH_2-N$⬡$N-CH_3$
Trifluoperazine	Stelazine	1	— CF$_3$	Same as above
Perphenazine	Trilafon	2	— Cl	$-CH_2-CH_2-CH_2-N$⬡$N-CH_2-CH_2OH$
Thiopropazate	Dartal	3	— Cl	$-CH_2-CH_2-CH_2-N$⬡$N-CH_2-CH_2-O-C=O$
Thioridazine	Mellaril	_ 6 _	— SCH$_3$	$-CH_2-CH_2-$⬡ (N—CH$_3$)

*Chemical name for chlorpromazine is 2-chloro-10-(3-dimethylaminopropyl)- phenothiazine.

Fig. 10-2. Phenothiazines.

practically specific: [It] produces marked quieting of the motor manifestations. Patients cease to be loud and profane, the tendency to hyperbolic associations diminishes, and the patients can sit still long enough to eat and to take care of normal physiological needs. . . .

In the more chronic psychotic states, the effect of the drug is much less immediately dramatic, but, for those experienced with the relief of psychotic symptoms from other measures, the use of the drug produces results that are equally gratifying when compared with results in the more acute situations.*

*From Goldman, D.: Treatment of psychotic states with chlorpromazine, Journal of the American Medical Association **157**(15):1276, 1955.

This early evaluation was well founded, as suggested by the following statement made in 1970:

Antipsychotic drugs have a profound beneficial effect on the symptoms of this family of disorders [schizophrenia]. . . . the acutely ill patient in the office and the chronically ill hospitalized patient both improve with drug treatment, differing only in degree.*

The tremendous impact of phenothiazine treatment on the management of hospitalized

*From Veterans Administration: Drug treatment in psychiatry, Washington, D.C., 1970, U.S. Government Printing Office.

psychotics is clear from a 1955 statement by the Director of the Delaware State Hospital.

> . . . we have now achieved . . . the reorganization of the management of disturbed patients. With rare exceptions, all restraints have been discontinued. The hydro-therapy department, formerly active on all admission services and routinely used on wards with disturbed patients, has ceased to be in operation. Maintenance EST [electroshock treatment] for disturbed patients has been discontinued. . . . There has been a record increase in participation by these patients in social and occupational activities.
>
> These developments have vast sociological implications. I believe it is fair to state that pharmacology promises to accomplish what other measures have failed to bring about—the social emancipation of the mental hospital.*

Even sharper contrast was drawn in 1957 between the pre- and post-tranquilizer era: "In the usual pathetically understaffed back ward, tranquilizing drugs have converted the zoo-smelling, dangerous bedlams into places fit for human beings to live and, at times, to recover from psychosis."[4]

Paralleling an increase in the use of phenothiazines in the treatment of the mentally ill was the increase in the sophistication of experimental programs designed to evaluate the effectiveness of various drugs. Two large-scale, long-term series of studies were those initiated by the Veterans Administration and those supported by the National Institute of Mental Health in public and private hospitals around the country.[5, 6] Results from these as well as other studies show clearly that phenothiazine-treated patients improve more than patients receiving placebo or no treatments. One summary of the double-blind, controlled studies found that 106 studies reported that phenothiazine treatment of psychotics was more effective than placebo treatment, while only twenty-four found it to be no better than placebo treatment.[3] In each of the twenty-four studies where phenothiazines were not shown

to be significantly better treatment than placebo, low doses of the drug were used. Even then there were nonsignificant trends favoring phenothiazine treatment.

Another aspect of evaluating the effectiveness of drug treatment is determining the incidence of relapse or symptom recurrence when treatment is discontinued. An excellent review[7] of such studies indicates that about 40% of the patients relapse when the drug is stopped, whether or not the drug is replaced with a placebo. Almost all studies report that when medication is resumed, there is again a reduction in symptoms. It has been shown that antipsychotic medication can be withdrawn 2 or 3 days a week without relapse occurring in "chronic schizophrenics on maintenance chemotherapy in mental hospitals."[7a] A contributing factor to the improvement seems to be the treatment milieu, including the physical aspects of the hospital as well as the attitudes of the personnel involved in treatment.

Since improvement is sometimes seen with placebo treatment, analysis was undertaken by a group at the National Institute of Mental Health to determine whether improvement during phenothiazine treatment was merely quantitatively or also qualitatively different from that seen during placebo treatment. In a multihospital double-blind study involving three phenothiazine and placebo treatments, evidence was obtained to support the view that results of phenothiazine and placebo treatment do differ qualitatively.

> . . . the group of symptoms on which there is no improvement on placebo, and the group on which there is the most improvement on placebo, correspond respectively to Bleuler's distinction between "fundamental" and "accessory" symptoms. . . .
>
> Although the fundamental symptoms seem not to improve with placebo, all but one of these are affected by drug treatment. While there may not be complete removal of symptoms while the patient is under the influence of phenothiazine therapy, the fundamental symptoms seem to be reduced in their intensity.*

*From Freyhan, F. A.: The immediate and long range effects of chlorpromazine on the mental hospital. In Chlorpromazine and mental health, proceedings of a symposium under the auspices of Smith, Kline and French Laboratories, Philadelphia, 1955, Lea & Febiger, pp. 83-84.

*From Goldberg, S. C., Klerman, G. L., and Cole, J. O.: Changes in schizophrenic psychopathology and ward behavior as a function of phenothiazine treatment, British Journal of Psychiatry 111:130, 1965.

What is the nature of this qualitative difference? A 1970 Veterans Administration publication, which summarized and integrated much of the work done with psychotherapeutic agents both within and outside the Veterans Administration, supported the idea that the action of phenothiazines is much more specific than the commonly used term "tranquilizer" implies.

> The inappropriateness of the term "tranquilizer" is evident when the pattern of response produced by antipsychotic drugs is examined. They certainly do more than simply calm patients or put them in a "chemical straitjacket." The core symptoms of schizophrenia are consistently improved: emotional withdrawal, hallucinations, delusions and other disturbed thinking, paranoid projection, belligerence, hostility and blunted affect. On the other hand, somatic complaints, anxiety and tension, symptoms which might ordinarily be favorably affected by a "tranquilizer," are not much changed. . .*

Many observers report that the most rapid change in symptomatology occurs in the first 4 to 6 weeks of treatment with the phenothiazines. From the sixth to twelfth week some improvement is still occurring, but beyond that there is little if any change. As might be expected, motor effects are usually the first to manifest themselves, while the psychological symptoms such as hallucinations show a more gradual decline. An interesting common finding is that all of the phenothiazines have about the same clinical effectiveness, but some patients will respond to one drug and not to another. Some patients do not respond to any of the phenothiazines, but recent work[8,9] using new techniques to monitor drug blood levels suggests that this may be because the drug is not absorbed from the gastrointestinal tract. Intravenous injections and the development of agents that improve phenothiazine absorption may drastically reduce the number of patients who do not improve with drug treatment.

Some studies point up two problems that seem to recur regularly. One is the use of drug levels inadequate to control the symptoms in the early stage of treatment. As the dosage of the phenothiazine administered increases, so does the clear superiority of drug treatment to placebo treatment. Another problem is the failure to reduce the daily dosage after the patient's behavior has been stabilized on the drug. Several of the reviewed studies suggest that adequate symptom control can be maintained by drug administration once or twice a day or every other day, rather than the presently used three or four times each day.

In evaluating antipsychotic drugs, the concern is not only on the decrease in symptoms but also on the patient's release from the hospital and his adjustment to the community. In some of the National Institute of Mental Health studies it was found: "Most (89%) of all patients still in the community after one year were judged to be functioning less well than the average person at their general social level and many were clearly not without psychopathology."[10] The Veterans Administration publication phrases it: "Few patients who have been hospitalized for any appreciable period as schizophrenics ever function in a completely 'normal' way thereafter, probably less than 15 percent. Accordingly, realistic efforts must be made to help the patient so that he can live in the community despite his handicap."

A 10-year study[11] of 1,300 hospitalized chronic schizophrenics that started in 1956 adds some significant data to the problem of release and adjustment. In this study it was found that about half the patients were released from the hospital (and stayed out at least 3 months) within 6 months of admission and over 80% were released within 2 years. Only 4% of the patients were never released from the hospital during the 10-year period. Of those released from the hospital 38% were readmitted within 1 year, and over the 10-year period about 77% were readmitted at some time. Taking into consideration the readmissions, these patients still spent about two-thirds of the 10 years outside the hospital. In spite of the time spent outside the hospital it was felt that ". . . these patients manifested a rather marginal level of community adjustment" and that ". . . the amount of change in average symptom and behavioral levels between the various rating timepoints, both in

*From Veterans Administration, op. cit., p. 4.

the community and in the hospital, is distinctly minimal. . . ."[11]

By comparing discharge rates from the various hospitals participating in the study, it was clear that the most important variable in determining the release of these phenothiazine-treated, chronic schizophrenics from the hospital was the philosophy of the hospital administrators and the attitudes of the staff. This may be a truism, but it is an important consideration since more of these patients could have been released from the hospital and remained in the community, albeit adjusting only marginally.

A well-controlled 1971 study[12] compared three groups of newly admitted schizophrenics on their readmission rate and community adjustment following varying treatment. One group was treated and discharged normally, that is, in the way most schizophrenics are when first hospitalized. The second group was discharged after 3 weeks' hospitalization but given intensified treatment after discharge. The third group was treated and discharged like the first group but given aftercare treatment similar to the second group. A few comments are of interest in again emphasizing that successful treatment is a combination of drug therapy and community-based rehabilitation programs.

> The brief-treatment group showed as much sustained improvement as those who stayed longer. . . . Both intensified aftercare groups manifested less pathological disturbance at 12 months.
> While sound aftercare programs would seem to constitute both medically and economically desired alternatives to prolonged hospitalization . . . implementation of such approaches requires the full utilization of community resources. . . . *

Finally, as a social statement of treatment effect:

> Chlorpromazine and other phenothiazines are not considered truly curative in psychotic disorders since most patients usually display some residual psychotic symptomatology, even

following considerable improvement. Individual patients may require phenothiazine medication for years, perhaps for a lifetime. It must be pointed out, however, that some patients are so benefited by the drugs that psychopathology is not detectable even by highly skilled observers.*

Side effects to phenothiazine treatment

Two very positive aspects of the phenothiazines are that they are not addictive and it is extremely difficult to use them to commit suicide. A few deaths have been reported following ingestion of high doses. In the early stage of phenothiazine treatment some allergic reactions are noted such as jaundice, photosensitivity of the skin, and skin rashes. These reactions have a low incidence and with a reduction in dose level decrease and/or disappear. Agranulocytosis, low white blood cell count of unknown origin, can develop in the early stages of treatment. It is extremely rare, but has a high mortality, perhaps 50%. The anticholinergic and antiadrenergic actions have such side effects as dry mouth, nasal congestion, and constipation. These can usually be satisfactorily controlled by reducing the dose of the drug.

Tardive dyskinesia, a motor disorder of any part of the body but particularly a bizarre muscular activity of the face, develops in some patients on long-term antipsychotic medication. The disorder persists after all medication is stopped, which suggests the possibility of permanent neurological damage.[12a] This syndrome is different from the extrapyramidal symptoms that frequently parallel the appearance of the antipsychotic effects. The major extrapyramidal effects include a wide range of signs from facial tics to the usual symptoms reported in Parkinson's syndrome, such as tremor-at-rest, rigidity, and a shuffling walk. All can usually be controlled by the use of anti-Parkinsonian drugs, which typically are anticholinergics.

Some workers believe that there is no antipsychotic effect of the phenothiazines without

---

*From Caffey, E., Galbrecht, C., and Klett, C.: Brief hospitalization and aftercare in the treatment of schizophrenia, Archives of General Psychiatry 24:81, 85, 1971.

*From Jarvik, M.: Drugs used in the treatment of psychiatric disorders. In Goodman, L., and Gilman, A., editors: The pharmacological basis of therapeutics, New York, 1970, The Macmillan Co., p. 167.

accompanying extrapyramidal effects. In fact, there are reports that the drug actions on the extrapyramidal system form the basis for the therapeutic effects. There is now no resolution of this problem since with increasing levels of medication there is both a decrease in psychotic behavior and an increase in extrapyramidal signs. Few authorities believe that the major extrapyramidal signs described are essential for antipsychotic effects, but there is dispute over the importance of very fine tremors. It is true, though that some individuals do not show even minimal extrapyramidal signs but are helped by the drugs.

Although there is no experimental basis for believing that one phenothiazine is more effective than another in controlling psychotic symptoms, there are some rather clear differences in the side effects common to the various drugs. One general rule is that the more potent phenothiazines result more often in the appearance of extrapyramidal symptoms than do the less potent agents, even though both are administered at doses equally effective against the schizophrenic behavior.

Pharmacology of phenothiazines

The phenothiazines are antieverything. They are antiadrenergic, antidopaminergic, anticholinergic, antihistaminic, and antiserotonergic. Their effects on these compounds vary, however, being strong adrenergic and dopaminergic blockers, mild cholinergic and weak histaminic blockers. Two more general effects are probably of crucial importance in their antipsychotic actions: depression of the hypothalamus and depression of input to the reticular activating system.

The reticular activating system, which controls cortical arousal, receives inputs from each of the sensory systems. The primary sensory pathways travel to the thalamus but send collaterals (branches) to the reticular system. Impulses via these collaterals activate the reticular system, which in turn sends alerting impulses to the cortex. The phenothiazines act to diminish activity in these collaterals, and this decreases the ability of sensory input to arouse the reticular system and the cortex.

This action is probably the basis for the observation by an early worker that with chlorpromazine "... there is not any loss in consciousness nor any change in the patient's mentality but a slight tendency to sleep and above all 'disinterest' for all that goes on around him." Following phenothiazine administration there is a slowing of the electroencephalogram, which may reflect the lowered arousal level of the individual. One group of scientists have suggested that schizophrenics are normally overaroused and that the phenothiazines return them to the normal range of reactivity.

The effects of the phenothiazines on the hypothalamus are ubiquitous and result in many minor changes in autonomic activities that are only incidental to the antipsychotic actions. One effect that may well be fundamental in this respect is the action on the reward system. There is good behavioral evidence that the phenothiazines diminish the effectiveness of the reward system. This is consonant with the finding that the neurotransmitter in the system is noradrenaline, which is blocked by the phenothiazines.

A decrease in the functioning of the reward system would agree with a decline in motor agitation, while the decrease in responsiveness to external stimuli may explain in part the decrease in hallucinations and confused thought that occurs after phenothiazine treatment. Blocking off minimal, irrelevant, sensory stimuli, which may be misinterpreted as voices, may be the basis for part of the antipsychotic action of these drugs. However, since there is no agreement on the biochemical, neurophysiological, or neuroanatomical basis for the symptoms of schizophrenia and there is no agreement on which action or set of actions of the phenothiazines are producing *the* antipsychotic effect, there are many theories about how these drugs have their effects but no consensus on any one of them.

The metabolism of the phenothiazines is not known, but at least 168 breakdown metabolites of chlorpromazine have been proposed, and many of them are already identified in the urine. The liver is the primary organ of detoxification and usually contains the highest drug level of any structure in the body following the administration of these drugs. The rate at which chlorpromazine leaves the body is extremely slow, and some investigators have reported breakdown products of chlorpromazine in the urine several months after termination of medication. These data are still debated but do agree with the general finding that when medication is stopped symptoms only slowly recur, perhaps not until 3 months after the last drug administration.

TREATMENT OF MOOD DISORDERS

Mood fluctuations are probably more common than disordered thinking in the general population and, in addition, there is also greater tolerance by society for this behavior. Only about 90,000 individuals enter mental hospitals each year because of depression[13] and, since most patients have recurring episodes of illness throughout life, probably fewer than 20,000 of these admissions are new patients. Hospitalization for mania is even more rare today. However, this low number of admissions results in part from the low incidence of mania in the general population. While there are no good data on the incidence of the illness, it is probably less than one-tenth that of depression.

There is some agreement that the disorders considered as mood disorders are closely related to impaired functioning of central adrenergic and cholinergic systems. The two systems that would seem a priori to be most relevant are the medial forebrain bundle and the periventricular system. As will be seen, the drugs that act to diminish the symptoms of mania and depression also have specific effects on these reward and punishment systems.

Depression

Depressive patients have been classified in many ways. Earlier it was mentioned that some patients are slowed down or retarded, while others are agitated. Another system groups these depressions not apparently related to a precipitating event, referred to as endogenous depressions, as contrasted to reactive depressions, in which there seems to be a precipitating event, such as death of a loved one, prior to the depression. One other classification divides the general class of depressed patients into the "anxious" (like the agitated), the "retarded," and the "hostile" and suggests that different drugs are effective in each of these groups.

Probably the single most effective treatment for the depressed patient is electroconvulsive therapy (ECT). One report[3] summarized the available good studies and showed that in seven of eight studies ECT was more effective in relieving the symptoms of depression than was placebo. Further, in four studies ECT was more effective than the most effective class of antidepressant drugs, and in three other studies the two treatments were equal. One factor that makes ECT sometimes the clear treatment of choice is its more rapid effect than that found with the antidepressant drugs. Reversal of the depression may not occur for 3 or 4 weeks with drug treatment, but with ECT results sometimes are noticed almost immediately. When there is a possibility of suicide ECT is thus the obvious choice, and there is no danger in pursuing both drug and ECT treatment simultaneously.

Drug treatment. The story of the antidepressant drugs starts with the fact that tuberculosis was a major chronic illness until about 1955. In 1952 preliminary reports suggested that a new drug, isoniazid, was effective in treating tuberculosis; isoniazid and similar drugs that followed were responsible for the emptying of hospital beds. One of these antituberculosis drugs was iproniazid, which was introduced simultaneously with isoniazid but was withdrawn as too toxic. Clinical reports on its use in tuberculosis hospitals emphasized that there was considerable elevation of mood in the patients receiving iproniazid. These reports were followed up, and the drug was reintroduced as an antidepressant agent in 1955 on the basis of early promising studies with depressed patients.

Iproniazid is a monoamine oxidase inhibitor (as well as many other things), and its discovery opened up a whole new class of compounds for investigation. As was mentioned in Chapter 5, monoamine oxidase is the only enzyme involved in the deactivation of serotonin and is also responsible for the deactivation of free noradrenaline within the neuron. Inhibition of this enzyme results in high levels

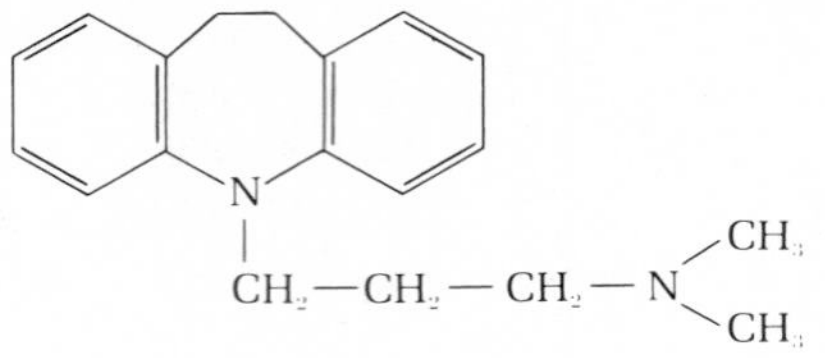

Imipramine
Tofranil (Geigy)
(5-[3-dimethylaminopropyl]-10,11-dihydro-5H-dibenz [b,f] azepine)

Fig. 10-3. Imipramine.

of functional serotonin, but the importance of the noradrenaline increase is not clear.

Despite the promise monoamine oxidase inhibitors held as antidepressant drugs, the number and severity of their side effects led to their demise. Iproniazid itself was removed from sale in 1961 after being implicated in at least fifty-four fatalities. Furthermore, a recent compilation of studies[14] showed that in fifteen of thirty-one well-controlled studies, the monoamine oxidase inhibitors were no more effective than placebo. Therefore, because of their dangerous side effects and their relative ineffectiveness, this group of agents is no longer widely used. If the ineffectiveness is true, then one must wonder about the basis of the original serendipity that "discovered" this class of antidepressants.

Chlorpromazine had been used and studied as an antihistaminic before its potential as an antipsychotic agent was appreciated. Imipramine, the next antidepressant to be discussed, left the animal testing laboratory as a phenothiazine-like antipsychotic. The similarity of the imipramine structure to that of the phenothiazines is clearly seen by comparing Figs. 10-2 and 10-3. In clinical tests, though, its outstanding characteristic was that it reduced the depression of depressed schizophrenics. Imipramine was the first of a series of compounds called tricyclics because of their chemical structure.

Tricyclic compounds have been shown to reduce depression better than placebo treatment in over 80% of the controlled studies.[3] This class of drugs is closely related to the phenothiazines but has weaker antiadrenergic and more potent anticholinergic properties

than the phenothiazines. Some suggestion of how close these family ties are can be seen in a 1970 Veterans Administration report on antidepressant drugs in which it was reported that controlled studies:

> ...have consistently revealed the superiority of tricyclics, both imipramine and amitriptyline, in depressions categorized as "retarded." Usually such patients compose less than 20 percent of a heterogeneous group of hospitalized depressions....
> ...antipsychotics have been consistently more effective in the most frequent depressive sub-type, the "anxious" category, which accounts for more than 50 percent of admission to hospitals.
> ...the third class of depressions, categorized as "hostile," seems to respond equally well to both tricyclic and phenothiazines.*

Both the phenothiazines and the tricyclics affect the reward and punishment systems. The tricyclics, with their greater anticholinergic effects, would be expected to have more blocking effect on the periventricular system, which would be congruent with a reduction in depression. Similarly, these drugs prevent presynaptic reuptake of released noradrenaline and may thus act to increase activity in adrenergic neurons such as those found in the reward system.

In spite of how well the actions of the antidepressant drugs fit into the prevailing beliefs about how the brain works, and with the chemistry of the reward and punishment systems, it is difficult to get too excited about them since there's something better!

*From Veterans Administration, op. cit., pp. 19-20.

Electroconvulsive treatment. As a general summary of the state of the art:

Many early publications provided enthusiastic testimonials for the efficacy of antidepressants, but the few controlled studies by the VA and others have provided only lukewarm support for belief in their effectiveness. From the confusion, however, a consistent pattern seems to be emerging. In the management of the depressed patient, treatments would fall thus: ECT, amitriptyline, imipramine, demethylated compounds, meprobamate, MAO inhibitors and placebo.

...It may very well be that the treatment of widely varying depressive syndromes requires a broad array of drugs. While it is still too early to recommend treating all anxious depressions with phenothiazines, a good case can be made for using antianxiety agents first and the traditional antidepressants last. On the other hand, tricyclics are clearly the drugs of choice in retarded depressions.*

Treatment of mania

The core symptoms of mania are an elated mood and hyperactivity. The manic person feels absolutely marvelous mentally and physically, but his normal judgments about the world and his own capabilities have disappeared. . . .

Although chlorpromazine and other antipsychotic drugs are not sedatives . . . they effectively suppress . . . mania by wrapping the patient's entire mind in a cocoon of stupefaction.

Lithium, on the contrary . . . is as if the manic symptoms were veins of porous limestone in a block of granite and lithium were water cascading through the block: Only the symptoms are leached out while the rest of the personality remains unaffected.†

Lithium is unlike any other drug discussed in this chapter. It is an element (but is administered as a salt), cannot be patented, and has been approved by the Food and Drug Administration for use in the treatment of mania only since April of 1970. There is no great amount of good clinical data available on lithium, but many investigators feel that it is a specific antimania agent and does not just control symptoms. Blood levels of the

*Ibid., pp. 19 and 20.
†From Gattozzi, A.: Lithium in the treatment of mood disorders, National Clearinghouse for Mental Health Information, Publication No. 5033, 1970.

lithium ion can easily be monitored to ensure a level high enough to yield a therapeutic effect but low enough to avoid the toxic side effects. Interestingly, its medical use may reach back to the fifth century in Greece where the use of alkaline mineral spring water was suggested for the treatment of mania!

Lithium was used about 100 years ago in the treatment of gout, but in the early part of the twentieth century its use was discontinued because of the side effects. In the late 1940's two medical uses and their results were reported almost simultaneously, and in the United States very nicely canceled each other out. Lithium chloride had been suggested and used with patients on low sodium diets. Unfortunately this use caused some fatalities, so no one was very interested in following up a report on lithium use that came out of Australia in 1949. The Australian report suggested strongly that mania and excitement were reduced when patients were given lithium carbonate. The lithium ion had been stumbled onto quite by accident but it seemed to work well, and some research programs on it began even before chlorpromazine was used with schizophrenics. Clearly the most comprehensive program is one still continuing in Denmark where in a well-controlled double-blind study good antimania effects were obtained in 80% of the cases.[15]

Treatment with lithium requires 5 to 10 days before symptoms begin to change. Lithium is both safe and toxic. It is safe because the blood level can be monitored routinely and the dose administered adjusted to ensure therapeutic but not excessive blood levels. It is a toxic agent but may be used with caution with patients with a kidney or cardiovascular disorder. The more minor side effects of gastrointestinal disturbances and tremor do not seem to persist with continued treatment. If excessively high blood levels persist, central nervous system and neuromuscular symptoms appear; these can progress to coma, convulsions, and death if lithium is not stopped and appropriate treatment instituted.

All the evidence is not yet complete on lithium but it seems to be very effective in reducing the symptoms of a mania state. Results to date suggest that, when continually given, the drug will prevent the recurrence of the manic episode.[16] Accumulating evidence hints that it may be useful also in those individuals who cycle between manic and depressed stages, but it will be a few years before the effectiveness of lithium can be evaluated unequivocally.[17] Equally unsettled at this time is the mechanism of action, although much research is directed toward answering that question.

TREATMENT OF NEUROSES

The neuroses are the most pervasive of the emotional disorders. Estimates are that about 10 million Americans could be diagnosed as neurotic. The actual classifying of an individual as neurotic is interesting in its own right, since for the most part it is a label that a person seeks for himself.

An individual is put into the large group of people society calls the emotionally disturbed under one of two conditions. His behavior may be disturbing or disruptive to others, and society then takes the responsibility for classifying, hospitalizing, and treating the individual. This is what is typically done with the psychotic, manic, and depressed individuals already mentioned.

Relatively few neurotics show behavior, thinking, or mood disorders of sufficient magnitude that require society's intervention. Usually an individual is labeled neurotic when he presents himself to a mental health professional and states directly or indirectly: "Help me, I'm unhappy, nothing seems right in my life, there must be some way in which you can make me feel more comfortable."

Interestingly, Galen, the second century Greek physician, estimated that about 60% of the patients he saw had emotional and psychological rather than physical illnesses. This is remarkably close to the present estimates of 50% to 60%. Treatments change but the patients don't. Perhaps though, the treatments don't change much either, just the brand names!

The treatment of neurosis, or of emotional problems, has never been shown to be very effective with any procedure. Psychotherapy,

whether individual or group and no matter what the training of the therapist, has never been shown to be reliably more effective than placebo or no treatment. About 60% of patients report improvement—that is, reduction in the aversive symptoms—whether treated or not. These facts are important because they make clear the base rate against which the effects of drugs must be measured. Also, most of the antianxiety drugs used by neurotics are used in situations and for symptoms that are very susceptible to influence by the nonspecific factors mentioned in Chapter 4.

Drug treatment

This section is labeled "Drug Treatment" for want of a better term or the use of six to ten pages listing the symptoms the drugs included here are supposed to control. Perhaps at the base of all of them is anxiety, but a better description of the kind of problem these agents aim to remedy is given by Shakespeare in *Macbeth*:

Raze out the written troubles of the brain,
and with some sweet oblivious antidote

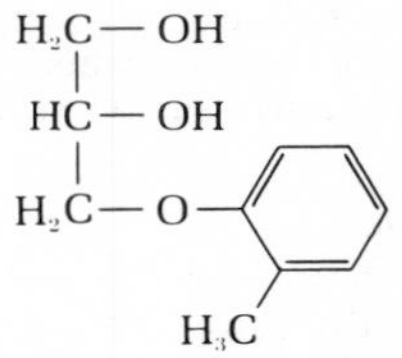

Mephenesin
Tolserol (Squibb)
(1,2-dihydroxy-3-[2-methylphenoxy] propane)

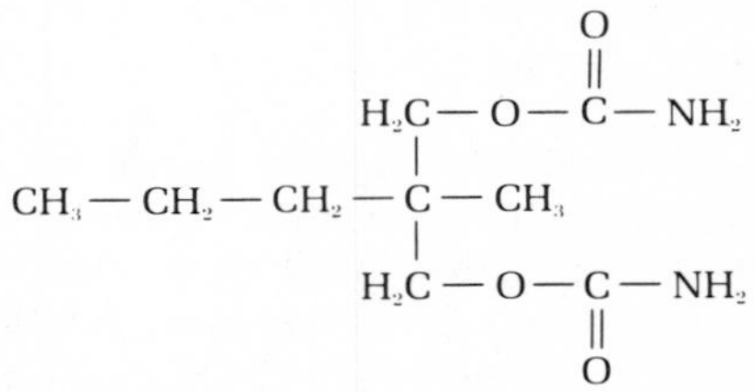

Meprobamate
Miltown (Wallace), Equanil (Wyeth)
(2,2-di [carbamoyloxymethyl] pentane)

Fig. 10-4. Mephenesin and meprobamate.

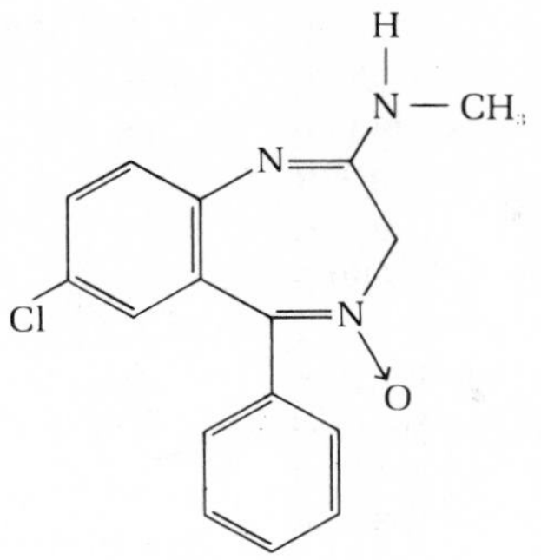

Chlordiazepoxide
Librium (Roche)
(7-chloro-2-methylamino-5-phenyl-3H-1,4-benzodiazepine 4-oxide)

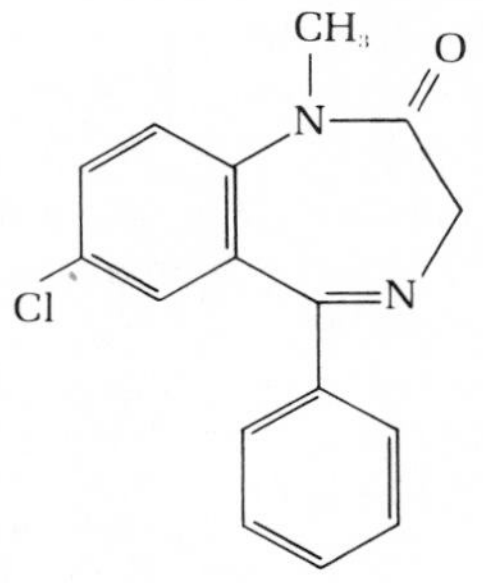

Diazepam
Valium (Roche)
(7-chloro-1,3-dihydro-1-methyl-5-phenyl-2H-1,4-benzodiazepin-2-one)

Fig. 10-5. Benzodiazepines.

Cleanse the stuff'd bosom of that perilous stuff
Which weighs upon the heart?

Since the early decades of the twentieth century the drugs used routinely with neurotic patients were the barbiturates (see Chapter 11), excluding of course alcohol, which has always been effective in controlling anxiety.

The modern antianxiety agents developed from a muscle relaxant called mephenesin, which was patented in 1946 and was a commercial success. The primary difficulty with mephenesin was its short duration of action. Extensive work was directed toward developing a longer-lasting, orally effective muscle relaxant. One compound patented in 1952 was not only longer lasting but believed to be a unique type of central nervous system depressant. Clinical trials in 1953 supported

this belief and after more work the compound was approved by the Food and Drug Administration and released for prescription use in 1955. Meprobamate, the generic name, became Miltown to the public, and it represented the drug revolution of the 1950's to most people. Fig. 10-4 shows the similarity of chemical structure of mephenesin and meprobamate.

The boom in meprobamate is difficult to see in perspective. In the year it was introduced sales of Miltown went from $7,500 in May to over $500,000 in December. The happy pills had arrived! A publicity agency and excessive prescribing by physicians combined to make Miltown a public nuisance ("Hello, I'm Miltown Berle!") as well as the unnamed object of comment concerning overuse by the

American Psychiatric Association and the World Health Organization in 1957. It became such a common word that physicians began prescribing meprobamate under its other brand name, Equanil.

It gradually became clear that meprobamate, like the barbiturates, is an addicting drug but only if taken at two to three times the normally prescribed therapeutic dose. As such, considerable care had to be used in prescribing it. In June of 1970 the Bureau of Narcotics and Dangerous Drugs brought meprobamate under the drug abuse control laws, which limited the number of times a prescription for it can be refilled. The real irony came in late 1970, however, when the NAS-NRC reported to the Food and Drug Administration that meprobamate was effective for the relief of anxiety and tension but was not effective as a muscle relaxant! Meprobamate has come a long way from its parent, mephenesin.

There is another class of compounds, the benzodiazepines, that is usually included along with the antianxiety agents. The best example of this class is the drug chlordiazepoxide, which is marketed under the trade name Librium. Chlordiazepoxide was synthesized in 1947, but it was 10 years before its value in reducing anxiety was suggested, and it was not sold commercially until 1960. Fig. 10-5 contains the chemical structure for chlordiazepoxide and for diazepam, another drug in the same class of compounds that is marketed under the brand name Valium.

With the two classes of antianxiety drugs (minor tranquilizers) established, the question is—are they effective? Do they work better than the much cheaper barbiturates? One summary[3] of the studies, in which these three groups of drugs (meprobamate, benzodiazepines, and barbiturates) were compared separately to the effectiveness of placebo treatment showed that each class was usually significantly better than placebo. When studies were summarized in which the two classes of minor tranquilizers were compared to the barbiturates, a predominance of results showed the minor tranquilizers were not more effective than the barbiturates.

A good summary of the clinical usefulness

of the benzodiazepine class of drugs was made in October, 1969:

> Librium and Valium are effective sedatives, but, except in potentially suicidal patients, it is still not clear that they have any important advantages over the barbiturates. Librium is useful in the management of the alcohol withdrawal syndrome and Valium is the preferred drug for the treatment of recurrent or prolonged seizures and similar disorders.*

A broader evaluation of all the minor tranquilizers was made in the 1970 report by the Veterans Administration:

> The new group of antianxiety agents has done little except to extend the range of available symptomatic treatment. Few psychiatrists regard them as having prime importance in treating psychoneuroses. But they can modify crippling anxieties and diminish the mounting tension that often precedes and accompanies impulsive and "acting-out" behaviors.†

A guarded but true statement about the clinical use of the minor tranquilizers is that:

> There is no very convincing evidence that these drugs are superior to shortacting sedatives, such as amytal, for the relief of manifest acute anxiety...But there is no doubt that these agents are superior to placebo in states of chronic anxiety.‡

Mechanism of action

Both classes of the minor tranquilizers are potent anticonvulsants and seem to have their primary action on the limbic system. The limbic system is seen as the intermediary between the hypothalamus, which controls changes in the autonomic nervous system, and the cerebral cortex, which is responsible for the experience of emotion. The important action of antianxiety drugs may be the result of depressing information exchange between two levels of emotional reaction. In this way experiences would elicit fewer body changes and, also, body changes would not be experienced with as great impact. By blunting this circle of action and reaction there may be a decrease in both the experience of emotion as well as the body changes that occur in

*From The Medical Letter on Drugs and Therapeutics 11(20):84, 1969.
†From Veterans Administration, op. cit., p. 15.
‡From Klein, D. F., and Davis, J. M., op. cit., p. 410.

emotional situations. This would certainly fit with the colloquial expression that these minor tranquilizers are the "I don't care" pills.

At therapeutic doses it may be that these agents do not cause as great a depression of cortical functioning as the barbiturates. This difference is still very much debated. Although more research is needed, it has been suggested that all these minor tranquilizers have their anxiety-reducing effect by selectively decreasing serotonin activity in the midbrain area.[18]

Initially, the hope was that the benzodiazepines would be successful in both the world of the antianxiety agents and the world of the antipsychotic drugs. This has not happened, although both classes of the minor tranquilizers do play a role in the reduction of anxiety symptoms in psychotics and anxious depressions.

Much has been said in the public press about the dangers of driving while using these compounds. The most sensible statement on the issue of these drugs and their influence on psychomotor skills is quoted here, and particular attention is directed to the last sentence.

With so many persons abroad in society under the influence of antianxiety drugs, it is unfortunate that we know so little about *adverse behavioral* effects, e.g., possible psychomotor impairment. The situation is complicated by the fact that laboratory experimental models may be quite inappropriate. Moreover, one can never be sure whether the person might not be more impaired from uncontrolled anxiety than from the drug used to treat it.*

A clear problem with these drugs is that tolerance develops and physical addiction can occur. The tolerance, addiction, and withdrawal are quite similar to that obtained with the barbiturates, and little comment will be made here except to note that abrupt withdrawal is quite dangerous. As mentioned, regular amounts of over twice the usual therapeutic dose of meprobamate may result in withdrawal symptoms when administration is stopped. The benzodiazepines are safer in this respect, and doses ten to twenty

*From Veterans Administration, op. cit., p. 17.

times the therapeutic level are needed to induce addiction and withdrawal signs.

Meprobamate and the barbiturates act on the liver microsomal enzymes to increase their activity. This will then increase the rate at which most drugs in the body are deactivated. There has been identification of the breakdown products and, using radioactively labeled meprobamate, it has been shown that some breakdown products appear in the urine about 30 minutes after oral intake and almost all of it in 24 hours. Peak blood levels are obtained 1 to 2 hours after intake and, with a single administration, almost all the meprobamate has left the bloodstream within 10 hours.

CONCLUDING COMMENT

This has been a varied chapter beginning with an understanding of the various classes of mental illness and moving on to the drug treatments that are used to control the symptoms of these illnesses. With the possible exception of Lithium, none of these drugs is seen as cures or even prophylactic for the illnesses mentioned—only symptoms are affected.

No one claims that these drugs return the patient to a normal level of functioning. The antianxiety agents may in fact decrease anxiety, but they also reduce all kinds of emotional responsiveness. In using any of the drugs discussed the real question that a physician asks is not whether the drug will return the individual to a state of normality, but will the use of the drug make it possible for the individual to better adjust to society and to himself.

PRECEDING QUOTES
1. Voltaire. In Esar, E., editor: The dictionary of humorous quotations, New York, 1953, p. 208.
2. Rush, B.: Talk to the managers of the Pennsylvania Hospital, 1810.
3. Joint Commission on Mental Illness and Health: Action for mental health, New York, 1961, Basic Books, Inc.
4. Veterans Administration: Drug treatment in psychiatry, Washington, D.C., 1970, U.S. Government Printing Office, pp. 26-27.

REFERENCES
1. Cited in Tourney, G.: A history of therapeutic fashions in psychiatry, 1800-1966, American Journal of Psychiatry **124**(6):784-796, 1967.

2. Mosher, L. R., and others: Special report on schizophrenia, U. S. Department of Health, Education and Welfare, National Institute of Mental Health, April, 1970.

3. Klein, D. F., and Davis, J. M.: Diagnosis and drug treatment of psychiatric disorders, Baltimore, 1969, The Williams & Wilkins Co., pp. 175, 185, 410.

4. Callaway, E.: Institutional use of ataractic drugs, Modern Medicine, January 15, 1957, p. 82.

5. Caffey, E., and others: Veterans Administration (VA) cooperative studies in psychiatry. In Clark, W., and del Giudice, J., editors: Principles of psychopharmacology, New York, 1970, Academic Press, Inc., pp. 429-442.

6. Goldberg, S.: Brief resume of the National Institute of Mental Health study in acute schizophrenia. In Clark, W., and del Giudice, J., editors: Principles of psychopharmacology, New York, 1970, Academic Press, Inc.

7. Prien, R. F., and Klett, C. J.: An appraisal of the long-term use of tranquilizing medication with hospitalized chronic schizophrenics, Schizophrenia Bulletin 5:64, 1972.

7a. Prien, R. F., Gillis, R. D., and Caffey, E. M., Jr.: Intermittent pharmacotherapy in chronic schizophrenia, Cooperative Studies in Psychiatry 93:145, 1973.

8. Curry, S. H., and others: Factors affecting chlorpromazine plasma levels in psychiatric patients, Archives of General Psychiatry 22:209-215, 1970.

9. Curry, S. H., and others: Chlorpromazine plasma levels and effects, Archives of General Psychiatry 22:289-296, 1970.

10. Cole, J. O., Bonato, R., and Goldberg, S. C.: Non-specific factors in the drug therapy of schizophrenic patients. In Rickels, K., editor: Non-specific factors in drug therapy, Springfield, Illinois, 1968, Charles C Thomas, Publisher, p. 124.

11. Gurel, L.: A ten year perspective on outcome in functional psychosis, Highlights of the 15th Annual Conference, Veterans Administration Cooperative Studies in Psychiatry, Houston, Texas, April 2-4, 1970, pp. 92-102.

12. Caffey, E., Galbrecht, C., and Klett, C.: Brief hospitalization and aftercare in the treatment of schizophrenia, Archives of General Psychiatry 24:81-86, 1971.

12a. Crane, G. E.: Clinical psychopharmacology in its 20th year, Science 181:124-128, 1973.

13. National Clearinghouse for Mental Health Information, Publication No. 5027, March, 1970.

14. Goldman, D.: Treatment of psychotic states with chlorpromazine, Journal of the American Medical Association 157(15):1276, 1955.

15. Schou, M.: New evidence of the prophylactic value of lithium carbonate, Highlights of the 15th Annual Conference, Veterans Administration Cooperative Studies in Psychiatry, Houston, Texas, April, 1970, pp. 108-118.

16. Prien, R. F., Caffey, E. M., Jr., and Klett, C. J.: Prophylactic efficacy of lithium carbonate in manic-depressive illness, Cooperative Studies in Psychiatry, Report Number 92, December, 1972.

17. Prien, R. F., Klett, C. J., and Caffey, E. M., Jr.: A comparison of lithium carbonate and imipramine in the prevention of affective episodes in recurrent affective illness, Cooperative Studies in Psychiatry, Report Number 94, April, 1973.

18. Wise, C. D., Berger, B. D., and Stein, L.: Benzodiazepines: anxiety-reducing activity by reduction of serotonin turnover in the brain, Science 177:180-183, 1972.

11 Stimulants and depressants

Like the morning cup of coffee, however, the drug produces a stimulation so pleasant that the problem of excessive use may arise quickly among individuals lacking medical control.

Air Surgeon's Bulletin, 1944

... amphetamine abuse is not confined to students. Our case files indicate that the most likely occupational group to be represented are medical personnel; housewives are next, and those engaged in nocturnal occupations follow. ... Addiction to amphetamine also occurs. ... direct observations of amphetamine addicts now make it clear that amphetamine addiction is more widespread, more incapacitating, more dangerous and socially disrupting than narcotic addiction.

John Griffith, 1970

Barbiturate abuse is an old and established vice of the American middle class and is related in many of its characteristics to our nation's number one drug problem—alcoholism.

D. Smith, D. Wesson, and R. Lannon, 1969

The drugs discussed in this chapter are those that alter an individual's activity and arousal level. Everyone has undergone considerable variation in arousal level from the deep sleep in the "wee small hours" to the hyperexcitability of an emotional situation. There seems to be an optimal level of arousal for most activities. If the activation level is too low, changes in the environment are not sensed nor will they lead to responding. If activation is too high, the nervous system fails to filter out many of the irrelevant sensory inputs. As a result, the information-processing system is overloaded and unable to integrate or discriminate multiple inputs. Such overloading has some of the same effects on the organism as does a lower than normal level of arousal, that is, failure to discriminate or respond to sensory changes.

Arousal level is primarily controlled by the reticular activating system. The cortex and other parts of the brain and body, as well as the external environment, send information to the reticular system to regulate it. The drugs considered here have been grouped as stimulants and depressants. The stimulants at proper dose levels increase the activity of the activating system as well as other brain areas. Activation of this system increases behavioral output as well as responsiveness to sensory input. The depressants are compounds that decrease activity level and sensitivity to the environment, usually through their actions on the reticular system.

Classically the stimulants are considered to be agents that improve mental and physical performance when they are impaired because of fatigue. There are three broad groupings of stimulants, one of which, the xanthines, was discussed in Chapter 8. Cocaine, a naturally occurring stimulant, is in a class by itself. The amphetamines are the best known stimulants and will serve as the prototype of the third group of agents.

The depressants are drugs that, by decreasing the activity of the reticular activating system, cause a reduction in behavioral output and in the level of awareness. Sometimes a differentiation is made among agents used as sedatives, hypnotics, and anesthetics, but these distinctions are only meaningful clinically. A sedative causes a mild depression of the central nervous system and decreases excitability and anxiety. Usually these effects can occur without excessive drowsiness or inefficiency. A larger dose of a sedative turns it into a hypnotic, that is, a drug used to induce sleep. By increasing the dose to still higher levels, an anesthetic state can be reached, and, with more drug and consequently greater depression of the central nervous system, death can occur.

Usually no distinction other than dose is made between sedatives and hypnotics. Rarely, though, is a compound used as both hypnotic and an anesthetic. Hypnotic (sleep-inducing) drugs are typically poor choices as anesthetic agents since they usually have a slow rate of elimination from the body and thus a long and not easily controlled duration of action. As with alcohol, some depressants have a narrow safety margin between the anesthetic and the lethal doses. Alcohol is one type of central nervous system depressant, and its use and misuse were discussed in Chapter 6. The remaining agents in this group are classed here as barbiturates and nonbarbiturates.

STIMULANTS
Coca and cocaine

History. A grave in Peru dating from about 500 A.D. contains the earliest record of use of coca leaves. Included along with other necessities for the afterlife were several bags of the leaves. Use of coca in this way gives no hint of the extent of cultivation or general use of the leaf at that time, but it certainly must have produced "exaltation of spirit, freedom from fatigue, and a sense of well being,"[1] even as it does today. By 1000 A.D. the coca shrub was extensively cultivated in Peru and today about 20 million pounds of coca leaves are used each year by the 2 million Peruvians who live in the highlands.

The terrain of the Andes in Bolivia and Peru is poorly suited for growing almost anything. *Erythroxylon coca*, however, seems to thrive at elevations of 2,000 to

8,000 feet on the Amazon slope of the mountains where there is over 100 inches of rain a year. The shrub is pruned to prevent it from reaching the normal height of 6 to 8 feet so that the picking, which occurs three or four times a year, is easier to accomplish. The shrubs are grown in small, 2- to 3-acre patches called cocals, some of which are known to have been under cultivation for over 800 years.

Before the sixteenth-century invasion by Pizarro, the Incas had built a well-developed civilization in Peru. The coca leaf was an important part of the culture, and although earlier use was primarily in religious ceremonies, it was treated as money by the time the conquistadors arrived. The Spanish adopted this custom and paid coca leaves to the native laborers for mining and transporting gold and silver.

The mountain natives at that time, as today, chewed coca leaves almost continually and kept a ball of them tucked in their cheek as they went about their business. The habit was so common that distances were measured by how far one could travel before it became necessary to stop and replenish the leaves. Even then, the leaf was recognized as increasing strength and endurance while decreasing the need for food. Early European chroniclers of the Inca civilization recorded and reported on the unique qualities of this plant, but it never interested Europeans until the last half of the nineteenth century.[2] At that time the coca leaf contributed to the economic well-being and fame of three individuals. They, in turn, brought the Peruvian shrub to the notice of the world.

One of these men was Angelo Mariani, a French chemist. His contribution was to introduce the coca leaf indirectly to the general public. Mariani imported tons of coca leaves and used an extract from them in many products. The quid of leaves was gone but you could suck on a coca lozenger, or drink coca tea, or obtain the coca leaf extract in any of a large number of products. It was Mariani's Coca Wine, though, that made him rich and famous. Assuredly, it had to be the coca leaf extract in the wine that prompted the Pope to present a medal of appreciation to Mariani. Not only the Pope but the royalty and the man in the street benefited from the Andean plant. For them, as it had for the Incas for 1,000 years and was to do for Americans who drank Coca-Cola (Chapter 8), the extract of the coca leaf lifted their spirits, freed them from fatigue, and gave them a general good feeling.

It was these three characteristics that led to the use of cocaine by Sherlock Holmes and Sigmund Freud. Coca leaves can contain a considerable amount (up to almost 2%) of the active ingredient, cocaine. Cocaine was isolated before 1860 but there is still debate over who did it and exactly when. An available supply of pure cocaine and the newly developed hypodermic syringe improved the drug delivery system, so that the following scene was easily conceived in 1890.

Sherlock Holmes took his bottle from the corner of the mantelpiece, and his hypodermic syringe from its neat morocco case. With his long, white, nervous fingers he adjusted the delicate needle and rolled back his left shirtcuff. For some little time his eyes rested thoughtfully upon the sinewy forearm and wrist, all dotted and scarred with innumerable puncture-marks. Finally, he thrust the sharp point home, pressed down the tiny piston, and sank back into the velvet-lined armchair with a long sigh of satisfaction.

Three times a day for many months I had witnessed this performance, but custom had not reconciled my mind to it. . . .

"Which is it to-day," I asked, "Morphine or cocaine?"

He raised his eyes languidly from the old black-letter volume which he had opened.

"It is cocaine," he said, "a seven-per-cent solution. "Would you care to try it?"

"No, indeed," I answered brusquely. "My constitution has not got over the Afghan campaign yet. I cannot afford to throw any extra strain upon it."

He smiled at my vehemence. "Perhaps you are right, Watson," he said. "I suppose that its influence is physically a bad one. I find it, however, so transcendently stimulating and clarifying to the mind that its secondary action is a matter of small moment."

"But consider!" I said earnestly. "Count the cost! Your brain may, as you say, be roused and excited, but it is a pathological and morbid process which involves increased tissue-change and may at least leave a permanent weakness. You know, too, what a black reaction comes upon you. Surely the game is hardly worth the candle. Why should you, for a mere passing pleasure, risk the loss of those great powers with which you have been endowed? Remember that I speak not only as one comrade to another but as a medical man to one for whose constitution he is to some extent answerable."

He did not seem offended. On the contrary, he put his finger-tips together, and leaned his elbows on the arms of his chair, like one who has a relish for conversation.

"My mind," he said, "rebels at stagnation. Give me problems, give me work, give me the most abstruse cryptogram, or the most intricate analysis, and I am in my own proper atmosphere. I can dispense then with artifical stimulants. But I abhor the dull routine of existence. I crave for mental exaltation.*

Sherlock Holmes! Perhaps even more surprising is the fact that the use of cocaine for these same purposes was advocated 6 years earlier by the father of psychoanalysis.

In 1884 Sigmund Freud wrote to his fiancée that he had been experimenting with "a magical drug." After dazzling success in treatment of a case of gastric catarrh he continues "If it goes well I will write an essay on it and I expect it will win its place in therapeutics by the side of morphium, and superior to it . . . I take very small doses of it regularly against depression and against indigestion, and with the most brilliant success." He urged his fiancée, his sisters, his colleagues, and his friends to try it . . . extolled the drug as a safe exhilarant which he himself used and recommended as a treatment for morphine addiction. For emphasis he stated, in italics, that "Inebriate asylums can be entirely dispensed with" . . .†

In an 1885 lecture before a group of psychiatrists, Freud commented on the use of cocaine as a stimulant, saying: "On the whole

it must be said that the value of cocaine in psychiatric practice remains to be demonstrated, and it will probably be worthwhile to make a thorough trial as soon as the currently exorbitant price of the drug becomes more reasonable." The first of the consumer advocates!

Freud was more convinced about another use of the drug, however, and in the same lecture said:

> We can speak more definitely about another use of cocaine by the psychiatrist. It was first discovered in America that cocaine is capable of alleviating the serious withdrawal symptoms observed in subjects who are abstaining from morphine and of suppressing their craving for morphine. . . . On the basis of my experiences with the effects of cocaine, I have no hesitation in recommending the administration of cocaine for such withdrawal cures in subcutaneous injections of 0.03-0.05 g per dose, without any fear of increasing the dose. On several occasions, I have even seen cocaine quickly eliminate the manifestations of intolerance that appeared after a rather large dose of morphine, as if it had a specific ability to counteract morphine.*

Even great men make mistakes. The realities of life were harshly brought home to Freud when he used cocaine to treat a close friend, Fleischl, to remove his addiction to morphine. Increasingly larger doses were needed, and "Freud spent one frightful night nursing Fleischl through an episode of cocaine psychosis and thereafter was bitterly against drugs. . . ."[3]

Even before Freud became aware of the problems with cocaine, Louis Lewin had attacked his proposal to use cocaine to cure morphine addiction and referred to Freud as "Joseph, the dream interpreter"! Although the biomedics were well aware of the dangers of using cocaine regularly, it was included unlabeled in all sorts of nerve tonics, patent medicines, and home remedies until the 1906 Pure Food and Drug Act was passed.

Therapeutic use and mechanism of action. The local anesthetic properties of cocaine—that is, the ability to numb the area to which it is applied—were discovered in 1860 soon after its isolation from coca leaves. It was not

*From Doyle, A. C.: The sign of the four. In The Complete Sherlock Holmes, New York, 1938, Garden City Publishing Co., pp. 91-92.

†From Holmstedt, B.: Historical survey. In Efron, D. H., editor: Ethnopharmacologic search for psychoactive drugs, Public Health Service Publication 1645, Washington, D.C., 1967, U.S. Government Printing Office, p. 17.

*From Freud, S.: On the general effects of cocaine, lecture before the Psychiatric Union on March 5, 1885. Reprinted in Drug Dependence **5:**17, 1970.

until 1884 that this characteristic was used medically, and the early applications were in eye surgery and dentistry. The use of cocaine spread rapidly since it apparently was a safe and effective drug. The potential for misuse soon became clear, and a search began for synthetic agents with similar anesthetic characteristics but little or no potential for misuse. This work was rewarded in 1905 with the discovery of procaine (Novocaine), which is still widely used. Many similar drugs have been synthesized since 1905 that have local anesthetic actions similar to that of cocaine but that do not have stimulatory effects on the central nervous system.

Local anesthetics probably block pain by preventing the generation and conduction of nerve impulses. They seem to act quite specifically on the cell membrane. By disrupting the membrane processes necessary for the initiation and generation of electrical impulses, impulse conduction and information processing is stopped.

Central stimulation effects and mechanism of action. Cocaine, compared to the other local anesthetics, is much more potent in causing increased electrical activity and arousal of the central nervous system. The evidence suggests that the initial effect is on the cerebral cortex (although perhaps via action elsewhere). Motor activity increases at low doses, but with higher doses convulsions may occur. At still higher dose levels, the respiration centers of the brain are affected and breathing rate will increase. Moderate doses also increase heart rate, but high levels of the drug delivered intravenously may stop the heart because of a direct action of cocaine on the heart muscle.

The central activation and the sympathomimetic actions are correlated with the action of cocaine at adrenergic synapses. Cocaine prevents reuptake of the released noradrenaline. The noradrenaline continues to act postsynaptically for an extended period and causes an enhancement of all adrenergic neurons and sympathetic nervous system effects. Fig. 11-1 shows the chemical structure of cocaine.

The effects of cocaine and its misuse are almost identical to those of amphetamine and will be discussed along with those actions of that drug. The major difference between the two agents is the duration of action. Cocaine must be injected every 15 minutes or snorted every hour to maintain the exhilaration, while amphetamine needs to be injected every 2 to 4 hours. Cocaine has emerged as the stimulant of the 1970's, and a 1973 government report estimated that almost 5 million Americans had tried cocaine — making its use more widespread than heroin.

Amphetamines

History. Amphetamine is a Johnny-come-lately in the stimulant world. The story of this stimulant starts with the search for a substitute for the naturally occurring sympathomimetic ephedrine. In the late 1920's two teams of researchers, one on the east coast and one on the west coast of the United States, synthesized and studied the effects of the amphetamine salts. Both groups applied for a patent on these amphetamine salts. The dispute was settled with the patent being issued to the California pharmacologist, Dr. Gordon Alles, in 1932. In exchange for royalties on sales he assigned the patent to Smith Kline

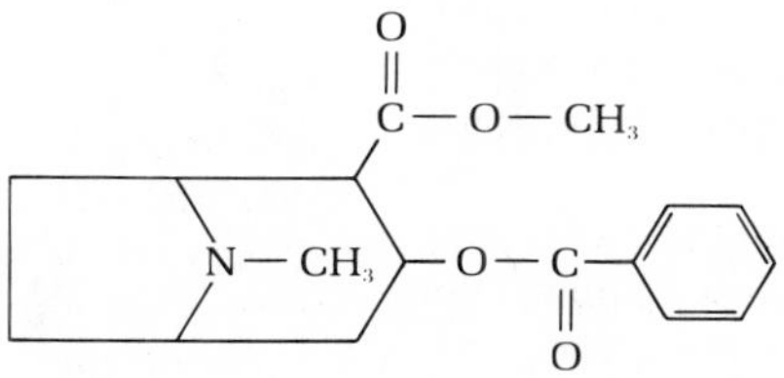

Cocaine
(3β-hydroxy-1αH,5αH-tropane-2β-carboxylic acid, methyl ester, benzoate [ester])

Fig. 11-1. Cocaine.

& French Laboratories, a Philadelphia pharmaceutical company.

All of the major effects of amphetamine were discovered in the 1930's, although some of the uses developed later. Quite early it was shown that amphetamine was a potent dilator of the bronchial tubes and could be efficiently delivered through inhalation. To capitalize on this effect of amphetamine, the Benzedrine (brand name) inhaler was introduced as an over-the-counter product in 1932. Some of the early work with amphetamine showed that the drug would awaken anesthetized dogs. As one writer put it, amphetamine is the drug that wouldn't let sleeping dogs lie!

Amphetamine was a central nervous system stimulant and in 1935 proved to be effective for the treatment of narcolepsy. This is a condition in which the individual spontaneously falls asleep five, ten, fifty times a day (even outside the classroom). Amphetamine enabled these patients to remain awake and function almost normally. In 1938, however, two narcolepsy patients treated with amphetamine developed acute paranoid psychotic reactions. The paranoid reaction to amphetamine and to cocaine has reappeared regularly and now is, unfortunately, a rather common reason for the arrival of individuals at psychiatric emergency wards.

In 1937 amphetamine became available as a prescription tablet, and a report appeared in the literature suggesting that amphetamine, a stimulant, was effective in reducing activity in hyperactive children. Two years later, in 1939, notice was taken of a report by amphetamine-treated narcolepsy patients that they were not hungry when taking the drug. This appetite depressant effect became the major clinical use of amphetamine, and the drug is still viewed as an effective short-term anorexient. Both the effect on hyperactive children and an appetite suppression are discussed later.

In 1939 amphetamine went to war, but it must have gone reluctantly since the research reports on its effects were not especially optimistic. One report in June of 1941 stated: "It seems clear . . . that benzedrine sulfate has no reliable or consistent facilitative or inhibitory effects upon higher mental functions."[4] The negative findings on the effects of amphetamine were offset, however, by many reports that Germany was using stimulants to increase the efficiency of their soldiers. One writer reported that the United States and Great Britain used almost 150 million amphetamine doses during World War II.[5]

A 1944 report in the Air Surgeon's Bulletin entitled "Benzedrine Alert" stated: ". . . this drug is the most satisfactory of any available in temporarily postponing sleep when desire to sleep endangers the security of a mission."[6] Some studies were reported including one in which:

> . . . one hundred Marines were kept active continuously for sixty hours in range firing, a twenty-five mile forced march, a field problem, calisthenics, close-order drill, games, fatigue detail and bivouac alerts. Fifty men received seven 10-milligram tablets of benzedrine at six hour intervals following the first day's activity. Meanwhile, the other fifty were given placebo (milk sugar) tablets. None knew what he was receiving. Participating officers concluded that the benzedrine definitely "pepped up" the subjects, improved their morale, reduced sleepiness and increased confidence in shooting ability. . . . It was observed that men receiving benzedrine tended to lead the march, tolerate their sore feet and blisters more cheerfully, and remain wide awake during "breaks," whereas members of the control group had to be shaken to keep them from sleeping.*

Although the blisters may have been in a different place, it was the same desire for increased alertness that resulted in the order in 1969 to astronaut Gordon Cooper to take an amphetamine prior to his manual control of reentry of his space capsule.

These alerting characteristics had already been well noted by truck drivers and college students. A group of psychology students at the University of Minnesota began experimenting with various drugs in 1937 and found that amphetamine was ideal for "cramming." (This experiment has probably been informally replicated more times than any other, except perhaps the one mentioned in *Macbeth* in Chapter 6!) College kids will try anything

*From Benzedrine alert, Air Surgeon's Bulletin **1**(2):19-21, 1944.

once (or twice, or . . .), but no real concern over nonmedical use of amphetamine came to the fore until later.

Concern over the nonmedical use of amphetamine developed after World War II. A 1946 article, "On a Bender with Benzedrine," appeared in a popular national magazine. It made explicit just how one could get his amphetamine without a prescription.

> . . . after I bought an inhaler, Hal worked off the perforated cap and pulled out the medicated paper, folded accordion-wise. . . . "Like this—" Hal took the innocent looking scrap of paper he had torn away and held it between thumb and finger. He alternately dunked and squeezed this paper into his glass of beer.*

Some of the medical and psychiatric problems that occurred when the contents of the benzedrine inhaler were used were discussed in a 1947 report[7] in the *Journal of the American Medical Association* entitled "Oral Use of Stimulants Obtained from Inhalers." Since each inhaler contained 250 milligrams of amphetamine, a considerable dose could be obtained if taken all at once. Of fifteen army prisoners using inhaler amphetamine, hallucinations and the feeling that others were talking about them were observed in four.

Misuse of oral amphetamine was widespread and common knowledge. This was the period of charm bracelets with an attached pillbox and the advertisement: "For 'Benzedrine' if you're having fun and going on forever; 'aspirin' if it's all a headache." Wearing your bracelet and singing one of the recently current pop tunes, "Who Put the Benzedrine in Mrs. Murphy's Ovaltine," who could care about inhaler eaters?

Smith Kline & French Laboratories, to some degree. They tried everything imaginable to make the amphetamine in the inhalers not suitable for oral use. Nothing succeeded, and a bill was introduced in Congress that would have made the Benzedrine inhaler a prescription item. However, the bill was not necessary, because in August, 1949, only 3 years after the problem was first discussed in a national magazine, the company replaced

*From On a bender with Benzedrine, Everybody's Digest 5(2):50, 1946.

the Benzedrine in the inhalers with Benzedrex! Benzedrex inhalers had equivalent nasal decongestant characteristics but not the stimulation of the Benzedrine inhalers. It was not until 1959 that the FDA banned the use of amphetamine in inhalers. Because of a loophole in the law one inhaler by another company, containing 150 milligrams of methamphetamine, was available as an over-the-counter item until 1965.[8]

The problem of the misuse of the inhalers was actually a minor one compared to the amphetamine problem, which began during World War II in Japan. Amphetamines were widely used in Japan to maintain production on the homefront and to keep the fighting men going. To reduce large stockpiles of methamphetamine after the war, the drug was sold without prescription and the drug companies advertised them for "elimination of drowsiness and repletion of the spirit." As a result "drug abuse grew as furiously as a storm."[9]

Medical problems developed and in 1948 stricter controls on amphetamine were put into force. Although they were tightened each year, the problem increased and in 1954 the Japanese Pharmacists Association estimated that 1.5 million people (about 2% of the population) were abusing the amphetamines. In that year the penal provisions were strengthened and treatment facilities expanded, and a year later, 1955, production was very tightly controlled. A massive public education program in 1954 to 1955 completed the triad of treatment, education, and penalties. These three factors eliminated the amphetamine abuse problem in Japan within 3 years.

In Sweden the amphetamine and stimulant misuse problem is probably greater than in any other country. Although there were some signs of amphetamine misuse in the 1940's in Sweden, the problem was diminished by educating the prescribing physicians and, in 1944, by placing the amphetamines under the same control as narcotics. Legal usage gradually increased, though, up to 1959, at which time the application of tighter controls on prescriptions reduced the legal sale of amphetamines.

The drug of choice for illegal use in the 1960's in Sweden was phenmetrazine (Preludin), which has almost identical central nervous system stimulation characteristics to methamphetamine. In 1965 Sweden experimented with giving legal prescriptions for narcotics and stimulants to some users. The plan was disastrous and was stopped in 1967. Drug misuse continued to increase at an unbelievable rate and Sweden, the country with the greatest illegal stimulant misuse problem, is now strongly urging tight international controls on production and use of these drugs. Central nervous system stimulants are now forbidden in Sweden except by special license for very selected medical cases.

There are no geographical restrictions in the misuse of drugs. There are, though, some unbelievably stupid behaviors because of separation in space. In 1952 the World Health Organization reported that amphetamine was being used by morphine addicts and that there was a possibility of amphetamine itself being addicting. Two years later, in 1954, when the Japanese pharmacists were expressing the same concern, the British Ministry of Health was saying:

> ... amphetamines have the advantage of being relatively non-toxic, addiction to them rare and there are no serious ill effects; they may, therefore, be given to patients without undue risk.*

Most of the misuse of amphetamines until the 1960's was through the legally manufactured, and sometimes legally purchased, oral preparation. Even today most amphetamine misusers take the drug orally. Those called "speed freaks," heavy users of the amphetamines intravenously, usually start with large oral doses. As recently as 1963 the AMA Council on Drugs could state: "At this time, compulsive abuse of the amphetamines (is) a small problem ..." As the later section on misuse will show, times have changed.

Therapeutic use. Until mid-1970, amphetamines had been prescribed for a large number of conditions including depression, fatigue, and long-term weight reduction. Acting on the recommendation of the NAS-NRC, the FDA in 1970 restricted the legal use of the amphetamines to three types of conditions: narcolepsy, hyperkinetic behavior, and short-term weight reduction programs.[10] Although the Kefauver Act of 1962 only mandated a reexamination of drugs introduced between 1938 and 1962 (amphetamine was introduced prior to 1938), the FDA felt it could evaluate and require changes in the approved uses for amphetamines because new uses for the drug had been added since 1938.

The use of amphetamine for the treatment of narcolepsy will not be discussed since its use for this condition is extremely infrequent. The value of amphetamine in the treatment of hyperkinetic children and in short-term weight reduction deserve comment for several reasons. There is dispute over the effectiveness of the amphetamines in *any* weight-control program, and there is considerable concern over the increasing tendency to routinely medicate the so-called hyperactive child.

Hyperactivity

> Hyperkinesis is a frequent behavioral disorder in children and adolescents, affecting boys more commonly than girls. It has been estimated that four out of every 100 grade school children and 40% of school children referred to mental health clinics because of behavioral disturbances are hyperactive. They have short attention and concentration spans, and their actions are irrelevant and without clear direction, focus, or object. Restlessness, impulsiveness, and garrulousness disrupt discipline in the home and in the classroom.*

Hyperkinetic children have frequently been referred to as having "minimal brain damage" but the evidence is mixed. Some have histories of difficult births or encephalitis when very young, and there are studies reporting a higher incidence of abnormal electroencephalographs (EEG's) in these children than in nonhyperactive children. There are many

---

*From Bloomquist, E. R.: The use and abuse of stimulants. In Clark, W. G., and del Giudice, J., editors: Principles of psychopharmacology, New York, 1970, Academic Press, Inc., p. 482.

*From Millichap, J. G.: Drugs in management of hyperkinetic and perceptually handicapped chilren, Journal of the American Medical Association **206:**1527-1530, 1968.

children, however, who do not show abnormal EEG's or medical histories, so the importance of these factors is not clear. There is also no evidence that all or even most of these children are mentally retarded, but their school achievement is usually quite poor. The difficulty seems to be self-limiting since, around the age of puberty, the symptoms decline and drug treatment is no longer needed.

In a recent review[11] of the studies that reported on the use of drugs in the treatment of the hyperactive child, it was found that methylphenidate (Ritalin) could be considered the drug of choice. Methylphenidate is a mild stimulant of the central nervous system that counteracts physical and mental fatigue while having only slight effect on blood pressure or respiration. In potency it is intermediate between the amphetamines and caffeine. When methylphenidate was used, 84% of the patients showed improvement (reduction of the hyperactive symptoms) while only 69% of the patients improved with amphetamine. There were annoying side effects in almost 15% of the patients regardless of which drug was used. Chlordiazepoxide and chlorpromazine have also been used in the treatment of hyperkinesis, with about 60% of the patients showing a reduction in symptoms.

Other drugs are clearly as effective or more effective than amphetamine in reducing hyperactivity, and they do not have as great, if any, appetite-depressing effects as does amphetamine. It may be that neither amphetamine nor methylphenidate will be widely used in the future. One report "showed that imipramine brought about the same improvement as amphetamines or similar drugs. However, imipramine caused fewer side effects and was easier to administer."[12] The FDA, however, has specifically warned against the use of this and similar drugs in children.[13]

Regardless of which drug is selected as the drug of choice for the treatment of hyperactivity, the therapeutic action of the drug upon the brain is not known.[14] Some work suggests that the effect of these drugs is more dramatic as the amount of stress becomes greater,[15] and frequently reports suggest that there is some brain malfunction at the level of emotional centers such as the hypo-thalamus. There is now neither an accepted physiological basis for hyperactivity nor an accepted pharmacological explanation for why the stimulant drugs are effective in reducing hyperactivity. In spite of this it is estimated that 150,000 to 300,000 children are being treated with psychoactive drugs for their hyperactive behavior.

As a final comment before leaving the problem of the handling of the hyperkinetic child, it should be emphasized that drug therapy is only one component of an effective treatment program. This was stated in 1970 by the Secretary of the Department of Health, Education and Welfare: ". . . hyperkinesis in children is a multifaceted problem which should be treated by all effective treatment modalities that are at our disposal. These would include remedial education, family counseling, many forms of psychotherapy and drug treatment where indicated."[16]

Obesity. Thirty-five percent of Americans are overweight by accepted medical and health standards.[17] This is a major health problem since statistics suggest that being overweight is an important factor in heart disease, coronary artery disease, and cerebrovascular disease.[18] Excess pounds must be a matter of concern to many individuals, since millions are spent each year for OTC diet aids and appetite suppressants.[19] This is the era of think young and think slim!

The reason why one-third of Americans are overweight and the means to lose weight or stay slim have been well studied. To this question, just as to the question of how to reduce the incidence of colds, science gives a hard, no-nonsense answer: eat less or work more. With the exception of thyroid compounds, there are no drugs that increase appreciably the rate at which we burn calories. Thyroid agents, by affecting the metabolic rate, will increase the rate at which our bodies use energy but have serious side effects and are used only to treat cases of hypothyroidism.

Amphetamine, as well as a host of similar compounds, is used for appetite control because it does decrease hunger. The drug does this in animals and in humans by a variety of mechanisms that have not yet been clearly specified. One partial basis is that amphetamine acts to suppress the appetite centers in the hypothalamus.[19a] Amphetamine does not affect blood sugar levels, but it does decrease food intake. Use of this drug for some weight loss programs is still legal in the U. S. but was banned in Canada as of 1973.

Many authorities feel that the euphoric effect of the amphetamines is the real basis for their continued use in weight-reduction programs. One physician phrased this attitude:

> There is very strong evidence, for example, that although they are effective in the short-term treatment of obesity, their effectiveness here relates not to a depression of the appetite control center but to the stimulant effect that they provide. In other words, fat people may be taking the drug for just the same reason that the young teenage speedfreak takes the drug—the stimulant effect, the euphoria effect.*

Two factors argue against the widespread, prolonged use of amphetamines for weight control. One is that tolerance develops rapidly to the appetite depressant characteristics of the drug. Even with moderate dosage increases, 4 to 6 weeks seems to be the limit before tolerance occurs to this effect of the drug. (With high doses tolerance can be overcome and, frequently, the speed freaks report little or no appetite and even an inability to swallow!)

The second reason for not relying on amphetamine-like drugs for long-term weight reduction is that overeating seems to be primarily controlled by psychological-behavioral factors, not by the physiology of the body. Overeating is a habit; unless the habit patterns are changed, overeating will occur as soon as the appetite-suppressing effects of the drug disappear.[20, 21]

A possibility is that if 4- to 6-week drug periods were altered with similar no-drug periods (to reduce tolerance), then a meaningful weight reduction program might be established. Drug periods could be used to teach new patterns of food intake. These new eating habits could be tested in the no-drug period before moving to more severe dietary restrictions in the next drug period. One major problem is that overweight individuals do not like the on-again, off-again schedule because the euphoria the amphetamines produce shows little tolerance. The amphetamine user would like to continue obtaining the euphoriagenic effect even though there is no suppression of food intake.

Basic pharmacology. There are three amphetamines, all of which have as a basic chemical structure the phenethylamine nucleus. Two of these are optical isomers of each other, while the third is a methylated form of either or both of the isomers. These two forms of amphetamines are shown in Fig. 11-2.

Amphetamine is usually manufactured as the sulfate salt and the chemical synthesized in 1927 was dl-amphetamine, a combination of both the d and the l isomers in a 1 to 1 ratio. In amphetamine the d form is more active (three to four times that of the l isomer) as a stimulant on the central nervous system. The l form, however, is slightly more active than the d form as a sympathomimetic and in its actions on the cardiovascular system. d-Amphetamine was first marketed in 1945 as Dexedrine for use as an antiappetite drug.

Methamphetamine, which has a methyl group added to the basic amphetamine structure, was previously marketed as Methedrine and in illegal use is called Meth, crystal, or speed. It has central nervous system stimulant effects about equal to d-amphetamine but is the drug of choice for euphoric effects. Perhaps the basis for intravenous users reports that methamphetamine is smoother than d-amphetamine is that it has fewer peripheral effects than the other amphetamines.

Amphetamine is rapidly absorbed when taken orally, and with the usual therapeutic dose of 10 milligrams peak effects are found 2 to 3 hours after ingestion. As mentioned, tolerance for amphetamine occurs to the appetite depressant effects within 4 weeks. Tolerance to the cardiovascular effects, increased heart rate, and elevated blood pres-

*From Crime in America—why eight billion amphetamines? Hearings before the Select Committee on Crime, House of Representatives, Ninety-first Congress, First Session, Washington, D. C., 1970, U. S. Government Printing Office, p. 44.

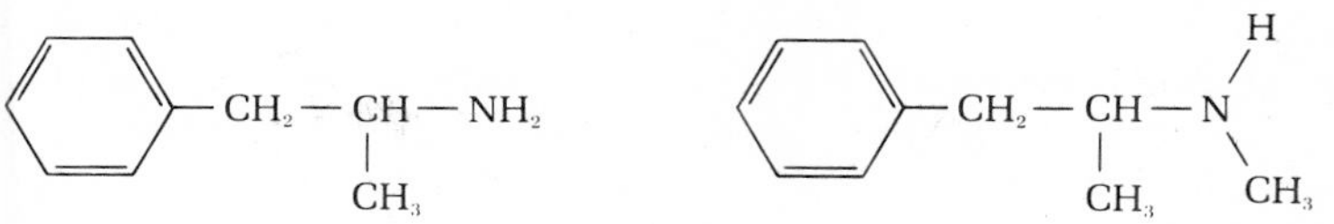

dl-amphetamine
Benzedrine (SKF)
(1-phenyl-2-aminopropane)

Methamphetamine
Methedrine (Burroughs Wellcome)
(1-phenyl-2-methylaminopropane)

Fig. 11-2. Amphetamines.

sure develop much more rapidly than tolerance to the central nervous system effects of arousal and euphoria.

The amphetamines have major effects on two brain systems that seem particularly relevant to their clinical use as well as their misuse. It should be clear, however, that no one can state for any psychoactive drug just which action is crucial in its effect. The reticular activating system is responsible for controlling the level of activation of the brain and is itself regulated by inputs from many areas of the brain as well as by sensory inputs. The reticular system in turn arouses the brain to prepare it to receive and process these sensory inputs. The degree of arousal is thus related to the amount of stimulus input and its meaning.

Amphetamine causes a biochemical arousal of the reticular activation system in the absence of sensory input. The activation is transmitted to all parts of the brain; the individual is aroused, alert, hypersensitive. Literally, the individual is "turned on." All circuits are go, even in the absence of external input. This activation may be itself a very pleasant experience, but there is some evidence that a continual high level of activation by itself may be anxiety arousing.

The other system on which amphetamines have potent effects is the medial forebrain bundle, the reward system. Increases in activity in this system are experienced as pleasurable—it feels good! This is, no doubt, the basis for the euphoria experienced even by those individuals who take only low doses of the amphetamines. The "flash" or sudden feeling of intense pleasure that is experienced when amphetamine is taken intravenously probably represents only the delivery of a very high blood concentration of the drug to the reward area of the brain. There are many other effects reported and sought by intravenous amphetamine users that are difficult to understand, let alone accept as pleasurable. One user reported that it "freezes my brain."

The pleasurable, rewarding characteristics of amphetamine have been shown in monkeys. These animals were given the opportunity to work (press a lever) to have amphetamines injected intravenously. When the chemical injected was amphetamine or cocaine, they worked cyclically for the drug just as human users inject at intervals. Data such as these support the idea that the drug itself has an action directly on the reward system.[22]

Mechanism of action. Until recently it was felt that amphetamine had its action at adrenergic sites by mimicking the neurotransmitters. That is, it was believed that amphetamine occupied and activated the receptor sites. Few authorities believe this today; the story is much more complicated.[23]

Amphetamine seems to have its adrenergic effects by acting on the axon terminal presynaptically. It has four major actions that form the basis for its effects as well as for the development of tolerance, which is regularly observed. First, amphetamine causes adrenergic neurotransmitters to leak spontaneously from the presynaptic sites. Such leakage will result in stimulation of the postsynaptic fiber in the same way as if normal information processing were occurring. It is quite important fundamentally, but of little significance here, that amphetamine has its action by causing the release of newly synthesized noradrenaline and not by emptying any of the storage depots of this compound.

Second, when electrical impulses do occur

in the presynaptic fiber, the presence of amphetamine increases the amount of transmitter substance released with each impulse. Third, amphetamine enhances its own effects as well as those resulting from electrical stimulation by blocking the presynaptic reuptake of noradrenaline so that the neurotransmitter will continue to act postsynaptically.

A fourth action of amphetamine may possibly be the mechanism for tolerance. Amphetamine is metabolized by liver-microsomal enzymes into p-hydroxynorephedrine. This metabolite, at least in the peripheral nervous system, functions as a false adrenergic transmitter. A false transmitter (see Chapter 5) is not as effective postsynaptically as the normal neurotransmitters, but it occupies space normally filled by the endogenous neurohumor. To offset this decrease in effectiveness of the released transmitter, larger doses of amphetamine would be needed to cause greater amounts of the transmitter substance to be released into the synaptic space.

Behavioral effects. Only the effects of low and moderate doses will be discussed here; the effects of high doses are detailed in the next section. The maximum effects of amphetamine seem to occur 2 to 3 hours after oral ingestion and, in terms of central nervous system potency, 5 milligrams of *dl*-amphetamine is about the equivalent of 150 milligrams of caffeine.

Amphetamine has several actions that may influence behavior. The clearest effect, as shown in many studies, has been to prevent the performance decrement caused by fatigue or boredom. In many studies amphetamine has been shown to prevent the fatigue-boredom performance decrement or to return impaired performance toward normal, rested levels. A 1968 review stated: ". . . amelioration of the feeling of fatigue developed by prolonged work is perhaps the most fully documented subjective affect of the amphetamines."[24]

However, one of the crucial and much-debated questions is: does amphetamine enhance normal performance, that is, can the performance—physical or intellectual—of rested individuals be improved above their normal nondrug levels? There are many

studies that report that amphetamine does not enhance optimal rested performance, although there is some evidence that at low doses, 5 milligrams, it may improve the attitude of individuals toward their work, even if they are rested. One 1959 experiment,[25] however, studied amphetamine effects on performance of swimmers, runners, and weight throwers and concluded: "This study has shown that the performance of highly trained athletes, of the classes studied, can be significantly improved in the majority of cases (about 75%) by the administration of amphetamine."[25]

Although not a particularly well-performed study by present standards, it is still the mainstay of those who feel that amphetamine does improve performance above that reached in the rested, nondrug state. The 1968 review of this area of research concluded:

> It is true that for a number of simple tasks there seemed to be little effect of amphetamine except in subjects whose performance had deteriorated as the result of prolonged work or sleep deprivation. On the other hand, data indicating a true enhancement are most convincing. Those on athletic performance obtained by Smith and Beecher found that the effects of amphetamine were more apparent in rested than in fatigued subjects.*

Since the 1959 Smith and Beecher study has not been repeated under better controlled conditions, it is unfortunate that so many writers cite it as having settled the question of the effects of amphetamines on athletic performance. It seems judicious, at this time, to withhold final judgment on the issue. The question, however, is very much alive.[26]

The use of drugs by athletes is not new, but professional organizations have hedged on the issue. The National Football League's effort was a locker room sign in the 1973 season that read in part: "It is League policy that the use by NFL players of any (nonprescribed) drugs . . . is not in your interest . . ."[26a] Not quite a hardline position on the problem of illegal drug use! Amateur organizations have begun steps to eliminate drug use by competitors.

*From Weiss, B.: Enhancement of performance by amphetamine-like drugs. In Sjöqvist, F., and Tottie, M., editors: Abuse of central stimulants, New York, 1969, The Raven Press, p. 57.

The Medical Commission of the International Olympic Organization conducted their first "doping" tests on a few of the athletes participating in the Winter Games at Grenoble in 1968. All tests were negative. In that same year, the Medical Commission indicated that doping consisted of the use of any of the following classes of drugs: sympathomimetic amines; central nervous system stimulants such as strychnine; pain pills, narcotics such as morphine, or any of the "caines" (cocaine, procaine, and so on); antidepressant agents; tranquilizers; and especially the phenothiazines. At the 1968 events in Mexico, the Medical Commission slightly(!) broadened the list to label the use of any and all medication as doping.

The problems involved in even spot-checking the urine of some athletes for drugs are unbelievable. Testing of all athletes or for all drugs cannot be realistically done, but some compromise system will certainly be developed. Considering the prestige attached to just being a participant in the Olympics, hopefully any system devised will include the also-rans as well as the winners. The difficulties in any system are pointed up in a 1958 book on the amphetamines:

> ... there seems to be no public condemnation of the use of coffee by athletes, either before an athletic contest, or in ordinary living. Nevertheless, caffeine produces the same general sort of central stimulation and reduction of fatigue that is characteristic of the amphetamines, the only difference being that the effects of caffeine are commonly less than those of the amphetamines, and coffee is an anciently used and long established social beverage. No one seems ever to have raised the question about athletes taking a large drink of coffee before an athletic contest or game. In contrast to public indignation at the use of amphetamines to increase physical performance, the situation regarding caffeine is an interesting commentary on what constitutes social acceptability. It seems that what has long been used, what is well established in social custom, and about which people think they know the facts generally, are sufficient to assure social acceptability.*

Misuse of amphetamines. There has been widespread misuse of legally manufactured amphetamine. In 1970 the Department of Justice was unable to account for 38% of the amphetamines produced. To decrease this problem and the overprescribing of amphetamines the FDA reduced the 1973 production of oral amphetamines to about 8% of the 1971 output. It also recalled and banned the production of injectable amphetamines and most amphetamine combinations with other drugs.

Even 782 kilograms of amphetamine (1973's quota) is far above the amount most authorities feel is necessary. Many physicians feel there are only two medical reasons for the amphetamines, narcolepsy and hyperactive children.[26b] In a Congressional hearing one physician felt that the number of amphetamines needed for these purposes was "in the thousands of pills,"[8] while another agreed it would be "a few hundred or a few thousand"![8] The basic issue in the legal use of amphetamine revolves around its prescription for short-term weight control.

Concern over the extensive prescribing of amphetamines is based both on the misuse of the drug by those for whom it is prescribed as well as on the resulting increased availability of the drug to those for whom it was not prescribed. One English expert phrased the latter concern:

> ... these latter meretricious agents of minimal therapeutic value, which should hardly ever be prescribed, are widely available, and may be stolen from factories, while in transit between factory and pharmacist, from pharmacists' shops, or from fat, tired women who have become dependent on them.*

Perhaps some of the amphetamine misusers are stealing their supply, but it is more likely that they are illegally buying 5- or 10-milligram tablets for a dime or quarter apiece. With many legally manufactured tablets available for illegal sales, there seems little point in stealing them. No one can estimate how much illegal amphetamine is manufactured and sold.

Truck drivers are usually the group most

---

*From Leake, C. D.: The amphetamines: their actions and uses, Springfield, Illinois, 1958, Charles C Thomas, Publisher, pp. 126 and 127.

*From Dunlop, D.: Abuse of drugs by the public and by doctors, British Medical Journal **26**(3):238, 1970.

singled out as misusing amphetamines in combating fatigue. The catch phrase seems to be the "Los Angeles Turnarounds"— enough amphetamines to make it possible for a driver to make a round trip from New York City to Los Angeles and back to New York City without sleeping. The concern, as always when drugs are used to combat fatigue, is that the fatigue will become so great that it will override the drug effect and result in accidents. This certainly is a possibility, although some old data make it unlikely that amphetamine misuse is a major cause of truck accidents.

> Truck accidents, commonly attributed to high rates of use by truckers, upon careful search reveal—using Senate hearing data as a base—that in 1957 (the year for which statistics were presented) of 40 truck accidents with amphetamine use by the driver implicated, only 13 were described as being due to driver-performance error presumably due to amphetamines. These 13 cases were out of 25,000 truck accidents filed for that year, .0005 percent.*

One widespread misuse is the oral use of amphetamines just for kicks. Ten to thirty milligrams of *d*-amphetamine will make people feel quite good, alert, talkative— a turned-on, it's good to be alive feeling. It will also probably make them hyperactive and nervous or jittery, and to combat these effects they may also use one of the barbiturates.

Speed is where the news is today in the amphetamine scene, although the number of speed users is relatively small. Speed is methamphetamine put into liquid for injection and used intravenously. It is readily but not too easily synthesized as a white powder crystal, and the mark-up from the manufacturer to the consumer is great enough to make its illegal production worthwhile. One estimate is that a pound of methamphetamine crystal can be manufactured for about $100 and sold in quarter or half ounce batches on the street for $2,500 a pound.

The street scene is changing in the world of amphetamines.

> Criminal traffic in commercially-produced amphetamines has existed since the 1930's and remains unchecked today. It was not until 1963 in California that illicitly produced methamphetamine or "speed" made its appearance, shortly after the injectable ampules of methamphetamine were voluntarily withdrawn from the market by the manufacturer . . .

> The marketplace of speed is currently undergoing rapid changes. As law enforcement pressures have increased, small amateur labs have started to disappear, with the traffic increasingly being handled by well-organized, and criminally-oriented groups. If this trend continues, we might well anticipate the entrance of organized crime into the production of speed.*

The slogans, *Speed Kills* and *Meth is Death*, contain enough truth to make them debatable. The two points of view are succinctly phrased in the preface to an excellent series of papers entitled *Speed Kills*. One author

> takes issue with the term "speed kills" indicating very few people die from direct overdosage of high dose amphetamine. The editor, however, points out that the secondary morbidity and mortality resulting from the use of amphetamines, including those deaths that occur from hepatitis, infection and violence certainly make the title *Speed Kills* appropriate.†

Intravenous amphetamine use may begin with only (!) 30 milligrams. In a long run (speed binge) of 3 or 4 days with injections occurring every 2 or 3 hours, tolerance develops rapidly and 500 to 1,000 milligrams may be injected at one time. The peripheral effects show greater tolerance than those of the central nervous system, so only moderate cardiovascular effects may occur even with high doses that still yield the euphoria. The effects of a single and repeated doses have been well described:

---

*From Task Force Report: Narcotics and drug abuse, The President's Commission on Law Enforcement and Administration of Justice, Washington, D. C., 1967, p. 30.

*From Smith, R.: Traffic in speed: illegal manufacture and distribution, Journal of Psychedelic Drugs 2(2):31, 40-41, 1969.
†From Smith, D. E.: Speed kills, Journal of Psychedelic Drugs 2(2):ii, 1969.

The physical effects of methamphetamine are quite variable depending on dose, duration of drug use, mental state and drug environment of the individual user. In general, however, after the intra-venous user injects the drug in sufficient quantity he experiences a "flash or rush" which he describes as orgasmic in nature. After this initial experience he usually becomes euphoric, with an increase in motor and speech activity. The individual may stay hyperactive for many hours with no signs of fatigue. . . .

The action phase of the "speed binge" is in effect repeated injection of the drug from one to ten times per day. With each "hit," the individual experiences the desired "flash" which the user often describes as a "full-body orgasm." Between "hits" the user is euphoric, hyperactive and hyperexcitable. This action phase of stimulation may last for several days in which the individual does not sleep and rarely eats.

For a variety of reasons this action phase terminates, however. The user may stop voluntarily because of fatigue, he may become confused, paranoid or panic-stricken and stop "shooting," or he may simply run out of drug.*

The "flash" or "splash" from amphetamine cannot be differentiated from that of cocaine, but both are uniquely distinct from that induced by heroin. The amphetamine rush produces "an abrupt awakening feeling as opposed to the drowsy, drifting effect of heroin."[27] Some individuals inject "speed balls" to obtain both effects. It is a little disconcerting to realize that this use has been around long enough so there are classic speed balls, cocaine and heroin, as well as modern speed balls, amphetamine and heroin. In both cases some people report the same effect: a brief period of intense pleasure followed by a longer, more moderate, good feeling.

If euphoria and orgasms followed by depression and hunger was the total story on the intravenous use of methamphetamine, it would not be more disturbing than other forms of drug misuse. Two additional interrelated factors make intravenous use of meth-

amphetamine particularly noteworthy. Some users develop a paranoid psychosis—so called because of the presence of hallucinations. Other heavy users only become suspicious and hostile, feelings that can lead to aggressive behavior. Because of this great potential for violence when speed users move into communes or into hallucinogen-using groups, the nonspeed users move out.

The development of a paranoid psychosis has been long known to be one of the effects of sustained cocaine use. The first amphetamine psychosis was described in 1938, but little attention was given this syndrome until the late 1950's. There have been many suggestions as to the reason for the psychosis—that heavy methamphetamine users have schizoid personalities[28] or that the psychosis is really caused by sleep deprivation, particularly dream-sleep deprivation. The question of the basis for the amphetamine psychosis was resolved by the demonstration that it could be elicited in the laboratory in individuals who clearly were not prepsychotic and who did not experience great sleep deprivation.[29] It seems, then, that the paranoid psychosis following high dose intravenous use of amphetamine is primarily the result of the drug and not the personality predisposition of the user.

The amphetamine psychosis has been studied and reported frequently and the consensus is that the psychosis is:

> . . . present as a well-defined syndrome of a paranoid state with auditory and visual hallucinations in a setting of clear consciousness. . . . two distinctive features of amphetamine psychosis are the prominence of visual hallucinations in some cases and the absence of thought disorder in all cases.*

Two other frequent effects of high doses of amphetamine deserve mention. One is the appearance of "cocaine bugs" (technically called formication). The individual feels something, bugs, crawling under his skin, and the sensation may become so great that he will use a knife to cut them out. Even without

*From Smith, D. E., and Fischer, C. M.: High dose methamphetamine abuse in the Haight-Ashbury. Section 4: Drug abuse of the stimulant type. In Smith, D. E., editor: Drug abuse papers 1969, ed. 2, Berkeley, 1969, University of California, p. 2.

*From Bell, D. S.: Comparison of amphetamine psychosis and schizophrenia, British Journal of Psychiatry **III**:706, 1965.

this extreme reaction the heavy amphetamine user may have many open sores as a result of his picking at the bugs. The basis for this experience is probably a drug-induced stimulation of nerve endings in the skin, but the mechanism is not yet clear.[30]

The other drug-induced behavior that appears is compulsive and repetitive actions. The behavior may be acceptable, the individual may compulsively clean a room over and over, or it may be bizarre. There is precedent for this stereotyped behavior in animal studies with high doses of amphetamine, and the suggestion has been made that it results from an effect of amphetamine on dopaminergic systems in the basal ganglia.[31]

Still being debated is the evidence that the use of intravenous amphetamines may be related to constriction of arteries in the brain, possibly causing strokes even in teen-agers.[31a, 31b] Also not settled is the question of physical addiction to amphetamines. Certain regular features occur in abstinence such as depression, overeating, and extreme fatigue, but usually go away in a week. Importantly, abrupt cessation of regular high doses of amphetamine is not life-threatening and convulsions never occur. In some instances the depression may persist; it is not clear whether this is a result of the amphetamine abstinence or a part of the personality of the individual that led him initially to use stimulants.[32]

Summary. Amphetamine can be misused in many ways, and it is. These different forms of misuse are not very closely related; the housewife using amphetamine regularly for "weight control" is as far from the speed freak as a heavy coffee drinker is from a cocaine user. The motivations, dosage form, social atmosphere, and end result are different. There is not an amphetamine problem, there are several amphetamine problems; the answer to one is not the answer to the others.[32a]

DEPRESSANT DRUGS

As mentioned at the beginning of this chapter, "sedatives and hypnotics are both depressants of the central nervous system, but in one case the intention is to relieve anxiety or restlessness and in the other it is to induce sleep. Many drugs may therefore be used in either capacity, depending upon the dose and the time of day that they are given."[33] The most widely used drug in this general category is alcohol. The second most commonly used depressant drugs are the barbiturates, with about 10 billion sedative doses being manufactured each year in the United States.[34]

Nonbarbiturates

Three other central nervous system depressants have a longer history than the barbiturates but are rarely prescribed today. Chloral hydrate and paraldehyde have chemical and pharmacological characteristics much like alcohol, while the bromides are different.

Chloral hydrate was synthesized in 1832 but was not used clinically until about 1870. It is rapidly metabolized to trichloroethanol, which is the active hypnotic agent. When taken orally, chloral hydrate has a short onset period (30 minutes), and 1 to 2 grams will induce sleep in less than an hour. This agent does not cause as much depression of the respiratory and cardiovascular systems as a comparable dose of the barbiturates and has fewer aftereffects. A disadvantage is that it is a gastric irritant and repeated use causes considerable stomach upset. Chloral hydrate in combination with alcohol is the famous Mickey Finn used before 1900 to knock out sailors so they could be shanghaied for the long trips to the Orient.

No such use ever occurred with paraldehyde, which was synthesized in 1829 and introduced clinically in 1882. Paraldehyde would probably be in great use today because of its effectiveness as a central nervous system depressant with little respiratory depression and a wide safety margin, except for one characteristic. It has a most noxious taste and odor that permeates the breath of the user.

The bromides are little used today except in OTC sleep preparations, and there is debate over whether the low amounts used have any sedative effect at all. Bromides do accumulate in the body, and the depression they cause builds up over several days of regular use. There are serious toxic side effects with repeated hypnotic doses of these agents. Dermatitis and constipation are minor accompaniments; with increased intake, motor disturbances, delirium, and psychosis develop.

Although the prescription drug methaqualone was introduced to the United States in 1965, it was 1971 before it began soaring in popularity to become *the* sedative of abuse for young people in 1974. Methaqualone is more addicting and more medically dangerous than the barbiturates, but not until 1973 did the government place it under Schedule II.[34a]

Barbiturates

History may not be strange, but records of history frequently are. On the fourth of December, 1862, one of the following things occurred in Munich, Germany. Dr. A. Bayer (yes, it's that Bayer) left the laboratory early to visit a tavern because he had successfully combined urea with malonic acid and made a new compound. A compound must have a name and perhaps "Barbara's urates" were so named by Bayer

> . . . because he wished to commemorate Barbara, a person he held in affectionate regard—a Munich waitress perhaps?—who gave him samples of urine for research purposes.*
> . . . Bayer celebrated the occasion of the synthesis of the new compound by visiting a nearby tavern frequented by artillery officers. It happened that it was the Day of St. Barbara, the patron saint of artillery officers, and in the ensuing festivities *Barbara* was amalgamated with *urea* to give the new compound its name.†

The new compound was barbituric acid, which is *not* a central nervous system depressant. The barbiturates, which are derived from it, are excellent central nervous system depressants. Over 2,500 barbiturates have been synthesized. Some of the best are among the oldest, although barbital (Veronal), the first to be used clinically in 1903, is little used today. It did start the practice of giving barbiturates names ending in -*al*. The second

barbiturate in clinical use, phenobarbital (Luminal), was introduced in 1912 and is still one of the widest used and best compounds in this class. Amobarbital (Amytal) in 1923, as well as pentobarbital (Nembutal) and secobarbital (Seconal), both introduced in 1930, are well-established and widely used examples of the barbiturates.

As Fig. 11-3 indicates, barbiturates are typically grouped on the basis of the duration of their activity. Some researchers do not feel that this categorization can be validated experimentally,[35] but other authorities report that the classification is meaningful. A standard reference book[36] indicates differences between the short, intermediate, and long-acting agents in both the delay to onset of action and the duration of action. The approximate time intervals are given in Table 11-1. The grouping of these agents on the basis of their duration of action is supported by their rate of metabolism. The short-acting barbiturates are very lipid soluble and are deactivated at a rate of about 2.5% per hour. Deactivation of the long-acting agents is at about one-third or one-fourth that rate (0.7% per hour).[37]

Deactivation occurs in the liver. The barbiturates are one of the classes of drugs that stimulate the activity of the microsomal enzymes of the liver. Perhaps some of the tolerance that develops to the barbiturates is the result of an increased rate of deactivation caused by this stimulation of microsomal enzymes. Tolerance does develop gradually and the dosage must be increased periodically to maintain a constant effect. Physical addiction dependence also occurs and, when the daily dose rises above 400 milligrams, some major withdrawal symptoms will occur following abrupt termination of use. Addiction and withdrawal will be discussed in the next section.

*From Hordern, A.: The barbiturates. In Joyce, C. R. B., editor: Psychopharmacology: dimensions and perspectives, Philadelphia, 1968, J. B. Lippincott Co., p. 118.
†From Sharpless, S. K.: Hypnotics and sedatives. In Goodman, L., and Gilman, A., editors: The pharmacological basis of therapeutics, New York, 1970, The Macmillan Co., pp. 98, 100, and 103.

Table 11-1

	Time to onset (hours)	Duration of action (hours)
Long	1	6 to 10
Intermediate	1/2	5 to 6
Short	1/4	2 to 3

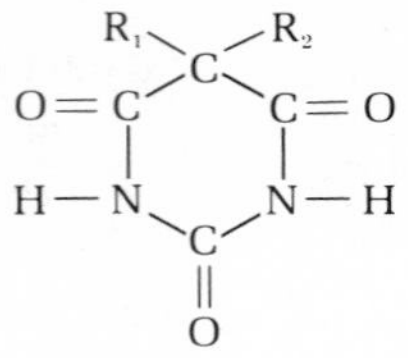

Generic name	Brand name	R₁	R₂
		R_1	R_2

Long-acting

| Barbital | Veronal | $-CH_2-CH_3$ | $-CH_2-CH_3$ |
| Phenobarbital* | Luminal | $-CH_2-CH_3$ | 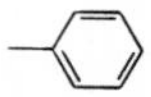 (phenyl ring) |

Intermediate-acting

| Amobarbital | Amytal | $-CH_2-CH_3$ | $-CH_2-CH_2-CH-CH_3$ with CH_3 |

Short-acting

| Pentobarbital | Nembutal | $-CH_2-CH_3$ | $-CH-CH_2-CH_2-CH_3$ with CH_3 |
| Secobarbital | Seconal | $-CH_2-CH=CH_2$ | $-CH-CH_2-CH_2-CH_3$ with CH_3 |

*Chemical name is 5-ethyl-5-phenylmalonylurea.

Fig. 11-3. Barbiturates.

The barbiturates have their primary effect on chemical transmission at the synapse, not on conduction in the neuron. The basic mechanism in the central nervous system has not yet been determined, but it is probably related to the depression of oxidative metabolism, which is one of the primary biochemical effects of these agents. A general lowering of brain excitability, as in the case of alcohol, sometimes releases behavior from inhibition. In the initial stages of these drugs' effects there may be some loss of inhibition, euphoria, and behavioral stimulation. The multisynaptic pathways such as the reticular system are among the first to be depressed. This occurs before the primary sensory or motor pathways are affected. At clinical doses:

> the CNS is exquisitely sensitive to the barbiturates, so that, when the drugs are given in sedative or hypnotic doses, direct actions on peripheral structures are absent or negligible.*

*From Sharpless, S. K., op. cit.

In normal therapeutic use, the barbiturates are not particularly toxic agents, but they have additive central nervous system effects with other depressants such as alcohol. There are many reported cases of death caused by respiratory failure resulting from the use of barbiturates as a sleeping aid at the end of an evening of alcohol intake.

Use and misuse. Barbiturates account for 20% of mood-changing prescriptions and are used for anxiety, insomnia, anesthesia, and epilepsy. Barbiturates for the treatment of anxiety have been in large part replaced by the antianxiety agents, even though there is no good evidence that they are more effective. For this antianxiety, sedative, purpose secobarbital or pentobarbital is prescribed at a dosage level of 25 to 35 milligrams three times a day.

Insomnia is a not uncommon problem. Most insomniacs have difficulty falling asleep as well as remaining asleep throughout the night. A dose of 100 or, at the most, 200 milligrams of secobarbital or pentobarbital before bed is usually effective in helping the insomniac get to sleep and stay asleep. Some problems do occur, however. One is the barbiturate hangover, the residual sedation that exists after the drug-assisted sleep ends. Even routine users sometimes require so great a dosage of a barbiturate to get and stay asleep that the drug effects are not gone in the morning. One study showed performance decrements 22 hours after 200 milligrams of secobarbital prior to bedtime, that is, the sedative effects were still measurable almost at bedtime the next evening.[38] As a result, an amphetamine or other stimulant is frequently used in the morning to counteract the remaining sedative effects.

Another problem may be that the barbiturates decrease the amount of sleep time spent in dreaming. The scientific study of dreaming behavior is just beginning, but some evidence suggests that it is psychologically healthy to dream three to six times each night. In addition, when an individual who has been using barbiturates regularly as a sleeping pill suddenly stops using them, he may over-dream or even have nightmares.

The evidence is difficult to obtain, but perhaps sometimes an accidentally fatal problem develops with the barbiturates or any hypnotic. After the regular sleeping dose has been taken, the individual may doze briefly and then awaken slightly sedated. In this condition he may be confused about whether he has taken his medication and may then take a second dose or even more—sometimes a fatal amount.

Since the effects of barbiturate intoxication are similar to those with alcohol, it is not surprising that the barbiturates are frequently misused. It has also been reported that under some conditions the barbiturates are not dissimilar in their effects from the opiates.[39]

Although the clinical use of the barbiturates began in 1903 and the first reference to barbiturate intoxication and withdrawal convulsions was in 1905, it was not until 1950 that a controlled study was published that conclusively showed physical dependency to the barbiturates.[40] There may be some anxiety and slight muscle twitches that develop when even a daily dose of 200 to 300 milligrams of pentobarbital or secobarbital is abruptly terminated. A level of 400 milligrams per day seems to be crucial for the development of convulsions and/or psychosis on withdrawal. As the daily dose increases above that amount, the probability of these symptoms increases. There is enough communality between alcohol addiction and barbiturate addiction that taking one drug can prevent the occurrence of withdrawal effects to the other agent.

Although it is probably more socially acceptable to be addicted to the oral use of the barbiturates than to require narcotics intravenously, the barbiturate addiction is medically more serious, as can be seen from the effects of abstinence. The barbiturate abstinence syndrome has been repeatedly described, but none has done better in summarizing the effects than one of the first American reports in 1953.

> Upon abrupt withdrawal of barbiturates from individuals who have been ingesting 0.8 gm. or more daily of one of the potent barbiturates (secobarbital, pentobarbital, amobarbital), signs of barbiturate intoxication disappear in the first 8-12 hours of abstinence, and, clinically, the patient seems to improve. Thereafter, increasing anxiety, insomnia, tremulousness,

weakness, difficulty in making cardiovascular adjustments on standing, anorexia, nausea and vomiting appear. One or more convulsions of grand mal type usually occur during the second or third day of abstinence. Following the seizures, a psychosis characterized by confusion, disorientation in time and place, agitation, tremulousness, insomnia, delusions and visual and auditory hallucinations may supervene. The psychosis clinically resembles alcoholic delirium tremens, usually begins and is worse at night, and terminates abruptly with a critical sleep.*

The world has taken little note of another misuse of the barbiturates—suicide. When a lethal dose is taken, there is little opportunity to change one's mind, since loss of consciousness occurs within a few minutes. The barbiturates are the single most frequently used class of drugs for suicide and in 1970 were taken in about 1,500 suicides.

Summary. The barbiturates are being used and misused greatly in the United States. Over 300 tons are manufactured each year and almost half probably end up in illegal channels. From the antianxiety pill popper to the heavy user for the induction of sleep, legal barbiturate misuse is second only to alcohol. Alcohol and the barbiturates are difficult drugs to use if one wishes to maintain a euphoric mood, since usually the user slips into sedation. In spite of the dangers and problems, depressant drug use by the young increased rapidly in the early 1970's, and 1972 was labeled the year of the "barbs."

CONCLUDING COMMENT

The uppers and the downers. It is perhaps worthwhile to reemphasize here that these drugs, especially the amphetamines and the barbiturates, are primarily misused by older individuals. Their misuse is not as spectacular as that of the speed freak, but the misuse is more consistent and more widespread. It is reassuring to know that all is not a series of fads in the world of drug misuse—there are some groups you can count on to misuse drugs: overweight and fatigued matrons and hyper-

*From Fraser, H. F., and others: Death due to withdrawal of barbiturates, Annals of Internal Medicine **38:**1319-1320, 1953.

excitable and anxious housewives and businessmen.

PRECEDING QUOTES
1. Benzedrine alert, Air Surgeon's Bulletin **1**(2):19-21, 1944.
2. Crime in America—why eight billion amphetamines? Hearings before the Select Committee on Crime, House of Representatives, Ninety-first Congress, First Session, Washington, D. C., 1970, U. S. Government Printing Office, p. 17.
3. Smith, D., Wesson, D., and Lannon, R.: New developments in barbiturate abuse. In Smith, D., editor: Drug abuse papers, 1969, University of California.

REFERENCES
1. Taylor, N.: Plant drugs that changed the world, New York, 1965, Dodd, Mead & Co., p. 12.
2. Taylor, N.: Flight from reality, New York, 1949, Duell, Sloan and Pearce.
3. Holmstedt, B.: Historical survey. In Efron, D. H., editor: Ethnopharmacologic search for psychoactive drugs, Public Health Service Publication No. 1645, Washington, D.C., 1967, U.S. Government Printing Office, p. 17.
4. Hecht, R., and Sargent, S. S.: Effects of benzedrine sulfate on performance in two tests of higher mental functions, Journal of Experimental Psychology **28:**532, 1941.
5. Bloomquist, E. R.: The use and abuse of stimulants. In Clark, W. G., and del Giudice, J., editors: Principles of psychopharmacology, New York, 1970, Academic Press, Inc., pp. 477-488.
6. Benzedrine alert, Air Surgeon's Bulletin **1**(2):19-21, 1944.
7. Monroe, R. R., and Drell, H. J.: Oral use of stimulants obtained from inhalers, Journal of the American Medical Association **135:**909-915, 1947.
8. Crime in America—why eight billion amphetamines? Hearings before the Select Committee on Crime, House of Representatives, Ninety-first Congress, First Session, Washington, D.C., 1970, U.S. Government Printing Office, p. 44.
9. Hemmi, T.: How we have handled the problem of drug abuse in Japan. In Sjöqvist, F., and Tottie, M., editors: Abuse of central stimulants, New York, 1969, Raven Press, p. 148.
10. FDA orders curbs on amphetamine claims, American Druggist **162:**16, August 24, 1970.
11. Millichap, J. G., and Fowler, G. W.: Treatment of "minimal brain dysfunction" syndromes: selection of drugs for children with hyperactivity and learning disabilities, Pediatric Clinics of North America **14**(4):767-777, 1967.
12. Drug slows over-activity in children, American Druggist **161:**66, January 26, 1970.
13. FDA warns against uses of "behavior" amphetamines, The Washington Post, September 30, 1970, p. A3.

14. Stimulants calm overactive kids, American Druggist **162**:37, August 24, 1970.

15. Conners, C. K.: The effect of dexedrine on rapid discrimination and motor control of hyperkinetic children under mild stress, Journal of Nervous and Mental Disease **142**(5):429-433, 1966.

16. Behavior changing drugs questioned, Associated-Press, November 8, 1970.

17. Wagner, M. G.: The irony of affluence, Journal of the American Dietetic Association **57**:311-315, 1970.

18. Obesity: a continuing enigma, Journal of the American Medical Association **211**(3):492-493, 1970.

19. Dwyer, J. T., and Mayer, J.: Potential dieters: who are they? Journal of the American Dietetic Association **56**:510-514, 1970.

19a. Cole, S.: Hypothalamic feeding mechanisms and amphetamine anorexia, Psychological Bulletin **79**(1):13-20, 1973.

20. Stunkard, A. J.: Environment and obesity: recent advances in our understanding of regulation of food intake in man, Federation Proceedings **27**(6):1367-1373, 1968.

21. Schachter, S.: Some extraordinary facts about obese humans and rats, American Psychologist **26**(2):129-144, 1971.

22. Thompson, T., and Pickens, R.: Stimulant self-administration by animals: some comparisons with opiate self-administration, Federation Proceedings **29**(1):6-12, 1970.

23. Sulser, F., and Sanders-Bush, E.: Biochemical and metabolic considerations concerning the mechanism of action of amphetamine and related compounds. In Efron, D. H., editor: Psychotomimetic drugs, New York, 1970, Raven Press, pp. 83-94.

24. Weiss, B.: Enhancement of performance by amphetamine-like drugs. In Sjöqvist, F., and Tottie, M., editors: Abuse of central stimulants, New York, 1969, Raven Press, p. 54.

25. Smith, G. M., and Beecher, H. K.: Amphetamine sulfate and athletic performance, Journal of the American Medical Association **170**(5):557, 1959.

26. Pierson, W. R.: Amphetamine sulfate and performance (a critique), Journal of the American Medical Association **177**(5):345-349, 1971.

26a. New York Times, June 28, 1973, p. C62.

26b. Use of d-amphetamine and related central nervous system stimulants in children, Pediatrics **51**:302-305, 1973.

27. Kramer, J. C., Fischman, V., and Littlefield, D. C.: Amphetamine abuse, Journal of the American Medical Association **201**(5):307, 1967.

28. Ellinwood, E. H.: Amphetamine psychosis: I. Description of the individuals and process, Journal of Nervous and Mental Disease **144**:273, 1967.

29. Griffith, J. D., and others: Experimental psychosis induced by the administration of d-amphetamine. In Costa, E., and Garattini, S., editors: Amphetamines and related compounds, Proceedings of the Mario Negri Institute for Pharmacological Research, Milan, Italy, New York, 1970, Raven Press.

30. Ellinwood, E. H.: Amphetamine psychosis: a multi-dimensional process, Seminars in Psychiatry **6**:208-226, 1969.

31. Ellinwood, E. H., and Cohen, S.: Amphetamine abuse, Science **171**:420-421, 1971.

31a. Rumbaugh, C. L., Bergerton, R. T., Fang, H. C., and McCormick, R.: Cerebral angiographic changes in the drug abuse patient, Radiology **101**:335-344, 1971.

31b. Rumbaugh, C. L., Bergerton, R. T., Scanlan, R. L., Teal, J. S., Segall, H. D., Fang, H. C., and McCormick, R.: Cerebral vascular changes secondary to amphetamine abuse in the experimental animal, Radiology **101**:345-351, 1971.

32. Connell, P. H.: The use and abuse of amphetamines, The Practitioner **200**:234-243, 1968.

32a. The politics of uppers and downers, Journal of Psychedelic Drugs **5**(2), Winter, 1972. Entire issue.

33. Hinton, J.: Sedatives and hypnotics, The Practitioner **200**:93, 1968.

34. Synthetic drugs used and abused, Chemical and Engineering News **48**:26, 1970.

34a. Perry, C.: Unconsciousness expansion: the Sopor story, Rolling Stone **131**:1, 1973.

35. Hinton, J. M.: A comparison of the effects of six barbiturates and a placebo on insomnia and motility in psychiatric patients, British Journal of Pharmacology **20**:319-325, 1963.

36. Martindale, W.: Extra pharmacopoeia, ed. 25, London, 1967, The Pharmaceutical Press, pp. 183-184.

37. Haddon, J., and others: Acute barbiturate poisoning, Journal of the American Medical Association **209**(6):893-900, 1969.

38. Sharpless, S. K.: Hypnotics and sedatives. In Goodman, L., and Gilman, A., editors: The pharmacological basis of therapeutics, New York, 1970, The Macmillan Co., pp. 98, 100, and 103.

39. Long, R. E., and Penna, R. P.: Drugs of abuse. In Drug abuse education, ed. 2, Washington, D. C., 1969, American Pharmaceutical Association, p. 8.

40. Essig, C.: Drug dependence of the barbiturate type, Drug Dependence **5**:24-27, 1970.

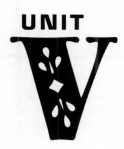

UNIT

V

The narcotic drugs

12 Opiates through the ages

...I cannot forbear mentioning with gratitude the goodness of the
Supreme Being, who has supplied afflicted mankind with opiates for their
relief; no other remedy being equally powerful to overcome a great
number of diseases, or to eradicate them effectually.

Dr. Thomas Sydenham, 1680

...thou hast the keys of Paradise, O just, subtle, and mighty opium!

Confessions of an English Opium-Eater
Thomas De Quincey, 1822

To tell a smoker in a continuous state of euphorion that he is degrading
himself, is equivalent to telling a piece of marble that it has deteriorated
through Michael Angelo, or a piece of canvas, that it has been stained
by Raphael, a piece of paper that it has been soiled by Shakespeare,
or silence, that it has been broken by Bach.

Opium: The Diary of an Addict
Jean Cocteau, 1933

"H" is for heaven; "H" is for hell; "H" is for heroin. In the life of the
addict, these three meanings of "H" seem inextricably intertwined.

The Road to H
Isador Chein, 1964

The thing about heroin is that it gives a human being a purpose in life.
It gives him an occupation, an identity, friends, a chance to be better at
something and above all it takes up time.

A 16-year-old junkie in the East Village, 1971

Heroin is a drug of despair. It fits in well with the growing pessimism
of the radical youth culture. The optimism of the flower children is gone.
The youngsters are moving from drugs that expand the consciousness
to ones that constrict it.

Dr. David E. Smith, 1970

...and soon they found themselves in the midst of a great meadow of poppies. Now it is well known that when there are many of these flowers together their odor is so powerful that anyone who breathes it falls asleep, and if the sleeper is not carried away from the scent of the flowers he sleeps on and on forever. But Dorothy did not know this, nor could she get away from the bright red flowers that were everywhere about; so presently her eyes grew heavy and she felt she must sit down to rest and to sleep.... Her eyes closed in spite of herself and she forgot where she was and fell among the poppies, fast asleep.... They carried the sleeping girl to a pretty spot beside the river, far enough from the poppy field to prevent her breathing any more of the poison of the flowers, and here they laid her gently on the soft grass and waited for the fresh breeze to waken her.*

From the land of Oz to the streets of Harlem the white poppy has caused much grief—and much joy. Opium is a truly unique compound. This juice from the plant *Papaver somniferum* has a history of medical use almost 6,000 years long. Except for the last century and a half, opium stood alone as the one agent physicians could use and obtain sure results. Compounds containing opium solved several of the recurring problems for medical science wherever used. Opium relieved pain and suffering magnificently. It induced sleep easily. Just as important in the years gone by was its ability to correct dysentery, the resulting constipation being one of the regular problems of opiate users today. Its reputation and use as an aphrodisiac have persisted through the ages, but its real effect is to prolong performance and thus increase the gratification of the user's partner.

Parallel with the medical use of opium was its use as a deliverer of pleasure and relief from anxiety. Because of these effects, extensive recreational use of opium also occurred. Soon after 1800 Frederich Serturner opened the alkaloid century by isolating morphine, the primary psychoactive agent in opium. Opium, smoked or eaten, and morphine, injected or oral, created the first period of widespread and frequent use of narcotics in this country before the turn of the twentieth

*From Baum, L. F.: The new wizard of Oz, New York, 1944, Grosset & Dunlap, Inc., pp. 69, 70, 72.

century. Heroin, which became available only three generations ago, is a more active form of morphine and, used by injection, has been the drug of choice in recent years.

With a history longer than that of all other psychoactive agents except alcohol, it should not be surprising that opium and the drugs related to it have been important in the medical and social history of the world. As the complexity of opium becomes apparent in the following pages, it will also be understandable that the actions it and its derivatives have on the brain are for the most part still a mystery.

EARLY HISTORY

The written story of opium begins 4,000 years before the birth of Christ with a reference to the "joy plant" on a Sumerian tablet. The same symbol appears 3,300 years later along with a description of the method used to harvest the opium: "Early in the morning old women, boys and girls collect the juice by scraping it off the wounds [of the poppy capsule] with a small iron scoope, and deposit the whole in an earthen pot."[1]

In a hot, dry, Middle East country several millennia ago, some unknown native discovered that for 7 to 10 days of its year-long life *Papaver somniferum* produced a substance that, when eaten, would ease pain and suffering. The opium poppy is an annual plant and opium is produced and available for collection for only a few days, between the time the petals drop and before the seed pod matures. Today, as before, to harvest the opium, workers move through the fields toward evening and use a sharp multiclawed tool to make shallow cuts into, but not through, the unripe seed pod. During the night a white substance oozes from the cuts, oxidizes to a red-brown color, and becomes gummy. In the morning the resinous substance is carefully scraped from the pod and collected in small balls. This raw opium forms the basis for the opium medicines used through history and is the substance from which morphine is extracted and then heroin is derived.

The importance and extent of use of the opium poppy in the early Egyptian and Greek cultures is still debated, but in the Ebers papyrus (circa 1500 B.C.) reference is made to a remedy "to prevent the excessive crying of children." Since a later Egyptian remedy for the same purpose clearly contained opium (as well as fly excrement), as does the western culture's remedy for this problem, paregoric (opium and alcohol), many writers report the first specific medical use of opium as dating from the Ebers papyrus.

Homer's *Odyssey* (1000 B.C.) contains a passage that some authors feel refers to the use of opium. A party was about to become a real bore since everyone was sad thinking about Ulysses and the deaths of their friends when:

> ... Helen, daughter of Zeus, poured into the wine they were drinking a drug, nepenthes, which gave forgetfulness of evil. Those who had drunk of this mixture did not shed a tear the whole day long, even though their mother or father were dead, even though a brother or beloved son had been killed before their eyes ...*

The drug could only have been opium.

The classical literature of Virgil and Ovid contains references to the sleep-producing poppy. The Greek god of sleep, Hypnos, as well as the Roman god of sleep, Somnus, usually was adorned with or carried poppies and sometimes an opium container. Unlike the sandman of today pouring sand into the eyes of children, Somnus was frequently pictured pouring juice from the container into the eyes of the sleeper. Greek mythology suggests that Ceres created the poppy so she could sleep and thus forget that her daughter had been given to Pluto. The Chinese legend has the poppy plant springing up from the earth where Buddha's eyelids fell when he cut them off to prevent sleep. Since seeds of the opium plant were carried to China only about 600 or 700 A.D., it would seem that the Greek legend has more validity!

Although Hippocrates was not an advocate of opium or the poppy, one of his remedies probably referred to it. A hundred years later, about 300 B.C., a Greek physician provided a

method for extracting poppy juice (meconium) by grinding the entire plant, but not until the first century A.D. was the extraction of opium clearly differentiated from meconium in Greek writings. Beginning around this period, the spread of opium use and poppy cultivation grew rapidly, and the Greek word *opius*, meaning "little juice," came into written records. Derivations and modifications of *opius* have been used as the term for the poppy sap in Arabic, Chinese, and English.

Opium was important in Greek medicine and Galen, the last of the great Greek physicians, felt that opium was almost a cure-all. It

> ... resists poison and venomous bites, cures chronic headache, vertigo, deafness, epilepsy, apoplexy, dimness of sight, loss of voice, asthma, coughs of all kinds, spitting of blood, tightness of breath, colic, the iliac poison, jaundice, hardness of the spleen, stone, urinary complaints, fevers, dropsies, leprosies, the troubles to which women are subject, melancholy and all pestilences.*

Recreational use even then must have been extensive, since Galen commented on the opium cakes and candies that were being sold everywhere in the streets. The medical use of opium was common in this period. Although the concepts of addiction and withdrawal had not yet been established, a recent writer suggests that the reports on the behavior and health of the Roman Emperor in this period, Marcus Aurelius, clearly indicate that he was addicted to opium and occasionally suffered withdrawal symptoms.[2]

Greek knowledge of opium use in medicine died with the decline of the Roman Empire and thus had little influence on the world's use of opium for the next 1,000 years. To the south in North Africa, though, the Arabic world clutched opium (and hashish) to its breast since the Koran forbade the use of alcohol in any form. Opium and hashish became the primary social drugs wherever the Islam culture moved, and it did move. The Mohammedans were active fighters, explorers, and traders. While Europe rested through the

---

*From Scott, J. M.: The white poppy: a history of opium, New York, 1969, Funk & Wagnalls, p. 6.

*From Scott, op. cit., p. 111.

Dark Ages the Arabian world reached out and made contact with India and China. Opium was one of the products they traded, but they also sold the seeds of the opium poppy and home cultivation began in these countries. By the tenth century A.D., opium was referred to in Chinese medical writings.

During this period when the Arabian civilization flourished, two Arabian physicians made substantial contributions to medicine and to the history of opium. Shortly after 1000 A.D., Biruni composed a pharmacology book. In his descriptions of opium was what some believe to be the first written description of addiction.[3] In this same period, the best-known Arabian physician, Avicenna, was using opium preparations very effectively and extensively in his medical practice. His writings, along with those of Galen, formed the basis of medical education in Europe as the Renaissance dawned, and thus the glories of opium were advanced. (Strange but true that a physician as knowledgeable as Avicenna, and a believer in the tenets of Mohammedanism, should die as a result of drinking too much of a mixture of opium and wine. Perhaps, as some suggest, he has been overrated as a physician.)

Early in the sixteenth century, European medicine had a happening by the name of Paracelsus. A true iconoclast and Renaissance man, he denounced all the famous medics of history—Hippocrates, Galen, Avicenna—as well as his contemporaries. He apparently was a successful clinician and accomplished some wondrous cures for the day. One of the secrets of Paracelsus was a potion called laudanum. Although it is not clear that his laudanum contained opium, he did use opium very extensively in his treatment of patients. Paracelsus was one of the early Renaissance supporters of opium as a panacea and referred to it as the "stone of immortality." According to a later writer (1701) Paracelsus believed that opium "... will dissolve Diseases, as Fire does Snow...."[1]

To this point in history there is no clear evidence that the regular use of opium was recognized as producing changes in the body that required continued use of the drug for normal functioning. Since the Roman period there had been incidental reports of tolerance to the drug so that larger and larger quantities were needed to obtain the same effect. There were also reports of discomfort at times in habitual opium users that could be relieved by the ingestion of more opium, but the concept of addiction was not delineated. Not until the last half of the sixteenth century was a clear association formed between discontinuing regular use of opium and the appearance of certain symptoms that we now call the withdrawal syndrome.

The first report of clearly addicted individuals appeared in 1563 when a Portuguese explorer, Garcia da Orta, commented on the use of opium in India. A better description, however, is from the German physician Rauwolf, who reported on his travels in the 1570's in the Middle East.

> Not least of all one finds there (namely in the bazaar of Aleppo) also a trade by pharmacists in opium (the inhabitants call it 'Ofiun'), which the Turks, Moors, Persians, and still other peoples are in the habit of taking—not alone during wars, to make them of good heart and strong courage at the time when they are to fight the enemy—but also at times of peace, to take away troubles and deliriums, or at least to alleviate them. Also their men of religion eat this, but particularly among others, the Dervishes; and they take so much of it that they thereupon immediately become sleepy and go out of their senses, so that when they, in their mad habit, cut, hack or burn themselves, they find the pains and sufferings much less. When now one or more thereby have thus begun (they in the habit of taking as much of it as the size of a pea without danger), then can they never more leave off therefrom, it being as if they sink into a sickness, or at least other new hazards are ready to excite them, as they themselves confess, if they leave off somewhat taking it, so that then they feel physically ill.*

Because of the increasing awareness of the broad effectiveness of opium as a result of Paracelsus and his followers, a variety of new opium preparations was developed in the sixteenth, seventeenth, and eighteenth centuries. Only two will be mentioned, partly

*From Sonnedecker, G.: Emergence of the concept of opiate addiction, Journal Mondial de Pharmacie: Federation Internationale Pharmaceutique 3:275-290, 1962; 1:27-34, 1963.

because of their importance in medical history and partly because they are still available today by the same names in many places. The first compound is laudanum, as prepared by Dr. Thomas Sydenham, the father of clinical medicine. (Although the name is the same as Paracelsus' compound, this seems to be the only similarity.) Sydenham's general contributions to English medicine are so great that he has been called the English Hippocrates. He spoke more highly of opium than did Paracelsus, saying that "without opium the healing art would cease to exist." His laudanum contained 2 ounces of strained opium, 1 ounce of saffron, and a dram of cinnamon and of cloves dissolved in 1 pint of Canary wine and taken in small quantities.

Thomas Dover, a resident of Sydenham's house and possibly his student, concocted an even more potent preparation of opium. Dover never did complete medical training, but he practiced medicine for 24 years before kicking over the traces in 1708 and commanding a ship on an around-the-world voyage. During his medical career, Dover made his claim to fame and fortune with Dover's Powder. Originally, it contained 1 ounce each of opium, ipecac, and licorice and 4 ounces each of saltpeter and tartar. The dose was about 100 grains of this mixture taken in wine. This quantity was so potent that even Dover admitted that the apothecaries wanted the patients to make their wills before taking the medicine. But it did provide relief from pain.

Thomas Dover can mark the end of an era. In the nineteenth century, big things happened to opium in the hands of the chemist that began to change the nature of the story. Also in the nineteenth century, opium and hashish became the touchstones for a number of famous writers in England and France. In this same period, Britain became the opium pusher for China and indirectly set the stage for the opiate addiction problem of today.

Writers and opium: liquid sky and the milk of paradise

In a momentous year for opium, 1805, Thomas De Quincey, a 20-year-old English youth who had run away from home at 17, purchased some laudanum for a toothache and received change for his shilling from the apothecary. His response to this dose was described:

> . . . I took it: and in an hour, O heavens! What a revulsion! what a resurrection from its lowest depths, of the inner spirit! what an apocalypse of the world within me! That my pains had vanished was now a trifle in my eyes; this negative effect was swallowed up in the immensity of those positive effects which had opened up before me, in the abyss of divine enjoyment thus suddenly revealed. Here was a panacea . . . for all human woes; here was the secret of happiness, about which philosophers had disputed for so many ages, at once discovered; happiness might now be bought for a penny, and carried in the waistcoat-pocket; portable ecstasies might be had corked up in a pint-bottle; and peace of mind could be sent down by the mail.*

For the rest of his life De Quincey used laudanum, although he probably was no longer addicted at his death. He did not try to conceal the extent of his addiction. Rather, his writings are replete with insight into the opiate-hazed world, particularly his article "The Confessions of an English Opium-Eater," which was published in 1821 (and in book form in 1823).

Several other famous English authors were also addicted to laudanum, including Elizabeth Barrett Browning and Samuel Taylor Coleridge.[4-6] Coleridge's magnificently beautiful "Kubla Khan" was conceived and composed in an opium reverie and then written down as best he could remember it. However, De Quincey is of primary interest here, as Baudelaire will be with hashish. His emphasis was on understanding the effects that opium has on consciousness, experience, and feeling, and as such he provided some of the most vivid accounts of the power of opium.

Opium does not produce new worlds for the user.

> If a man, "whose talk is of oxen," should become an opium-eater, the probability is, that (if he is not too dull to dream at all)—he will dream about oxen: whereas, in the case before him [De Quincey], the reader will find that the opium-eater boasteth himself to be a philosopher; and accordingly, that the phan-

*From De Quincey, T.: Confessions of an English opium-eater, New York, 1907, E. P. Dutton & Co., Inc., p. 179.

tasmagoria of *his* dreams (waking or sleeping, day-dreams or night dreams) is suitable to one [of] that character. . . .*

Opium does, however, change the way the world is perceived. For example, ". . . an opium eater is too happy to observe the motion of time."[7] De Quincey wrote about the added dimensions to sounds and music that occurred when he attended the opera while using opium.

> . . . It is by the reaction of the mind upon the notices of the ear (the *matter* coming by the senses, the *form* from the mind) that the pleasure is constructed. . . . Now opium, by greatly increasing the activity of the mind, generally increases. . . its activity by which we are able to construct out of the raw material of organic sound an elaborate intellectual pleasure.†

The contrast between the feelings, effects, and experiences that result from alcohol were discussed extensively and sharply contrasted with those accompanying the use of opium.

> . . . crude opium . . . is incapable of producing any state of body at all resembling that which is produced by alcohol . . . it is not in the quantity of its effects merely, but in the quality, that it differs altogether. The pleasure given by wine is always rapidly mounting, and tending to a crisis, after which as rapidly it declines; that from opium, when once generated, is stationary for eight or ten hours . . . the one is a flickering flame, the other a steady and equable glow. But the main distinction lies in this—that, whereas wine disorders the mental faculties, opium, on the contrary (if taken in a proper manner), introduces amongst them the most exquisite order, legislation, and harmony. Wine robs a man of his self-possession; opium sustains and reinforces it. Wine unsettles the judgment . . . opium, on the contrary, communicates serenity and equipoise to all the faculties . . .‡

In spite of all the good things De Quincey said about opium and the effects it had on him, he suffered from its use. For long periods in his life he was unable to write as a result of his addiction. As with most things: "Opium gives and takes away. It defeats the *steady*

*From Turk, M. H.: Selections from De Quincey, Boston, 1902, Ginn and Company, p. 156.
†From De Quincey, op. cit., p. 189.
‡ Ibid., pp. 180-181.

habit of exertion; but it creates spasms of irregular exertion. It ruins the natural power of life; but it developes preternatural paroxysms of intermitting power."[8]

Publication of De Quincey's book in 1823 and its first translation into French in 1828 were events that spurred the French Romantic writers into exploration with opium and hashish in the 1840's and later. Baudelaire's famous book *The Artificial Paradises*[9] was composed of two parts, the first being an original account of the effects of hashish and the second his translation of *The Confessions of an English Opium-Eater*. Baudelaire was to repeatedly comment that much of what he wrote at various times about the effects of opium could equally be said about hashish.[10] The only associated American article of note in this period, *An Opium Eater in America*,[11] appeared in an American magazine in 1842.

An 1854 article in *The Journal of Psychological Medicine* on the addiction of Coleridge and De Quincey was at times almost as lyrical in describing the effects of opium eating as were the writers of this period. The paper also clearly indicated the difficulty of dealing with the problem of opiate addiction, a difficulty that existed then as well as now, over 100 years later.

> How extraordinary is the human mind! how elevated in comprehension—how godlike in sympathy—and yet the human mind may be rendered joyous or fierce, wild or torpid—foolish or entranced, by such agents as alcohol or opium! Spiritual, indeed, we are, but how curiously is our spirituality mixed up with the gross and material. A miserable and despairing being, shall, under the influence of such an agent, be transferred to a paradise of joy, and yet his real condition be not a whit the less destitute. After all, there is something more in this than our philosophy can reach, but it teaches one piece of philosophy, that it is the state of mind, rather than external circumstances, which constitutes happiness.*

The opium wars

While literary figures experimented, merchants made money with opium. Although

*From Harrison, J. B.: The psychology of opium eating, The Journal of Psychological Medicine 7:240, 1854.

opium and the opium poppy had been introduced to China well before the year 1000, there was only a moderate level of use by a select, elite group. Spreading much more rapidly after its introduction was tobacco smoking. It is not clear when tobacco was introduced to the Chinese, but its use had spread and become so offensive that in 1644 the Emperor forbade tobacco smoking in China. The edict did not last long (as is to be expected), but it was in part responsible for the development of opium smoking.

Up to this period the smoking of tobacco and the eating of opium had existed side by side. The restriction on the use of tobacco and the population's appreciation of the pleasures of smoking led to the subterfuge of combining opium and tobacco for smoking. The amount of tobacco used was gradually reduced and soon omitted altogether. Very rapidly the smoking of opium spread, although opium eating had never been very attractive to most Chinese,[12] perhaps, at least partly, because smoking results in a rapid effect compared to oral use of opium.

In 1729 China's first law against opium smoking mandated that opium shopowners were to be strangled. Once opium for non-medical purposes was outlawed, it was necessary for the drug to be smuggled in from India where poppy plantations were abundant. Smuggling opium was so profitable for everyone—the growers, the shippers, and the customs officers—that unofficial and illegal, but formal and binding, rules were gradually developed for the game.[13] The background to the Opium Wars is too lengthy and complex to even attempt to sketch adequately. However, some points must be made to explain why the British went to war so they could continue pouring opium into China against the wishes of the Chinese national government.

Since before 1557, when the Portuguese were allowed to develop the small and remote trading post of Macao, pressure had been increasing on the Chinese Emperors to open the country up to trade with the "Barbarians from the West." Not only the Portuguese but the Dutch and the English repeatedly knocked on the closed door of the Chinese. Near the end of the seventeenth century the port of Canton was opened under very strict rules to foreigners. The primary import trade was opium, even after it became illegal. Tea was the major export, paid for with the profit from selling opium.

Toward the end of the eighteenth century the British East India Company was able to obtain a monopoly on Indian opium but did not feel it could openly engage in the illegal business of smuggling. A gentleman's agreement was reached so that the East India company sold its Indian opium to private (but selected) firms who "smuggled" the opium into China. All went well, with everyone making much money. The number of chests of opium imported to China increased from 200 in 1729, to about 5,000 at the century's end, to 25,000 chests in 1838.

The following year, 1839, the Emperor of China made a fatal mistake—he sent an honest man to Canton to suppress the opium smuggling. Commissioner Lin made everyone nervous. He demanded that the barbarians deliver all their opium supplies to him and subjected the dealers to confinement in their houses. After some haggling, the representative of the British Government ordered the merchants to deliver the opium, which was then destroyed and everyone set free. Pressures mounted, though, and an incident involving drunken American and British sailors killing a Chinaman started the Opium War in 1839. The British Army arrived 10 months later and in 2 years 10,000 British soldiers won a victory over a country of more than 350 million citizens! As victors, the British were given the island of Hong Kong, broad trading rights, and $6 million to reimburse the merchants whose opium had been destroyed.

Through it all, the smuggling of opium continued. There was another Opium War in the 1850's, but the British imports of illegal opium continued and increased until 1908, when Britain and China agreed to limit imports of opium from India.

The Chinese opium trade posed a great moral dilemma for Britain.[14-16] The East India Company protested until its end that it was not smuggling opium into China, and technically it was not. Although the 1839 Opium War was precipitated by opium-related incidents, the primary British motivation in both wars was to open the vast country of China to world, and especially British, trade. From 1870 to 1893 motions in Parliament to end the extremely profitable opium commerce failed to pass. In 1893 a moral protest against the trade was supported, but it was not until 1906 that the government supported and passed a bill that started the process that ended the opium trade by 1913.

MIDDLE HISTORY

In 1805 in London, England, a 20 year old eased a toothache and fell into the abyss of divine enjoyment. In Hanover, Germany, a 20 year old worked on the experiments that were to have great impact on science, medicine, and the pleasure seekers. In 1806, this German youth, Frederich Sertürner, published his report of over fifty experiments that clearly showed that he had isolated the primary active ingredient in opium. In doing this he also opened the door to the new field of alkaloidal chemistry, actually an even more important and amazing achievement.

The active agent was ten times as potent as opium. Sertürner named it morphium after Morpheus, the god of dreams. Use of the new agent developed slowly, but by 1831 the implications of his chemical work and the medical value of morphine were so overwhelming that this pharmacist's assistant was given the French equivalent of the Nobel Prize. Later work into the mysteries of opium found over thirty different alkaloids, with the second most important one being isolated in 1832 and named codeine, the Greek word for poppy head.

The availability of a clinically valuable, pure chemical of known potency is always capitalized on in medicine. The major increase in the use of morphine came as a result of two nondrug developments, one technological and one political. The technological development was the perfection of the hypodermic syringe in 1853 by Dr. Alexander Wood. This made it possible to rapidly deliver relief from pain and suffering by injecting morphine directly into the blood or tissue rather than the much slower process of eating opium or morphine and waiting for absorption to occur

from the gastrointestinal tract. A further advantage of injecting morphine was thought to exist. Originally it was felt that morphine by injection would not be as addicting as the oral use of the drug. However, this belief was later found to be false.

The political events that sped the drug of sleep and dreams into the veins of people worldwide were the American Civil War (1861-1865), the Prussian-Austrian War (1866), and the Franco-Prussian War (1870). Military medicine was, and to some extent still is, characterized by the dictum "first provide relief." Morphine given by injection did work rapidly and well, and it was administered regularly in large doses to many soldiers for the reduction of pain and relief from dysentery. The percentage of returning veterans from these wars who were addicted to morphine was so high that the illness was called the "soldier's disease" or the "army disease."

In this second half of the nineteenth century there were three forms of opiate addiction developing in the United States. The long-useful oral intake of opium, and now morphine, increased greatly as patent medicines became a standard form of self-medication. After 1850 Chinese laborers were imported in large numbers to the west coast, and they introduced opium smoking to this country. The last form, medically the most dangerous and ultimately the most disruptive socially, was the injection of morphine.

Around the turn of the century the percentage (and perhaps the absolute number) of Americans addicted to one of the opiates was very probably greater than at any other time before or since. Several authorities, both then[17] and more recently[18] agree that no less than 1% of the population was addicted to opium, although accurate statistics are not available. In spite of the high level of addiction, it was not a major social problem. In this period:

> Little emphasis was placed on the effects of evil association, and dope peddlers were not mentioned because they were rare or nonexistent.

> The public then had an altogether different conception of drug addiction from that which prevails today. The habit was not approved,

but neither was it regarded as criminal or monstrous. It was usually looked upon as a vice or personal misfortune, or much as alcoholism is viewed today. Narcotics users were pitied rather than loathed as criminals or degenerates—an attitude which still prevails in Europe.*

The opium smoking the Chinese brought to this country never became widely popular. Perhaps it was because the smoking itself only occupied about 1 minute and was then followed by a dream-like state or reverie that may last 2 or 3 hours, hardly behavior that is conducive to a continuation of daily activities or consonant with the outward, active orientation of most Americans in that period. Another reason why opium smoking did not spread was that it originated with Orientals, who were scorned by whites. Similarly, the opium smoking that did occur among whites was found within the asocial and antisocial elements of this culture.[19] Amusingly, even the underworld has its standards of morality and opium smokers looked down on those who used their drugs via injection. In a New York opium-smoking joint early in this century: "One of the smokers discovered a hypodermic user in the bathroom giving himself an injection. He immediately reported to the proprietor that there was a 'God-damned dope fiend in the can'. The offender was promptly ejected."[19] Those who used morphine, and later heroin, via injection will be reported later, but brief mention must be made of one of the major sources of addiction in this period, patent medicines.

The growth of the patent medicine industry after the Civil War has been well documented.[20-22] Everything seemed to be favorable for the industry and it took advantage of each opportunity. There were few government regulations on the industry, and as a result addicting drugs were an important part of many tonics and remedies, although this fact did not have to be indicated on the label. Since labeling of ingredients was not required, a user who had become aware that he was addicted and who wanted to purchase a cure could be sold a remedy labeled as a cure

*From Lindesmith, A.R.: Addiction and opiates, Chicago, 1968, Aldine Publishing Co., p. 211.

that contained almost as much of the addicting drug as he had been receiving in the original tonic.

The generally poor level of health care in the country and a large number of maimed and diseased veterans created a need for considerable medical treatment. Patent medicines promised, and in part delivered, the perfect self-medication. They were easily available, not too expensive, socially acceptable, and, miracle of miracles, they did work. The amount of alcohol and/or opiates in many of the nostrums was certain to relieve the user's aches, pains, and anxieties.

Two other points help explain the increase in the sales of patent medicines. One was the lack of sophistication and education of most Americans during this period, and the other was the use of fantastic advertising campaigns. The two elements worked together, the first explaining the great appeal and effectiveness the active advertising campaigns had in selling the merchandise. Medicine shows, testimonials, songs, newspaper and magazine ads, all said the same thing: You feel ill! *This* product will cure. People believed and bought!

Gradually some medical concern developed over the number of people who were addicted to opiates, and this concern was a part of the motivation that led to the passage of the 1906 Pure Food and Drugs Act. In 1910 a government expert in this area made clear that this law was only a beginning.

The thoughtful and foremost medical men have been and are cautioning against the free use of morphine and opium, particularly in recurring pain. The amount they are using is decreasing yearly. Notwithstanding this fact, and the fact that legislation, federal, state and territorial, adverse to the indiscriminate use and sale of opium and morphine, their derivatives and preparations, has been enacted during the past few decades, the amount of opium per capita imported and consumed in the United States has doubled during the last forty years. . . . It is well known that there are many factors at work tending to drug enslavement, among them being the host of soothing syrups, medicated soft drinks containing cocaine, asthma remedies, catarrh remedies, consumption remedies, cough and cold remedies, and the more notorious so-called "drug addiction cures." It is often stated that medical men are frequently the chief factors in causing drug addiction.*

Data were presented in that paper that tended to support the belief that medical use of opiates initiated by a physician was one, if not *the*, major cause of addiction in this country at that time. A 1918 government report clearly indicted the physician as the major cause of addiction in addicts of "good social standing."

That physicians widely used opiates as drugs in treatment is understandable in light of articles that had been published, such as one in 1889 entitled "Advantages of Substituting the Morphia Habit for the Incurably Alcoholic." The author stated:

> The only grounds on which opium in lieu of alcohol can be claimed as reformatory are, that it is less inimical to healthy life than alcohol, that it calms in place of exciting the baser passions, and hence is less productive of acts of violence and crime; in short, that as a whole the use of morphine in place of alcohol is but a choice of evils, and by far the lesser. . . . if a person has got to the stage of abnormity that he cannot do without a pathological nutrient, particularly of the alcoholic kind, is it better to allow him to go on, or to endeavor to have him substitute morphine for it? After years of experimental trial and observation I have arrived at the conclusion that the latter is immeasurably the best, or by far the least of the two evils.†

The author justifies at length the exchange of oral morphine addiction for alcohol addiction since:

> In this way have I been able to bring peacefulness and quiet to many disturbed and distracted homes, to keep the head of a family out of the gutter and out of the lock-up, to keep him from scandalous misbehavior and neglect of his affairs, to keep him from the verges and actualities of delirium tremens horrors, and above all, to save him from committing, as I veritably believe, some terrible crime.‡

*From Kebler, L. F.: The present status of drug addiction in the Unites States. In Transactions of the American Therapeutic Society, Philadelphia, 1910, F. A. Davis & Co., pp. 105-106.
†From Black, J. R.: Advantages of substituting the morphia habit for the incurably alcoholic, The Cincinnati Lancet—Clinic 22:538, 1889.
‡Ibid., p. 540.

The article concludes:

> I might, had I time and you space, enlarge by statistics to prove the law-abiding qualities of opium-eating peoples, but of this any one can perceive somewhat for himself, if he carefully watches and reflects on the quiet, introspective gaze of the morphine habitue, and compares it with the riotous, devil-may-care leer of the drunkard.*

This middle history period, 1806 to 1914, is rich in material on the use of opiates that gives background to the thesis that if drugs are widely used it is because they meet the needs of a culture. The typical opiate addict in this period was a 30- to 50-year-old white woman who functioned well and was adjusted to her life as a wife and mother. She bought opium or morphine legally at the local store, used it orally, and caused few, if any, social problems. An 1880 report called addiction a "vice of middle life."[23] The picture changed completely with the passage of the Harrison Act in 1914, which virtually removed opiates from the nonprescription market.

One other factor helped change the opiate addiction scene to the one we have today. Toward the end of this period, a chemical transformation of the morphine molecule was put on the market. In 1874 two acetyl groups were attached to morphine, yielding heroin, which was placed on the market in 1898 by Bayer Laboratories as a nonaddicting substitute for morphine and/or codeine. The chemical change was important because heroin is about three times as potent as morphine. The pharmacology of heroin and morphine are identical except that the two acetyl groups increase the lipid solubility of the molecule and thus the molecule enters the brain more rapidly. The additional groups are detached, yielding monoacetylmorphine, which is then converted to morphine. Therefore, effects of morphine and heroin are identical except that heroin is more potent and acts faster.[23a]

The history of heroin is interesting in that it provides strong support for those who argue for extended experimental study of new therapeutic agents before they are marketed. Heroin, marketed as a nonaddicting

*Ibid., p. 541.

substitute for morphine and codeine, seemed the perfect drug, more potent yet less harmful. Although not introduced commercially until 1898, heroin had been long studied and many of its pharmacological actions were reported in 1890.[24] By January, 1900, a comprehensive review article started with the statement:

> A sufficiently long period having elapsed since the introduction of heroine, the new substitution product for codeine, during which it has been used very extensively, we are now enabled to pass judgment upon its real value, and to definitely determine in what manner this drug has fulfilled the expectations raised in its behalf.*

The author then proceeded to extensively survey the pharmacological and clinical literature, after which he concluded that tolerance and addiction (habituation) to heroin were only minor problems.

> Habituation has been noted in a small percentage... of the cases.... All observers are agreed, however, that none of the patients suffer in any way from this habituation, and that none of the symptoms which are so characteristic of chronic morphinism have ever been observed. On the other hand, a large number of the reports refer to the fact that the same dose may be used for a long time without any habituation.†

Many other articles and letters expressed the same attitude. They generally echoed the following sentiment: "... he finds heroine an excellent sedative for the respiratory tract, devoid of the narcotic effect of codeine and morphine, and therefore in physiological doses entirely uninjurious."[25] Slowly the situation changed, and a 1905 text on *Pharmacology and Therapeutics* took a middle ground on heroin by saying it: "... is stated not to give rise to habituation. A more extended knowledge of the drug, however, would seem to indicate that the latter assertion is not entirely correct."[26] In a few more years everyone knew that heroin was the most addicting of the opiates.

Toward the end of this era the 1906 Pure Food and Drugs Act made it necessary for man-

ufacturers to place on the label of their products the kind and amount of opiates the compound contained. The 1909 Exclusion Act restricted the importation of opium for nonmedical purposes, but it was the Harrison Narcotic Act of 1914 that finally resulted in a decrease in the percentage of people addicted to the opiates. However, this same act produced the conditions that led to opiate addiction becoming an increasing social problem.

THE MAKING OF A CRIMINAL ADDICT

In 1908 Great Britain and China agreed to stop the importation of opium into China. At the time about 25% of the Chinese population was estimated to be addicted to opium smoking. President Theodore Roosevelt recognized that no single country (such as China) could control its internal use of these drugs without some international regulations. To that end President Roosevelt called the First Opium Conference in 1909. By 1912 some agreements had been reached and, in considerable part, to honor and support the international commitments the Harrison Narcotic Act was passed in 1914.[23, 27]

The Harrison Act was a regulatory and revenue measure. As is true of most laws, it is not the law itself that becomes important in the ensuing years, but the court decisions and government regulations that evolve around the law.

> The passing of the Harrison Act in 1914 left the status of the addict almost completely indeterminate. The Act did not make addiction illegal and it neither authorized nor forbade doctors to prescribe drugs regularly for addicts. All that it clearly and unequivocally did require was that whatever drugs addicts obtained were to be secured from physicians registered under the act and that the fact of securing drugs be made a matter of record. While some drug users had obtained supplies from physicians before 1914, it was not necessary for them to do so since drugs were available for purchase in pharmacies and even from mail-order houses.*

In 1915 the United States Supreme Court decided that possession of smuggled opiates was a crime and thus users not obtaining the

*From Manges, M.: A second report on the therapeutics of heroine, New York Medical Journal **71:**51, 1900.
†Ibid., pp. 82-83.

*From Lindesmith, A. R.: The addict and the law, Bloomington, 1965, Indiana University Press, p. 5.

drug from a physician became criminals with the stroke of a pen. An addict could still obtain his supply of drugs on a prescription from a physician until this avenue was removed by the 1920 Webb and the 1922 Behrman Supreme Court decisions. The ruling in these cases prevented the prescribing of drugs to an addict unless he was institutionalized and the daily dose gradually decreased, that is, withdrawal initiated. Even though the Lindner case in 1925 reversed these earlier decisions and said that a physician could prescribe drugs to a nonhospitalized addict just to maintain him, the doctors had been harassed enough. Though it was legal to prescribe drugs to an addict, few physicians would do so. Attempts in the early 1920's to maintain clinics for the treatment of opiate addicts failed for a number of reasons, including poor management and disapproval by law enforcement officials.[28]

During the early 1920's law enforcement agencies and the popular press brought about a change in the attitudes of society toward the addict. A 1925 article by a recognized authority in the field of drug addiction said:

> There is a widespread popular belief that narcotic-drug addiction has in recent years been responsible for much violent crime. . . . In so far as its influence on crime is concerned, addiction to opium or any of its preparations creates two tendencies directly opposed to each other. The immediate effect of excessive indulgence in all forms of the drug is to soothe abnormal impulses, while the ultimate effect is to create a state of idleness and dependency which naturally enhances the desire to live at the expense of others and by anti-social means. The effect of addiction on the psychopathic murderer is to inhibit his impulse to violent crime. . . . He, therefore, becomes less a murderer and more a thief.*

Thus in the 1920's:

> . . . the addict was no longer seen as a victim of drugs, an unfortunate with no place to turn and deserving of society's sympathy and help. He became instead a base, vile, degenerate who was weak and self-indulgent, who contaminated all he came in contact with and who deserved nothing short of condemnation and society's moral outrage and legal sanction.

*From Kolb, L.: Drug addiction in its relation to crime, Mental Hygiene 9:74-75, 1925.

The law enforcement approach was accepted as the only workable solution to the problem of addiction.*

A brief review may help in appreciating the changes that had taken place between 1850 and 1940. Opium smoking always stayed out of the mainstream of American life and was condemned in part as a generalization from the negative attitudes in this country toward Orientals in the nineteenth and early twentieth centuries.[28] The use of patent medicines containing opiates increased greatly during the period from 1850 to 1906, when the labeling requirements of the Pure Food and Drugs Act caused many preparations to be withdrawn. The individuals addicted to these medicines were primarily middle-aged and female, rural as well as urban dwellers. In general they carried out their normal duties even though addicted. After 1906 many of these users switched to prescriptions from physicians or to opiate-containing medicines that were freely available from the druggist. There seems to be no general picture of the addict who used the hypodermic in this period, but many of these had apparently been introduced to the drug through a physician's treatment of an illness.

The 1914 law and the ensuing court decisions changed the pattern. The oral opiate users began to decline after the Harrison Law was passed, and the primary remaining group were those who injected morphine or heroin. By 1920, about the only source of opiates for a nonhospitalized addict was an illegal dealer. The cost through this source was thirty to fifty times the price of the same drug through legitimate sources, which no longer were available to the addict. As a consequence, then, of the 1914 law and the Supreme Court decisions in the early 1920's, the opiate user was forced to either stop using the drug or buy from an illegal dealer. To maintain a supply of the drug in this way was expensive. Many addicts resorted to criminal activity, primarily burglary and other crimes against property, to finance their addiction.[28a-c]

*From Smith, R.: Status politics and the image of the addict, Issues in Criminology 2(2):172-173, 1966.

ILLEGAL OPIATE USE TODAY
The changing population

The change in the type of addict population in the United States from the 1920's to the 1970's is easier to specify than the number of addicts in this country after 1914. After the Harrison Act, there almost certainly was a decline in the number of addicts using opiates orally and thus a drop in white middle-aged users. The transition from the 1930's to the 1950's in the United States has been well described by an internationally recognized expert who worked in the area of drug addiction through this period.

> If you go back to 1935 the other problems, apart from alcohol, were primarily the opiates and cocaine, usually taken together in the form of the so-called "speed ball" and then as now . . . drug use was multiple. These individuals that I know used morphine, cocaine, heroin, bromides, phenobarbital or whatever happened to come along but they preferred the opiates and cocaine. The people of those days were really predominantly white individuals, they were on the whole members of various criminal trades, pickpockets and so on, and in fact most of them had been involved in these criminal trades either before or after their onset of their career of using drugs. These people more or less disappeared during the Second World War which practically made these drugs unavailable . . . the old fashioned addict, the expert pickpocket, the short change artist couldn't get drugs. This group was succeeded, after the war was over, by a new kind of opiate taker. These were primarily individuals from the minority groups in the big city slums and in contrast to the older addicts who got good drugs, who knew good stuff when they got it, this new group were getting drugs extremely diluted, full of all kinds of other poisons and were a very different kind of people. They were not expert thieves, in fact very inexpert.*

With the growth of the urban black ghettos, there was an increase in the use of intravenous heroin by the inhabitants. The story has not changed with the new ghetto dwellers, in-cluding Puerto Ricans. As recently as 1968 one authority stated:

> Heroin addicts are regarded by most as relics of the past; as weak minded individuals who are untrustworthy and incapable of relating to other people. It would seem that this assessment is generally correct. The heroin addict of today is little different from the addict of ten or twenty years ago. He is still a product of a slum environment, he is still a dependent, inadequate individual, unable to cope with the challenges of everyday life.*

It is still true today that many addicts, white and black, come from slum environments. Of more concern, however, are the trends that may well specify the addict of tomorrow. Three changes seem to be of primary importance.

Some experts feel that the incidence of deaths directly and clearly related to heroin (mostly overdose deaths) has been relatively constant over a number of years at about 1% to 2% of the addict population.[29] With this figure as a base, the 1969 total for the country would have been about 200,000 addicts.[30, 31]

Throughout the 1960's and early 1970's the number of heroin users skyrocketed. A plateau seemed to be reached, and by 1973 most signs pointed to a decrease in heroin use: the number of deaths due to overdose and to serum hepatitis, the number of arrestees showing narcotics in their urine, and the number of new heroin users all decreased.[28d-f] There is no way to accurately estimate the number of heroin users, but the Bureau of Narcotics and Dangerous Drugs estimated total narcotic addicts in 1972 at over 500,000.

With the trend to a plateau or decrease in heroin addiction was a change in the age at which heroin use was initiated. As heroin use expanded in the 1960's the age of first use decreased. There are now some signs that the age is increasing at which heroin use starts. It's about time. In New York City from 1966 to 1969, the average age of the arrested new addicts dropped from 28 to 22 years. Reports by the New York City Board of Education of 22,000 heroin users in its public

*From Isbell, H.: Discussion, Symposium on Problems of Drug Dependence, 14th Annual Conference Veterans Administration Cooperative Studies in Psychiatry, Houston, Texas, April 1, 1969, Highlights of the Conference, Veterans Administration, Washington, D. C., 1969, U. S. Government Printing Office, pp. 32-35.

*From Smith, R.: U. S. marijuana legislation and the creation of a social problem, Journal of Psychedelic Drugs 2(1):101, 1968.

schools become more believable when heroin-related deaths are studied. In 1960 less than 10% of heroin-related deaths were among teenagers. By 1969 the percentage was 30% and, for the first time, heroin-related deaths were reported in individuals under 15 years of age, twenty in all. Heroin killed more teenagers in New York, 224, in 1969 than anything else, including automobile accidents.[32, 33]

In 1972 New York City reported 1,409 deaths attributable to addiction, with half occurring in individuals 23 years old or less. Most (about 70%) of the heroin-related deaths in New York and elsewhere result from overdoses of the drug. The other deaths have a variety of causes including hepatitis and other illnesses from dirty needles.

The third direction opiate addiction seems to be taking is toward the white, middle-class youth. The youth drug culture is probably nowhere more advanced than in California. A 1971 report from San Francisco forecast what was to flow over the country. The three trends came, peaked, and now seem to be on the wane.

> Within the last two years there has evolved a new style of heroin addict consisting largely of alienated white youth suffering from disillusionment, disaffiliation, frustration, and despair.... The newer addicts are predominantly of urban white middle class extraction. ...[They] entered the drug subculture at a time of beginning frustration and despair, and therefore, engaged in less drug experimentation before "settling" on heroin. He is more aware of some of the dangers of the "street" drugs.... These young people are now turning to heroin abuse as the most effective escape mechanism available to them. As one of our patients noted: "It's like a finance-plan which allows you to consolidate all of your problems into one — Junk! and then the injection in your arm makes them all go away."*

In summary, the rate at which new users are appearing is slowing, and the total number of addicts is now steady or perhaps decreasing. Also changing are the characteristics of the new addict. The number of urban, ghetto,

*From Sheppard, C. W., Gay, G. R., and Smith, D. E.: The changing patterns of heroin addiction in the Haight-Ashbury subculture, Journal of Psychedelic Drugs 3(2):22, 29, 1971.

minority group addicts has increased from the 1950's but some of the increase is the result of alienated white middle-class youths turning to heroin. The third trend is less definite, but age at first narcotic use may be on the rise. Whatever the causes, there are more, and younger, addicts today than a decade ago. A forecast for tomorrow is impossible; 1974 is a borderline year in narcotic use.

Production and delivery of the drug

Until 1973 about 80% of all illegal heroin entering the United States originated in the poppy fields of Turkey. In the late 1960's Turkey came under increasing pressure from the United States to restrict or eliminate the cultivation of poppies. In June, 1971, the government of Turkey announced: "ALL OPIUM cultivation and production throughout Turkey will be banned by the end of fall, 1972, definitely and totally. . . ." In return for this action the United States agreed to give $35 million to the poppy farmers and the government for their financial loss and to help develop new crops.[34, 34a]

Up to 1972 Turkey accounted for about 9% of the world's legal supply of opium, with India supplying all the rest. Concern over adequate opium for medical use led the French government to encourage the cultivation of opium poppies in the Loire Valley and Yugoslavia to increase its opium production fourfold. The world turns. In 1974 Turkey announced that the ban against opium poppy cultivation was abolished! What will it cost to stop that?

Why worry? For a brief period in 1973 heroin *was* in short supply on the streets of New York, but there are many sources other than the fields of Turkey. Burma, Laos, and Thailand — the Golden Triangle of Southeast Asia — produce more than half of the world's illicit opium, mostly now for home consumption. An American Cabinet-level report in 1972 said there was no way in which the smuggling of narcotics in Southeast Asia could be controlled since the involved countries were not interested. Things change. A sharp rise in 1973 in the number of middle and upper class Burmese youths addicted to heroin resulted in the government deciding to increase enforcement against opium cultivation and smuggling![34a] (Déjà vu? See pp. 18 and 27.)

Temptation is great for an opium farmer.[35] In Turkey 1 kilogram of legal opium yielded about $10. The same amount sold illegally for three times as much. Many farmers grew extra poppies just for the illegal market, and in 1970 at least 60 tons of Turkish opium were sold illegally. Illegal opium is converted to its primary active ingredient, morphine. This relatively simple chemical procedure reduces the bulk by 90% without losing any pharmacological activity.

Changing 10 kilograms of opium worth $300 into 1 kilogram of morphine increased its value to $500. Delivery to the contact in southern France doubled the value of the kilogram of morphine. At this stage the morphine is converted into heroin, which is about three times as potent as morphine. This is a sophisticated technique and requires a well-equipped laboratory and some chemical expertise. There is little change in the bulk when the morphine is transformed to heroin, but the appearance changes from the light fluffy powder of morphine to the crystal-like form of heroin.

The kilogram of heroin is worth $4,000 to $6,000 in France and $10,000 to $15,000 delivered in the United States. It is then sold to distributors who may pay $30,000 to $40,000 for the heroin and then mix it with milk sugar or quinine and sell small amounts to street pushers. The pushers will adulterate the drug still more so that a user might pay $5 for a bag containing 5 to 50 milligrams of heroin. The dilution is so great that a kilogram of heroin sold at the street level may retail for a quarter of a million dollars, $300 of which was received by the farmer in Turkey. It is estimated that organized crime takes in about $2.2 billion a year from the illegal narcotic trades. Clearly there is money to be made in illegal opiate traffic.

The world's largest market for illegal heroin is the United States, and the primary problem is getting the drug past the American customs agents. The job of the customs officials seems almost insurmountable. There are nearly 400 official ports of entry into the United States and over 220 million travelers enter this country each year. In spite of the difficulties, or perhaps because of the great increase in the drug traffic and the concomitant increase in the number of amateur smugglers, heroin seizures in 1971 were greater than the 10 previous years combined. Only about 5% of the seizures occurred as a result of tips to the customs officials.[36]

Turkey had many competitors for the illegal trade. Estimates are that Mexico now supplies 15% of America's heroin, and Afghanistan has started cultivating illegal opium poppies in quantity. Southeast Asia, especially Burma, is beginning to export considerable quantities of opium, morphine, and/or heroin. The morphine content, however, is not as high in Asian opium as it is in Turkish opium. One Asian country, India, has a large number of poppy farmers (almost 200,000) and the best system in the world for paying for legal opium. The more opium a farmer produces from his land, the more he is paid for each kilogram. This system encourages high yields per acre and also rewards putting all of the opium crop into legal channels, since the more he sells legally the more he gets for each kilogram.

It is doubtful whether shutting off, if possible, illegal narcotics from Turkey or any other country will have much lasting influence on the street market in this country. It has increased the cost by causing a temporary shortage, but other suppliers are available and willing. Increasing the cost of the drug to the user only makes the social consequences of addiction even greater.

Street use

The street scene is changing as rapidly in heroin use as with other drugs. The addict encounters many problems in his daily drug-oriented life, and only a glimpse of some of the mechanics can be offered here. Since the initial withdrawal signs begin about 4 hours after the last use of the drug, many addicts are on a 4-hour schedule that requires six injections a day. Each injection may require about 15 milligrams of heroin, and the problems begin here.[37]

No one seems to be sure why heroin is the drug of choice for addicts. Possibly it is because of the belief that heroin delivers more euphoria than morphine, although most addicts cannot differentiate the effects of equipotent doses. Some authorities have reported differences in the experienced effects of heroin and morphine when administered intravenously, but not subcutaneously.[38]

The addict buys heroin usually in small packets costing $5 to $10. Using a number of these "bags" each day requires an outlay of $20 to $100. Most male addicts steal to maintain themselves and their habit, while female addicts resort to either prostitution or shoplifting. Stolen property is worth one-third to one-fifth of its retail value, so to keep even a small $25 a day habit, goods worth about $100 must be stolen each day—7 days a week, 52 weeks a year. No vacations for the addict! If only 100,000 of the addicts engage in this kind of activity to support their addiction, the total yearly cost to this country would be $3.6 billion. There are not that many thefts and burglaries and holdups, so something is wrong. In fact, there is no clear relationship between heroin addiction and crime.[38a-c]

There is no FDA watching over the illegal sale of heroin, so the buyer is never quite sure what he is getting. One survey in New York City showed 10% of the bags purchased on the street contained no active drug at all. The concentration of heroin in the remaining equisize packets ranged from 1% to 77%.[39] This variability is a problem since it increases the possibility of an overdose. The variability is of recent origin and may represent only a problem of quality control in an expanding market. The higher amounts of heroin per bag may be an effort on the part of the sellers to speed up the addiction process.[32]

Because of the variability of doses, the addict must live in fear of an overdose (OD) with each new batch of drug he uses. A sophisticated user buying from a new or questionable source will initially try a much smaller than normal amount of the powder to evaluate its potency. An overdose may not be fatal, but if fatal it may be so rapid that the user is found with the needle still in his arm. Whether fast or slow, death seems to result from asphyxiation caused by acute congestion and edema of the lungs, the basis of which is still unknown.[40, 40a,b]

Once the user has acquired the drug, he prepares it for injection. Usually, he

...mixes the powder with unsterile water, heats the mixture briefly in a spoon or bottle cap with a match or lighter, then draws the heroin into a syringe or eyedropper through cotton, thus filtering out the larger impurities. The heroin is then injected intravenously without any attempt at skin cleansing.*

Under these conditions it is not surprising that infections do occur. The preferred equipment today for injection is the eyedropper with a hypodermic needle attached, since the rubber bulb of the dropper is easier to operate than the plunger of a syringe.

The most usual form of heroin use by male addicts is to inject the drug intravenously, that is, to "mainline" the drug. A convenient site is the left forearm (for right-handed users) and the frequent use of dirty needles will leave the arm marked with scar tissue. If the larger veins of the arm collapse, then other body areas will be used. Many beginning addicts start by "skin-popping"—subcutaneous injections—and this method remains the preferred one for most women. "Skin-popping" increases the danger of tetanus but decreases the risk of hepatitis compared to mainlining.

Because of the lack of sterility or even cleanliness, hepatitis, tetanus, and abscesses at the site of injection are not uncommon in street users who inject drugs. The common practice of sharing needles and droppers is bringing back a danger that has not been associated with heroin use in this country since the 1930's. In the spring of 1971 some veterans returning from Vietnam shared their unclean injection equipment and thus were responsible for the worst outbreak of malaria California had seen for 20 years. The malaria parasite from the blood of infected veterans was transmitted to nonveterans who used the same equipment. This incident was no doubt one of the factors that resulted in increased screening for drugs and drug equipment of the veterans returning from Southeast Asia.[41]

If the addict survives the perils of an overdose, escapes the dangers of contaminated equipment, and avoids being caught, there are still some dangers. Since heroin is a potent analgesic, its regular use *may* conceal

---

*From Louria, D. B., Hensle, T., and Rose, J.: The major medical complications of heroin addiction, Annals of Internal Medicine **67**(1):1, 1967.

the early symptoms of an illness such as pneumonia. The addict's lack of money for, or interest in, food frequently results in malnutrition. With low resistance from malnutrition and the symptoms of illness unnoticed as a result of heroin use, the addict becomes quite susceptible to serious disease.[42] If all of these dangers are overcome the addict may continue to use opiates to an advanced age. Sometimes, though, the addict who avoids illness, death, or arrest and who does not enter and stay in a rehabilitation program or withdraw himself from the drug may no longer feel the need for the drug and gradually stop using it. The data are still very much debated, but this "maturing out" is probably what happens to a large number of addicts. One authority reports that if an addict lives, he remains addicted for only about 8 or 9 years. This is an average, however, and according to this report the earlier a user starts, the longer he remains addicted, with maturing out generally occurring in the 35- to 45-year age period.[43] Even if he lives, the street life of an addict isn't a rose garden.

The Southeast Asia scene

> It is ironic indeed that in the last two years of the war our biggest casualty figures will come from heroin addiction, not from combat.*

The Department of Defense established a Task Force on Drug Abuse in 1967, and since then there has been growing awareness of the rapidly developing problem of illegal drug use by American soldiers in Vietnam. Initial reports emphasized concern over the widespread use of marijuana by troops in combat zones as well as in rest and rehabilitation areas. In 1970 public and federal concern began to focus on the problem of heroin addiction among service personnel stationed in Southeast Asia.[44]

Opium poppies grow widely in Burma, Laos, and Thailand in areas far removed from governmental control. It is estimated that these three countries produce about 1,000 tons of opium

each year—over half of the world's illegal production. Much of this is consumed as opium, but the available evidence indicates that the amount converted to heroin was increased as the demand for heroin increased among Americans in South Vietnam. Although the governments of these countries verbalize willingness to fight the illegal production of opium and heroin with American money, it is unlikely that significant impact can be made on such an excellent money crop.

Heroin is about 95% pure and almost openly sold in South Vietnam. Purity in the United States has declined from 5% in 1969 to about 2% in 1973. Not only is the Southeast Asia heroin undiluted, it is inexpensive. Ten dollars will buy about 250 milligrams, an amount that would cost over $500 in the United States. The high purity of the heroin makes it possible to obtain psychological effects by smoking or sniffing the drug. This fact, coupled with the completely wrong belief that addiction occurs only when the drug is used intravenously, has resulted in about 40% of the users sniffing, about half smoking, and only 10% mainlining their heroin.[45] An addict accustomed to sniffing heroin in Vietnam would be forced to inject the diluted United States drug to obtain the same effects.

Some early 1971 reports estimated that 10% to 15% of the American troops in Vietnam were addicted to heroin. As a result of the increased magnitude and visibility of the heroin problem, the United States government took several rapid steps in mid-1971. One of the first moves initiated by a new Special Action Office on Drug Abuse was to initiate a urine testing program for opiates in those servicemen ready to leave Vietnam. The testing program, which tested only for opiates, was later expanded to include other American personnel. In addition to those permanently leaving, servicemen who travel outside Vietnam for 1-week rest-and-recreation leaves are tested, as well as those who volunteer to extend their tour in Vietnam.

As the result of the poor facilities and the speed with which the testing program was initiated, there were varied reports, but in October of 1971 the Pentagon released figures for the first 3 months of testing. These data

*From The World Heroin Problem, Committee Print, House of Representatives, Committee on Foreign Affairs, Ninety-second Congress, First Session, May 27, 1971, Washington, D. C., 1971, U. S. Government Printing Office, p. 18.

showed that 5.1% of the 100,000 servicemen tested showed traces of opiates in their urine. The army had a higher incidence of users, 6.4%, than either the air force, 1.3%, or the navy, 1.7%, and most of the opiate users were concentrated in the lower ranks. To deal with the problem of drug-using soldiers and veterans, the Department of Defense and the Veterans Administration prepared massive rehabilitation programs.

Until July of 1971, soldiers identified as drug users could be, and frequently were, released from the service under less than honorable conditions. Without an honorable discharge these ex-soldiers were not eligible for veterans' benefits, which included treatment for their drug abuse. In July, 1971, the Department of Defense made mandatory an amnesty program that had previously been optional. The amnesty program held that if a drug user turned himself in for treatment he would be placed in a rehabilitation program, retained in the service for his normal tour of duty, and not be given a less than honorable discharge on the basis of illegal drug use by itself. This procedure has not always worked smoothly in the army.[45a] The amnesty program was later made retroactive, so that any veteran given a dishonorable discharge because of drug use would be told he could have his case reviewed and possibly changed to an honorable discharge.

The Veterans Administration prepared to meet the drug problems of the returning Vietnam veteran and the increasing incidence of illegal drug use among veterans in the community. In July, 1971, the Veterans Administration initiated a program that increased its expenditures for drug treatment fiftyfold.

There is still debate about the success of rehabilitating veterans who became drug users while in Vietnam. Some individuals misused drugs, or had a high potential for misuse, prior to their service. Those veterans with a background of economic frustration, personal hopelessness, and low-level job skills will probably respond to various treatments the same as their non-veteran counterparts. Some Vietnam addicts may be individuals who would not have become heroin users elsewhere. In Vietnam they may have tried heroin because of its availability and low cost, boredom, and the general unpopularity of the war. These individuals possibly have a better potential for rehabilitation than those whose history does not forecast an easy integration into meaningful positions in the community. That this differentiation is real is suggested by one follow-up study. It found that being in Vietnam did *not* result in an increased number of addicted veterans. About 1.3% of the returnees were addicted in 1972, the same as the percentage of individuals found to be using narcotics when examined for induction into the service.[28f, 45b] Of those soldiers addicted when they left Vietnam and then rehabilitated, only 7% became readdicted in their first 8 months in the United States. Not all agree with these conclusions.[45c]

PHARMACODYNAMICS

Pain has long been one of society's and medicine's primary concerns. Second only to curing an illness or preventing death and disability has been the reduction of pain. Opium, its constituents such as morphine and codeine, its semisynthetics such as heroin, and the purely synthetic opiate-like agents such as methadone and meperidine (Demerol), are the most effective analgesics known today. In spite of the great research activity on the problem and the ability of the biochemist to build molecules that have very much the same effect as morphine, the mechanism by which these drugs reduce pain is still unknown. Collectively, the opiates and the synthetic compounds with similar activity are classed as narcotic analgesics.

Tolerance develops to most of the effects of these drugs, which means the dose must be regularly increased to maintain a constant effect. Concomitant with tolerance is the establishment of physiological dependency, which is manifested as a consistent pattern of physiological responses when regular drug use is discontinued. These agents also have the capability to induce a sense of euphoria in many people. The euphoria seems to be more than just the reduction of tension and suffering. For years pharmacologists and biochemists have sought to develop compounds that would make possible a separation of

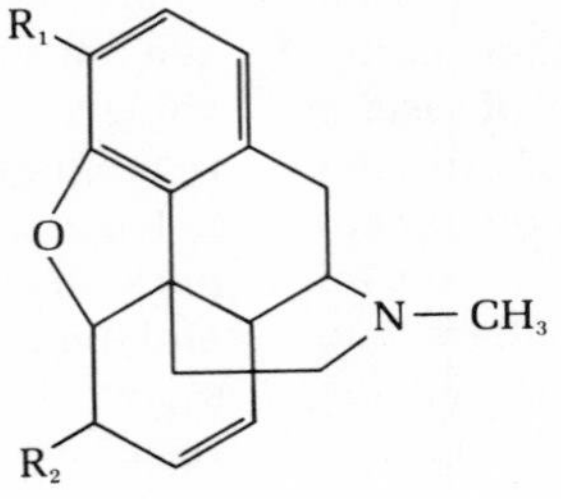

	R₁	R₂
Morphine	$-OH$	$-OH$
Codeine	$-O-CH_3$	$-OH$
Heroin	$-O-\overset{\displaystyle O}{\underset{\parallel}{C}}-CH_3$	$-O-\overset{\displaystyle O}{\underset{\parallel}{C}}-CH_3$

Fig. 12-1. Narcotic agents isolated or derived from opium.

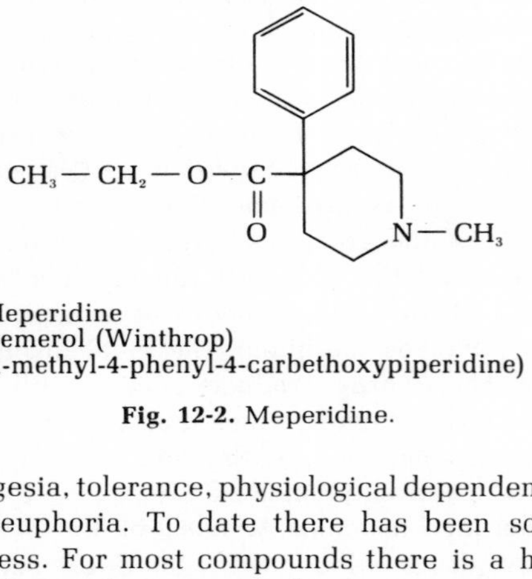

Meperidine
Demerol (Winthrop)
(1-methyl-4-phenyl-4-carbethoxypiperidine)

Fig. 12-2. Meperidine.

analgesia, tolerance, physiological dependency, and euphoria. To date there has been some success. For most compounds there is a high correlation between analgesic potency and the euphoriant effects the agent elicits. In some synthetic narcotics, however, analgesia, euphoria, and physical dependency have been dissociated. Considering the many narcotic agents in the marketplace, they offer little advantage for the most part over the primary active ingredient in *Papaver somniferum*, and so morphine remains the standard against which other narcotics are judged.[45d] For this reason, the pharmacological and physiological effects of morphine in man will be emphasized.

Pharmacological effects

"Morphine and its surrogates produce their major effects on the central nervous system (CNS) and the bowel."[46] The major therapeutic indications for morphine are the reduction of pain and relief from dysentery and diarrhea. The effect on pain is clearly a central nervous system action of morphine. Many laboratory reports suggest that morphine has no effect on the threshold to pain. Experimental work supporting this comes from the fact that morphine does not impair conduction in peripheral nerves. In line with these results is the finding that the other sensory systems are not affected by therapeutic doses of morphine.

Following the administration of an analgesic dose of morphine some patients report that they are still aware of the pain, but the pain is no longer aversive. Frequently, though, the pain stimulus is not attended to by the drug user. He is not aware of the pain stimulus until it is pointed out to him, and when made aware of the stimulus he does not perceive it as aversive. The narcotic agents seem to have their effect in part by diminishing the awareness the individual has of the aversive stimulus and in part on his response to the stimulus. Morphine, then, primarily reduces the emotional response to pain, the suffering, and to some extent also decreases knowledge of the pain stimulus. The effect of narcotics on pain is relatively specific. Fewer effects on mental and motor ability accompany analgesic doses of these agents than with equipotent doses of other analgesic and depressant drugs. As mentioned in Chapter 9 (pp. 121 to 122), most types of pain are reduced following administration of narcotic agents.

It is probable that morphine reduces suffering primarily through two actions on the brain. One action decreases the effectiveness of the cortical arousal system, but there is still debate over whether this effect is mediated via the reticular activating system. A pain-reducing dose of morphine disrupts the electrical activity of the brain (measured by an EEG) seen in dream and nondream sleep. Although one of the characteristics of the narcotic agents is their ability to reduce pain without inducing sleep, drowsiness is not uncommon after a therapeutic dose. (In the addict's vernacular, the patient is "on the nod.") The patient is readily awakened if he sleeps, and dreams during the sleep period are frequent. The second action that may be important here is one on the limbic system, which is a general term for several of the brain areas important in emotional responses. Some investigators report that morphine decreases the electrical activity in the limbic system that normally follows painful stimulation. The combination of these two actions— a general decrease in brain arousal to painful stimulation and a specific decrease to it in the emotional center of the brain—may be the basis for the decrease in suffering and diminished awareness of the pain that occurs following morphine-induced analgesia. These effects possibly form the basis for morphine's primary therapeutic effect, but the complete explanation must await more information on both the brain systems involved and the specific actions of morphine on the systems.

Another very specific effect of morphine is to depress the respiratory centers in the brain so that respiration slows and becomes shallow. This is perhaps the major side effect of the narcotic agents and one of the most dangerous, since death resulting from respiratory arrest can easily follow an excessive dose of these drugs. The basis for this effect is that the respiratory centers become less responsive to carbon dioxide levels in the blood, but again the mechanism of morphine is not known. Not nearly so dangerous but almost as common is another effect of the narcotics: constriction of the pupils of the eyes. In complete darkness there is some constriction and, even in moderate light, the pupils are reduced to little more than pinpoints. Tolerance to the pupillary response is minimal.

Morphine also stimulates the brain area controlling nausea and vomiting, which are other frequent side effects. Usually, nausea occurs in about half of the ambulatory cases given a 15-milligram dose of morphine. Still other side effects result from morphine-induced decreases in the response of the hypothalamus to external input, which impairs its regulation of many homeostatic functions. For example, body temperature decreases slightly and fluid is retained in the body. In addition, the hormonal output from the pituitary gland is generally depressed.

To summarize the central nervous system effects of therapeutic levels of morphine: sensory pathways function normally but the response to pain stimuli is diminished; respiration is depressed and nausea is induced via effects on lower brain centers; the hypothalamic response to external input is decreased and pituitary gland functioning is depressed. In spite of these seemingly selective actions, work with radioactively labeled narcotics does not show specific localization of the drug anywhere in the central nervous system.

The effects of morphine on the gastrointestinal system have been well studied, although, again, the mechanisms remain elusive. Morphine impairs digestion by decreasing the secretion of essential digestive juices. The narcotic agents also slow the passage of food through the gastrointestinal tract by decreasing the number of peristaltic contractions. At the same time, however, there may be an increase in other gastrointestinal contractions, with the result that there is much activity but little movement of the material in the intestines. Considerable water is absorbed from the intestinal material; this fact, plus the near absence of contractions to move material through the intestine, results in constipation. Tolerance to these effects develops very slowly.

Both the central and the peripheral effects described are generally true for all the narcotic agents. Differences between these compounds are primarily in their speed and duration of action and their potency. When given intravenously the latency to onset of action of most of the narcotics is about the same. Since 10 milligrams of morphine is effective in providing relief to about 70% of patients with moderate to severe pain (such as postoperative pain), that dose is generally used as the standard. The data in Table 12-1 present a partial comparison of some characteristics of the most frequently used narcotic analgesics. These data are only approximations, since many factors determine the effects in a particular person.[47]

Mechanism of action

There is no generally accepted concept about the biochemical mechanism(s) through which the narcotics have their effects. Most researchers, though, have accepted the idea that there are specific receptors on neurons that are sensitive to narcotic agents. These agents have their effects as a result of combination with these receptors. These receptors are not those affected by the neurotransmitters and, in the absence of narcotics, presumably are unused throughout life. The combination of a narcotic with the receptor does not directly or immediately affect the metabolism of neurons, so the analgesic effect of these drugs is more likely via some action on synaptic transmission. However, the development of tolerance does not seem to be mediated by such a synaptic effect but rather by a metabolic effect. Work with protein synthesis inhibitors have made possible a separation of the analgesic effects and the development of tolerance. The protein synthesis inhibitors modify the metabolism of the neurons by preventing the building of proteins. These inhibitors do not effect the analgesic potency of morphine or similar compounds, but they do prevent tolerance. A possibility, then, is that an alteration in general neuronal metabolism is directly responsible for tolerance and physiological addiction but not analgesia.

Some authorities feel that the narcotics may function by affecting the enzymes responsible for the synthesis of one or more neurotransmitters. The data are far from complete and no definite position can be taken, although some of the present hypotheses may be correct. Serotonin, for example, is implicated in the action of morphine, since as tolerance develops the synthesis but not the accumulation of serotonin doubles. Relevant also is the finding that a decrease in brain serotonin level increases the sensitivity of the animal to painful stimuli and decreases the analgesic effect of morphine. Noradrenaline levels in the brain change in some species following the administration of morphine, but no general pattern seems clear.

Other work suggests that dopaminergic neurons show an increase in activity following the administration of morphine but are not

Table 12-1. Partial comparison of some characteristics of frequently used narcotic analgesics

	Equianalgesic doses (milligrams)	Time to onset of action (subcutaneous injection)	Duration of analgesic action (hours)
Morphine	10	30-60 minutes	4-5
Codeine	120		2-4
Heroin	3-4	15 minutes	4-5
Methadone	8-10	30 minutes	4-6
Meperidine	80-100	10 minutes	2-4

affected by withdrawal. Acetylcholine has been studied to a lesser degree, but it seems clear that morphine addiction and withdrawal has little effect on the total brain level of this transmitter. Clearly none of these studies indicates which are the crucial elements for the analgesic or other actions of the narcotic agents. The major current general hypothesis is that some serotonergic functioning is responsible for the analgesic and sedating effects of the narcotics, while the euphoria and excitation are related to noradrenergic processes.

The hypothesis of specific narcotic receptors fits with the fact that there are narcotic antagonists, drugs that specifically block the effects of a narcotic drug when given to an individual. Most investigators feel that these drugs compete with the narcotic agents for the hypothesized narcotic receptor, although some research suggests separate receptor sites for the antagonists. The presently dominant hypothesis is that the antagonists have two important characteristics. They have a greater affinity for the receptor site than the narcotic drugs and thus displace the narcotic molecule from the receptor. Additionally, the antagonists have less activity at the receptor than do the narcotics, that is, they combine with the receptor but do not initiate a response of it. Whether the hypothesis about the mechanism of action is correct or not, the administration of an antagonist to an individual using narcotics causes the narcotic effect to very rapidly decrease to almost no effect. Narcotic-induced analgesia will diminish and, if the individual is an addict, administration of an antagonist will rapidly induce severe withdrawal symptoms. Furthermore, pretreatment with an antagonist will prevent subsequent doses of a narcotic from being effective, a fact that is the basis for one of the experimental treatment programs for narcotic addicts. Although administration of most antagonists to an individual who is not using narcotics could induce some narcotic effects, these effects occur only at doses producing severe side effects. Thus their usefulness for these purposes is severely limited.

To briefly summarize the actions of the narcotic antagonists, they appear to have a greater affinity than do the narcotic drugs for the narcotic receptor site and thus will displace the narcotic drug at the receptor or prevent its combination with the receptor. Because of the much lower activity of the antagonist at this receptor, narcotic effects will greatly diminish if they are present or appear only minimally if not already present.

THE ADDICTIVE AND WITHDRAWAL PROCESSES

Addiction is a unique symptom in medicine. It is a symptom of comfort rather than discomfort, providing relief from emotional as well as physical pain. Its comfort goes even further, by lessening the tensions of psychic and biologic drives.*

Addiction to a drug is more than a habit of regularly using a drug. The term "addiction" is restricted to those conditions where physiological symptoms occur when the regular use of the drug is discontinued. The evidence is clear that addiction can occur to alcohol, the barbiturates, the antianxiety agents, and the opiates. These are all depressant drugs. The evidence is not yet convincing that addiction can occur to stimulant drugs.

Some writers feel that addiction should be defined as a personal and social concept rather than a biomedical one. In such a definition, addiction includes recognition by the individual that the physical symptoms he is experiencing are caused by a low level of the drug in the body and that he must take steps to correct the situation.

. . . One can only be addicted when he experiences physiological withdrawal symptoms, recognizes them as due to a need for drugs, and relieves them by taking another dose. The crucial step of recognition is most likely to occur when the user participates in a culture in which the signs of withdrawal are interpreted for what they are. When a person is ignorant of the nature of withdrawal sickness, and has some other cause to which he can attribute his discomfort (such as a medical problem), he may misinterpret the symptoms and thus escape addiction. . . .†

*From Jurgensen, W. P.: Problems of inpatient treatment of addiction, N. Y. State Narcotic Addiction Control Commission Reprints 1(1):2, 1968.
†From Becker, H. S.: History, culture and subjective experience: an exploration of the social bases of drug-induced experiences, Journal of Health and Social Behavior 8:175, 1967.

Such an explanation is offered for why hospitalized patients can receive large doses of morphine regularly without showing drug-seeking behavior after the drug is stopped.

Addiction to a drug is characterized by three features: a tendency to increase the dose (since tolerance occurs); appearance of physiological changes when drug use is discontinued (withdrawal symptoms develop); and a strong desire to continue taking the drug, frequently stronger than any other desire the addict has known. A recent article states: "In susceptible persons they [narcotics] produce a pathological hunger of such intensity that the drive for narcotics displaces all other responsibilities."[48]

Still not resolved is the basis for the "pathological hunger." There are two basic positions.[49] One is that the primary drive is euphoria.

> The primacy of euphoria, as asserted by the addict, is central to the elaboration of addiction. The addict seeks to limit tolerance and avoid abstinence, but he also urgently demands the recovery of his capacity for the "high."*

The other point of view holds that avoidance of withdrawal is fundamental.

> ... the hook in addiction arises, not from the euphoria which the drug initially produces, but from the beginner's realization that the discomfort and misery of withdrawal is caused by the absence of the drug and can be dispelled almost magically by another dose of it.†

Neither theory is complete. One study[49a] indicates that addicts who can afford it always go for the euphoria. Those who work primarily to avoid withdrawal are those less adept at hustling on the street.

The middle ground presented here suggests (1) learning to be an addict is a separate and distinct stage from being an addict; (2) learning to be an addict can result from either an approach to pleasure or an escape from discomfort; (3) being an addict has multiple motivations and rewards; and (4) the same nonspecific factors that help determine other forms of drug taking operate in addiction.

*From Scher, J.: Patterns and profiles of addiction and drug abuse, Archives of General Psychiatry **15**:543, 539-551, 1966.
†From Lindesmith, A. R.: Addiction and opiates, Chicago, 1968, Aldine Publishing Co., pp. 73-74.

Some of the misconceptions surrounding addiction and withdrawal deserve comment before expanding slightly these four points. None of the opiates fits the fantasized drug: one shot and you are hooked for life. Becoming an addict takes some time, perhaps a week, and persistence on the part of a beginner. Regular use of the drug seems to be more important in establishing physiological addiction than the size of the dose used. Becoming physiologically addicted *is* possible on a weekend, but it frequently requires a longer period with three or four injections a day.[49b]

Another of the misconceptions about mainlining heroin or morphine is that it induces in everyone an intense pleasure unequalled by any other experience. Addicts talk in glowing terms of the "rush" or "kick" they frequently experience.[50] Often it is described as similar to a whole-body orgasm that persists up to 5 or more minutes. Some addicts report that they try with every injection to reexperience the extreme euphoria of the first injection, but they always have a lesser effect. There are studies, however, as well as clinical and street reports, that many people experience only nausea and discomfort following the intravenous administration of morphine or heroin.[51] For whatever reasons, some of these users persist and the discomfort decreases, that is, shows tolerance more rapidly than the euphoric effects. Under these conditions the injections soon result primarily in pleasant effects. To maintain these pleasurable feelings, though, the dose level must gradually be increased. There is no resolution of what type of individual—socially, psychologically, or biochemically—readily experiences pleasure in contrast to those whose initial symptoms are unpleasant. It is true, however, that even with the narcotics the addict must partially learn which experiences are defined as pleasurable.[52, 53]

One final cautionary statement has to do with the development of withdrawal symptoms. The addict undergoing withdrawal without medication is always portrayed as being in excruciating pain, truly suffering. It depends. With a large habit, withdrawal without medication is truly hell. The opiate addiction scene is changing too rapidly to be definite about today's user, but a few years ago most addicts were described as having "ice cream habits," that is, they used a low daily drug dose. On this basis some hospitals provide no medication during withdrawal, while others operate on the assumption that if any discomfort exists it should be relieved. The experience of the withdrawal syndrome from even a small habit (such as 60 milligrams of morphine per day) can be very uncomfortable. It is probably true, however, that the amount of withdrawal discomfort from small habits depends to a considerable degree on the attitude, personality, and other characteristics of the individual. The actual intensity of the symptoms, however, is directly related to the daily dose of the drug. One ex-addict described his withdrawal from a moderate habit. "Remember when you had a bad case of the 24-hour virus. You're coming out both ends—vomiting and diarrhea—and every joint in your body hurts. You wish you could die but feel too badly to do anything about it. Take that, double it, and spread it over 4 or 5 days. That's cold turkey." (Cold turkey because the goose bumps that occur in abrupt withdrawal resemble a plucked turkey.)

The sequence of appearance of some of the abstinence syndrome symptoms are included in Table 12-2[37] along with the time of their appearance after the last dose of the indicated drugs. In general, the longer it takes for the initial symptoms to develop, the less intense the withdrawal effects will be. The muscle twitches appearing about 12 hours after the last dose of heroin are primarily in the legs and feet and increase in intensity over the next day or so. The foot twitches are particularly severe and are the basis for the phrase "kicking the habit."

It has been suggested that becoming and staying an addict are separate stages. The acquisition of addiction requires some steady behavior on the part of the individual. It seems clear that the behavior in this initial stage is maintained either by the delivery of positive feelings or the reduction of unpleasant feelings. Some individuals probably persist in the use of the drug for one reason, some for the other, and a third group for a combination of the reasons. It is meaningless to look for a single type of individual who has an "addict personality."

In the second stage of use of the opiates the individual acquires an additional motivation for using the drug. No longer is he only looking for pleasure or to decrease the tensions and stresses of his nondrug life. This stage is marked by the clear development of withdrawal symptoms when the drug level in the body drops too low. It is at this stage that the behavior of the addict becomes truly routinized. The drug-taking behavior becomes very closely and directly tied to the removal of specific symptoms. The regularity of drug use is no doubt controlled by the appearance of withdrawal symptoms, but the amount of drug used is probably related to the positive

Table 12-2. Sequence of appearance of some of the abstinence syndrome symptoms

Signs	Approximate hours after last dose		
	Heroin	Morphine	Methadone
Craving for drugs, anxiety	4	6	12
Yawning, perspiration, running nose, teary eyes	8	14	34 to 48
Increase in above signs plus pupil dilation, goose bumps (piloerection), tremors (muscle twitches), hot and cold flashes, aching bones and muscles, loss of appetite	12	16	48 to 72
Increased intensity of above, plus insomnia; raised blood pressure; increased temperature, pulse rate, respiratory rate and depth; restlessness; nausea	18 to 24	24 to 36	
Increased intensity of above, plus curled-up position, vomiting, diarrhea, weight loss, spontaneous ejaculation or orgasm, hemoconcentration, increased blood sugar	26 to 36	36 to 48	

pleasure it delivers, since usually much lower doses, or doses taken orally, would be adequate to prevent withdrawal discomfort.

Another variable develops throughout the addiction process. Each drug administration is followed by a decrease in discomfort, increase in pleasure, or both. As a result the behavior itself of preparing and injecting the drug acquires pleasurable, positive characteristics via learning mechanisms. The best example of this acquired pleasure is the needle freak who, when he injects, always withdraws and reinjects blood several times and between injections is preoccupied with his injection equipment. The ultimate is the addict who has a "needle habit" and will insert the needle into a vein frequently even though he injects nothing.

Only the drug-centered bases for addiction have been mentioned. The addict lives, however, in a heroin centered subculture that provides support for his behavior and the means and opportunity to engage in drug-taking behavior. All three factors—drug, individual, setting—contribute to making an addict. This has been convincingly demonstrated with animals as well.

Two brief points will close this section. One deals with the 4- to 6-hour period between the possible euphoria of the injection and the beginning of withdrawal signs. The effects will vary. In some addicts all drives feel satisfied: sex, hunger, aggression. These feelings are muted to the point where they no longer cause anxiety. Anxiety and stresses from other sources also diminish into nothing, as does any physical pain the individual may have. In other addicted individuals these drives are not blunted at all and they continue without change. For this 4 to 6 hours heroin acts as the perfect tranquilizer for some chronic users. If the dose is correct the individual is able to function well in a job; many addicts, however, do as little as possible for a large portion of this interval.[54]

The second point follows from the previous one but also expands the idea. There is nothing in the drug or the addiction process itself to prevent a controlled addict (one whose dosage is carefully adjusted to the appropriate level) from working normally.

Neither are there any necessary negative physiological or medical effects from heroin or being addicted. The usual medical and vocational problems that are correctly associated with opiate addiction today stem neither from the drug nor its regular use but from the drug delivery system and the subculture that surrounds this illegal drug use. Many physicians and other biomedical people become addicted and continue their normal activities for years. Physicians have the highest addiction rate of any group, about thirty to one hundred times that in the general population.[55]

TREATMENT AND REHABILITATION OF THE OPIATE ADDICT

> ...I am absolutely certain that no substitute exists which, without containing opium or any of its derivatives, can cure the morphinist of his passion or even alleviate it.*

When Dr. Lewin wrote the above, his statement was almost certainly true. Until the late 1950's few people believed that a modern opiate addict who injected heroin intravenously could ever be successfully weaned from his drug and rehabilitated into society. The data well into the 1960's seemed to be on the side of those who argued that opiate addiction is a chronic disease and that the addict patient can never be considered cured or rehabilitated. Studies of relapse rates in this period showed that many heroin addicts became readdicted following release from hospitals or institutions after treatment for the addiction.[56]

Times have changed. There are several forms of treatment in use today that seem to deliver positive results, that is, social rehabilitation of the addict. Although there are many names used for the various, probably effective, treatment modes, there are only two basic types. One approach is primarily psychosocial and emphasizes the necessity of the addict relearning certain patterns of living. There are two subgroups in this approach, with one group emphasizing the necessity for lifetime treatment and the

*From Lewin, L.: Phantastica narcotics and stimulating drugs: their use and abuse, New York, 1931, E. P. Dutton & Company, Inc., p. 69.

other feeling that it can accomplish true social rehabilitation and move the ex-addict completely back into the community. The second basic type of approach is pharmacological. The crucial element is the use of drugs to block the pleasurable, tension-reducing effects of heroin while also preventing the discomfort of withdrawal. There are two subgroups here also, with the methadone maintenance procedure being the best known. The other pharmacological approach involves the use of opiate-blocking drugs such as cyclazocine. The structures of these two drugs are shown in Figs. 12-3 and 12-4.

In 1958 an ex-alcoholic felt that an organization such as Alcoholics Anonymous should be able to help narcotic addicts who want to be rehabilitated. From quite meager beginnings Synanon has grown into an apparently successful rehabilitation program and philosophy. The Synanon concepts and practices are extensive but a few points seem crucial.

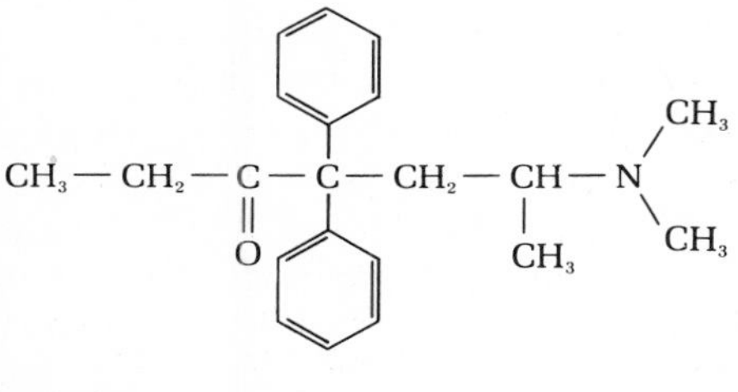

One is the belief that a narcotic addict is never cured (as AA believes an alcohol addict is never cured). Thus he should continue forever to live in the Synanon center or, after being clearly stabilized as an ex-addict, move into nearby living quarters and stay affiliated and involved with the Synanon program. In line with this belief Synanon counts the success of its program in terms of drug-free days. It expects relapses, since the addict is never cured, but emphasizes the time the ex-addict is free of drugs.

A second premise of this organization is that the addict must really want to be helped to discontinue drug use. To assure this motivation, there is an open door policy; a member is free to leave at any time. A third practice is the use of only ex-addicts as staff, with professionals being involved only for emergency medical service. Use of ex-addicts has two advantages, one being that he's "been there" and he's beaten addiction. Thus new members have someone to relate to who understands their problems. The ex-addict also has the advantage of knowing the tricks of the trade. As a result, he is able to structure the situation such that the living style of the street is rapidly shown to be not effective at Synanon.[57, 58]

Several things do make living at Synanon, and thus staying off drugs, effective. One is work; the ex-addict is kept busy. Another is faith, a religious-like belief of any sort. A third practice is to relate the type of work, the freedom, and the responsibility the individual has to the degree of his acceptance of

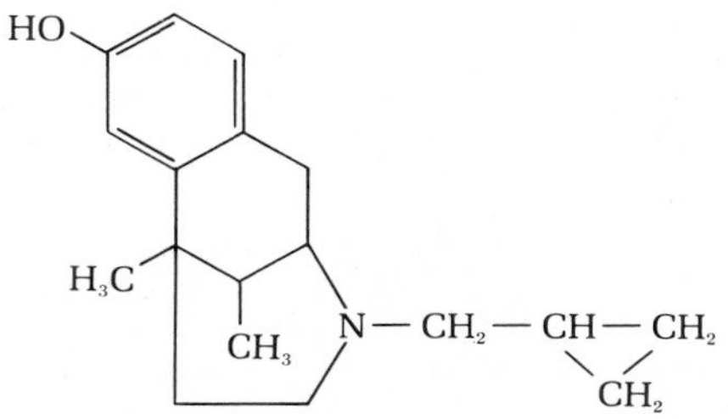

Methadone
Dolophine (Lilly)
(*dl*-6-dimethylamino-4,4-diphenyl-3-heptanone)

Fig. 12-3. Methadone.

Cyclazocine
WIN 20,740 (Winthrop)
(3-[cyclopropylmethyl]-1,2,3,4,5,6-hexahydro-6,11-dimethyl-2,6-methano-3-benzazocin-8-ol)

Fig. 12-4. Cyclazocine.

a nondrug life style and thus, in their terms, to his emotional maturity. Last is the assumption that an addict has difficulty in expressing his emotions and in identifying his own and others' emotions. The formal group encounters, which occur three to five times a week, are often psychologically violent but are the arena in which the ex-addict learns to stop using destructive guards to protect himself and above all learns to see himself and others as they really are.

The major objection raised to Synanon is the belief that an addict can never be cured. This means he may stay in residence for a long period and even after (if) he moves to live nearby, his world still must be centered on Synanon if he is to stay off drugs. People do leave Synanon to live *in* the community, but they are only members *of* the Synanon community. This idea is now being carried to its ultimate with the construction of a self-sustaining Synanon City, which the ex-addict will never have to leave. It is this lifelong commitment and absence of reentering the community that makes some wonder whether the Synanon program is moral or ethical.

The many other types of moderately effective psychosocial rehabilitation programs have similar kinds of residential treatment, and most are run by ex-addicts. They are also similar to Synanon in their emphasis on the necessity of the ex-addict's learning a new set of social and living skills. The major difference seems to be that programs other than Synanon see themselves as waystations in the individual's life rather than a permanent home. These centers operate to make the ex-addict a member of the community where he lives when he leaves the center. These centers want to give the ex-addict an involvement in something outside the center, and their programs are geared toward social rehabilitation.[59-61]

The pharmacological methods of treatment are better studied than the psychosocial methods, because the drugs used are classed as experimental for this use and the FDA requires that data be collected on their use.

The use of the synthetic opiate methadone on a continuing maintenance schedule is unquestionably the most successful and most widely applicable treatment for the control of opiate dependence.*

Methadone maintenance is receiving the most action and money today. Although there are variations, the basic procedures today are the same as those reported in the first paper on this procedure.[62] Methadone is an addicting drug and is given orally once a day in treatment programs. In the first stage of treatment of a heroin addict the daily dose of methadone is increased from about 10 milligrams to 40 or 50 milligrams. At this level, the desire (craving, drive) for the use of opiates disappears. That is, there is no motivation to seek and/or use opiates. At still higher doses, 80 to 100 milligrams, a blocking of the effects of mainlined heroin occurs. At the daily maintenance dosage (80 to 140 milligrams) methadone has three effects: it prevents withdrawal symptoms; it stops the desire for opiates; and it blocks the pleasurable effects of opiates.

The results of this form of treatment are even more impressive when it is appreciated that most centers use methadone maintenance only for addicts with a long history and a substantial level of addiction. Frequently addicts are not admitted unless they have tried other modes of rehabilitation and failed. No one is now suggesting that methadone maintenance be used with young, short-term addicts. Also, few people believe that methadone should be prescribed by individual physicians. All supporters of methadone maintenance emphasize the need for its use in a clinical setting where the addict does not control his own supply. A recent article summarized the results of this form of treatment.

There are now six years of experience with methadone maintenance. There are now perhaps 10,000 patients in about 50 programs. Results have uniformly been good. In round numbers, about 80 percent of the patients who have started remain in the program and free of dependence on the use of opiates other than methadone. Of these 80 percent, most have resumed productive lives; the remainder, though unemployed, no longer engage in illicit enterprise. . . . The 20 percent who

*From Kramer, J. C.: Methadone maintenance for opiate dependence, California Medicine **113**(6): 6, 1970.

must be removed from standard programs fail either because they abuse non-opiate drugs, particularly alcohol, choose to discontinue, usually in order to move elsewhere, or though freed from the costs of daily heroin use, persist in criminal activities, while a few may be so disruptive that their behavior cannot be tolerated.*

For many opiate addicts methadone maintenance is the road to social rehabilitation.[63] Many who oppose the expanded use of this drug in treatment programs do so on the grounds that a person using methadone is still an addict and may have to continue taking the drug for the rest of his life. Some argue that this treatment is immoral, some that it is just unethical. A "Letter to the Editor" stated it nicely.

> ...although there is no question that methadone maintenance treatment is an effective way of reducing the criminalistic activities of drug addicts, it is a question who is being treated: society or the drug takers. There is no doubt that the citizens of New York who are the victims of criminal addicts will be benefited by methadone maintenance programs, especially if applied to 5000 drug addicts. On the other hand, each individual addict who is given this narcotic is still an addict, and all the problems that he had that led up to addiction remain unsolved. In this sense methadone maintenance as a treatment program is highly anti-individualistic... each physician who prescribes methadone to a narcotic addict has this moral question to answer: Is he maintaining the patient on drugs for the good of society or for the good of his individual patient? Is he encouraging a kind of "cop out" by reinforcing the hopeless feeling of drug addicts when he wonders whether he can renounce drug use?†

Some who oppose the expansion of methadone maintenance programs do so on the basis that there is not adequate evidence to support the belief that methadone blocks the euphoria from intravenous heroin use. One study[64] found that over half of a long-term (2 years), high-dose (140 milligrams or more daily) methadone maintenance group of patients was still using heroin.

*Ibid., p. 8.
†From Myerson, D. J.: Methadone treatment of addicts, The New England Journal of Medicine **281**(7):390, 1969.

Some oppose methadone because from 1972 to 1974 it became a major drug of abuse and illegal sales of legally manufactured methadone boomed. Spending $10 a day on methadone could prevent withdrawal from a $30 to $50 a day heroin habit. Closer government controls reduced the availability of illegal methadone, but the message was clear: if a drug can be misused, it will be misused![64a] (See p. 189.)

These concerns should certainly be openly debated, but most authorities feel that certain facts support the expansion of methadone clinics. First, traditional therapies have not been effective in the social rehabilitation of narcotic addicts. Second, the psychosocial therapies, even though possibly effective, cannot be expanded rapidly enough to meet the needs of society or the demands of the addicts. Third, the methadone addict is not the same as the heroin addict and is, in fact, more like the diabetic who needs insulin on a regular basis.

The methadone addict and the diabetic view their drug use as incidental to their everyday living rather than focusing on it as the prime reason for living, which is the attitude of the heroin user. Almost 100 years ago a physician expressed what seems to be the crucial point about the morality of the methadone maintenance program.

> Is it not the duty of the physician when he cannot cure an ill, when there is no reasonable ground for hope that it will ever be done, to do the next best thing—advise a course of treatment that will diminish to an immense extent great evils otherwise irremediable?*

The final experimental treatment program that is developing rapidly is the use of narcotic antagonists. These programs have two phases, the substitution of oral methadone for heroin and the gradual withdrawal of all methadone, which results in a narcotic-free individual. This withdrawal phase is followed by the administration of a narcotic antagonist. Although several antagonists have been used, the one that has been studied most extensively is cyclazocine. The daily oral dose is gradually increased to a level where injected heroin has no effect. Mechanically the use of cyclazo-

*From Black, op. cit., p. 540.

cine has the same advantages as the use of methadone in that it can be orally administered once a day after a stabilization dose level has been reached.

Cyclazocine has one characteristic that is both a boon and a bane. Because of its low activity at the narcotic receptor site, it does not decrease the addict's desire for heroin. This may be a disadvantage and result in a higher failure rate than found with methadone programs. However, proponents of the narcotic antagonist treatment method emphasize the positive aspect of this characteristic. An addict on a narcotic antagonist program may continue to use heroin since the desire to use narcotics remains high. But the heroin in this case will have no effect. Thus these proponents suggest that the addict will learn that heroin does not give pleasurable effects, and all of the behaviors associated with its use will become less likely to occur. (In learning terms, these other behaviors will lose their pleasurable characteristics and extinguish.) When this occurs, perhaps the regular use of the antagonist can be stopped. The concept is interesting but clear evidence of the effectiveness of this type program is not yet available.[65-67]

No one of these treatment modes will be effective for all addicts. A 1972 government-supported study of all types of treatment programs concluded: "If society should decide to eliminate coercion as a means of controlling addiction, then heroin maintenance is the appropriate treatment. . . . If the goal is to achieve a given level of control with minimum . . . coercion, then it seems necessary to integrate . . . coercion and treatment into a single cooperative effort."[67a, p. 56] In other words, only the threat of prolonged confinement will bring addicts into, and keep them in, treatment.

One addict who dropped out of a methadone program indicated the complexities of the problem: "Methadone did the trick. . . . The reason I didn't stay on it was that I missed the excitement of using dope. I missed all the glamour of hustling and beating on people."[68]

CONCLUDING COMMENT

Narcotic use is slowing but is still spreading to new groups of users. Treatment programs have expanded but only partially solve the problem. As with most drug use the concern is not with the direct effects of the drug on the individual. Rather, the present patterns of addiction to narcotic agents result in indirect harm to both the individual and society.

> . . . harm to the individual is, in the main, indirect, arising from preoccupation with drug-taking; personal neglect, malnutrition and infection are frequent consequences. For society also, the resultant harm is chiefly related to the preoccupation of the individual with drug-taking; disruption of interpersonal relationships, economic loss, and crimes against property are frequent consequences.*

*From Eddy, N. B., and others: Drug dependence: its significance and characteristics, Bulletin of the World Health Organization 32:721-733, 1965.

PRECEDING QUOTES
1. Sydenham, T., 1680. Quoted in Gibson, M. R.: Botanicals: a factor in 50% of drug products, American Professional Pharmacist, February, 1969, p. 48.
2. De Quincey, T.: Confessions of an English opium-eater, New York, 1907, E. P. Dutton and Co., Inc., p. 194.
3. Cocteau, J.: Opium: the diary of an addict, London, 1933, Allen and Unwin, p. 72.
4. Chein, I., and others: The road to H, New York, 1964, Basic Books, Inc.
5. McCabe, P.: School days, Rolling Stone, February 18, 1971, p. 24.
6. Smith, D. E. Quoted in Nelson, H.: "Speed freaks" turning to heroin as antidote, Los Angeles Times, September 24, 1970.

REFERENCES
1. Sonnedecker, G.: Emergence of the concept of opiate addiction, Journal Mondial de Pharmacie; Federation Internationale Pharmaceutique 3:275-290, 1962; 1:27-34, 1963.
2. Africa, T. W.: The opium addiction of Marcus Aurelius, Journal of the History of Ideas 22:97-102, 1961.
3. Quoted in Hamarneh, S.: Sources and development of Arabic medical therapy and pharmacology, Sudhoffs Archiv fur Geschichte der Medizin und der Naturwissenschaften 54:34, 1970.
4. Abrams, M. H.: The milk of paradise, Cambridge, Massachusetts, 1934, Harvard University Press.
5. Lowes, J. L.: The road to Xanadu, Boston, 1927, Houghton Mifflin Company.
6. Ober, W. B.: Drowsed with the fume of poppies: opium and John Keats, Bulletin of the New York Academy of Medicine 44(7):862-881, 1968.
7. De Quincey, T.: Confessions of an English

opium-eater, New York, 1907, E. P. Dutton & Co., Inc.

8. De Quincey works, Vol. 206. Quoted in Lowes, J. L.: The road to Xanadu, Boston, 1927, Houghton Mifflin Company, p. 424.

9. Baudelaire, C.: Les paradis artificiels, Paris, 1961, Le Club du Meilleur Livre.

10. Mickel, E. J.: The artificial paradises in French literature, Chapel Hill, 1969, The University of North Carolina.

11. Blair, W.: An opium-eater in America, The Knickerbocker (New York Monthly Magazine) 20:47-57, 1842.

12. Hahn, E.: The big smoke, The New Yorker, February 15, 1969, pp. 35-43.

13. Scott, J. M.: The white poppy; a history of opium, New York, 1969, Funk & Wagnalls.

14. Fry, E.: China, England, and opium, Contemporary Review 27:447-459, 1876.

15. Fry, E.: China, England, and opium, Contemporary Review 30:1-10, 1877.

16. Fry, E.: China, England, and opium, Contemporary Review 31:313-321, 1878.

17. Kebler, L. F.: The present status of drug addiction in the United States. In Transactions of the American Therapeutic Society, Philadelphia, 1910, F. A. Davis Co., pp. 105 and 106.

18. Seevers, M. H.: Drug addiction problems, Sigma XI Quarterly 27(1):91-102, 1939.

19. Lindesmith, A. R.: Addiction and opiates, Chicago, 1968, Aldine Publishing Company.

20. Cook, J. G.: Remedies and rackets, New York, 1958, W. W. Norton and Company, Inc.

21. Holbrook, S. H.: The golden age of quackery, New York, 1959, The Macmillan Co.

22. Young, H. H.: The toadstool millionaires, Princeton, New Jersey, 1961, Princeton University Press.

23. Lindesmith, A. R.: The addict and the law, Bloomington, 1965, Indiana University Press.

23a. Bassett, C. A., and Pawluk, R. J.: Blood-brain barrier: penetration of morphine, codeine, heroin and methadone after carotid injection, Science 178:984-986, 1972.

24. Dott, D. B., and Stockman, R.: Proceedings of the Royal Society of Edinburgh, 1890, p. 321.

25. Floeckinger, F. C.: Clinical observations on heroin and heroin hydrochloride as compared with codeine and morphine, New York Medical Journal 71:970, 1900.

26. Wilcox, R. W.: Pharmacology and therapeutics, ed. 6, Philadelphia, 1905, P. Blakiston's Son and Co., p. 860.

27. Historical background of the existing system of international narcotics control, International Control of Narcotic Drugs, United Nations, New York, October, 1965.

28. Smith, R.: Status politics and the image of the addict, Issues in Criminology 2(2):157-175, 1966.

28a. Kramer, J. C.: Controlling narcotics in America, Drug Forum 1(1):51-69, 1971.

28b. Kramer, J. C.: Controlling narcotics in America, Drug Forum 1(2):153-167, 1972.

28c. Markham, J. M.: The American disease, New York Times, sec. 7, April 29, 1973.

28d. District of Columbia reports drop in abuse of heroin; trend seen, U. S. Medicine, p. 15, June 15, 1973.

28e. "Turnabout" seen in nation's epidemic of heroin abuse, U. S. Medicine, p. 2, Aug. 1, 1973.

28f. Harris, T. G.: As far as heroin is concerned, the worst is over, Psychology Today, pp. 68-85, August, 1973.

29. DuPont, R. L.: Profile of a heroin-addiction epidemic, The New England Journal of Medicine 285(6):320-324, 1971.

30. Richards, L. G., and Carroll, E. E.: Illicit drug use and addiction in the United States, U. S. Public Health Reports 85(12):1035-1041, 1970.

31. Hess, J. L.: U. S. and France sign antidrug accord, The New York Times, February 27, 1971, p. 3.

32. Drug abuse and the young, The Attack, Winter, 1970, pp. 5-8.

33. Sutton, H.: Drugs: ten years to doomsday? Saturday Review, November 14, 1970, p. 18.

34. Thomas, H.: Turkey agrees to '72 ban on poppies, United Press International, July 1, 1971.

34a. Spong, W.: Heroin: can the supply be stopped? Report to the Committee on Foreign Relations, U. S. Senate, Sept. 18, 1972.

35. A series of articles in the Christian Science Monitor beginning May 29, 1970.

36. Booming traffic in drugs: the government's dilemma, U. S. News and World Report, December 7, 1970, pp. 40-44.

37. Bewley, T. H.: The diagnosis and management of heroin addiction, The Practitioner 200:216, 218, 1968.

38. Jaffe, J. H.: Treatment of drug abusers. In Clark, W. G., and del Giudice, J., editors: Principles of psychopharmacology, New York, 1970, Academic Press, Inc., pp. 547-570.

38a. Powers, T.: What do you do for somebody who shoots smack? Rolling Stone 140, Aug. 2, 1973.

38b. Markham, J. M.: Heroin hunger may not a mugger make, New York Times Magazine, pp. 39-42, March 18, 1973.

38c. A perspective on "get tough" drug laws, The Drug Abuse Council, Inc., May, 1973.

39. Louria, D. B., Hensle, T., and Rose, J.: The major medical complications of heroin addiction, Annals of Internal Medicine 67(1):1, 1967.

40. Wilson, C. W. M., editor: The pharmacological and epidemiological aspects of adolescent drug dependence, New York, 1968, Pergamon Press, Inc.

40a. Brecher, E. M.: Licit and illicit drugs, Mt. Vernon, N. Y., 1972, Consumers Union, chap. 12.

40b. Helpern, M.: Heroin as a killer, New York Times Magazine, p. 29, Dec. 10, 1972.

41. Altman, L. K.: New outbreak of malaria in California traced to heroin users, The New York Times, March 17, 1971, p. 45.

42. Mason, P.: Mortality among young narcotic

addicts, Journal of Mt. Sinai Hospital **34**:4-10, 1967.

43. Winick, C.: Maturing out of narcotic addiction, Bulletin on Narcotics **14**(1):1-8, 1962.

44. Inquiry into alleged drug abuse in the armed services, Report of a special subcommittee of the Committee on Armed Services, House of Representatives, Ninety-second Congress, First Session, April 23, 1971, Washington, D. C., 1971, U. S. Government Printing Office.

45. Quoted in The World Heroin Problem, Committee Print, House of Representatives, Committee on Foreign Affairs, Ninety-second Congress, First Session, May 27, 1971, Washington, D. C., 1971, U. S. Government Printing Office, p. 18.

45a. Whitney, C. R.: Army drug plan in Germany hinges on court suit, New York Times, p. 10, Jan. 31, 1974.

45b. Finny, J. W.: Veteran addicts few, army finds, New York Times, p. 10, April 24, 1973.

45c. Addicted veterans fail to kick drug habit, U. S. Medicine, p. 6, June 15, 1973.

45d. Eddy, N. B., and May, E. L.: The search for a better analgesic, Science **181**:407-414, 1973.

46. Jaffe, J. H.: Narcotic analgesics. In Goodman, L. S., and Gilman, A., editors: The pharmacological basis of therapeutics, New York, 1970, The Macmillan Co., p. 238.

47. Osol, A., Pratt, R., and Altschule, M. D., editors: The United States dispensatory and physician's pharmacology, ed. 26, Philadelphia, 1967, J. B. Lippincott Co.

48. Dole, V. P.: Biochemistry of addiction, Annual Review of Biochemistry **39**:821, 1970.

49. Kolb, L.: Pleasure and deterioration from narcotic addiction, Mental Hygiene **9**:699-724, 1925.

49a. McAuliffe, W. E., and Gordon, R. A.: A test of Lindesmith's theory of addiction. I. The frequency of euphoria among long-term addicts, American Journal of Sociology. In Press.

49b. Powell, D. H.: A pilot study of occasional heroin users, Archives of General Psychiatry **28**:586-594, 1973.

50. Mathis, J. L.: Sexual aspects of heroin addiction, Medical Aspects of Human Sexuality **4**(9):98-109, 1970.

51. Isbell, H., and White, W. M.: Clinical characteristics of addictions, The American Journal of Medicine **14**(5):558-565, 1953.

52. Willis, J. H.: Some problems of opiate addiction, The Practitioner **200**:220-225, 1968.

53. Eddy, N. B.: Analgesic and dependence-producing properties of drugs. In Wikler, A., editor: The addictive states, Baltimore, 1968, The Williams & Wilkins Co., pp. 1-12.

54. Wilner, D. M., and Kassebaum, G. G., editors: Narcotics, New York, 1965, McGraw-Hill Book Co.

55. Simon, W., and Lumry, G. K.: Alcoholism and drug addiction among physicians—chronic self-destruction? Drug Dependence **3**:11-14, 1969.

56. O'Donnell, J. A.: The relapse rate in narcotic addiction: a critique of follow-up studies, New York State Narcotic Addiction Control Commission Reprints **2**(1):1-21, 1968.

57. Deissler, K. J.: Synanon—its concepts and methods, Drug Dependence **5**:28-35, 1970.

58. Yablonsky, L., and Dederich, C. E.: Synanon: an analysis of some dimensions of the social structure of an antiaddiction society. In Wilner, D. M., and Kassebaum, G. G., editors: Narcotics, New York, 1965, McGraw-Hill Book Co., p. 194.

59. Wolfe, R. C., and Boriello, R.: Drug addiction: an effective therapeutic approach, Medical Times **98**(9):185-193, 1970.

60. Casriel, D., and Deitch, D.: Permanent cure of narcotics addicts, The Physician's Panorama, October, 1966, pp. 4-12.

61. Sanders, M. K.: Addicts and zealots, Harper's Magazine, June, 1970, pp. 71-80.

62. Dole, V. P., and Nyswander, M.: A medical treatment for diacetylmorphine (heroin) addiction, Journal of the American Medical Association **193**(8):646-650, 1965.

63. Blachly, P. H.: A venture into medical treatment of crime, Medical Record News, February, 1971, pp. 24-29.

64. Taylor, W. J. R.: Addiction and the community: narcotic substitution therapy, a paper presented at the American Medical Association Annual Convention, Atlantic City, New Jersey, June 24, 1971.

64a. Drug abuse: methadone becomes the solution and the problem, Science **179**:772-775, 1973.

65. Freeman, A. M., and others: Clinical studies of cyclazocine in the treatment of narcotic addiction, American Journal of Psychiatry **124**:1499-1504, 1968.

66. Fink, M.: Narcotic antagonists in opiate dependence, Science **169**:1005-1006, 1970.

67. Zaks, A., and others: Naloxone treatment of opiate dependence, Journal of the American Medical Association **215**(13):2108-2110, 1971.

67a. Narcotic antagonists: the search accelerates, Science **177**:249-250, 1972.

67b. McGlothlin, W. H., Tabbush, V. C., Chambers, C. D., and Jamison, K.: Alternative approaches to opiate addiction control: costs, benefits and potential, Bureau of Narcotics and Dangerous Drugs, U. S. Department of Justice, June, 1972.

68. Quoted in Medicine, Time, January 4, 1971, p. 60.

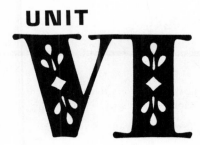

UNIT VI

The phantasticants

13 Introduction to the hallucinogens

It is remarkable that one characteristic which seems to separate man from the allegedly lower animals is a recurring desire to escape from reality.

> *The Food of the Gods*
> C. H. W. Horne and J. A. W. McCluskie, 1963

These substances have formed a bond of union between men of opposite hemispheres, the uncivilized and the civilized; they have forced passages which, once open, proved of use for other purposes; they produced in ancient races characteristics which have endured to the present day, evidencing the marvellous degree of intercourse that existed between different peoples just as certainly and exactly as a chemist can judge the relations of two substances by their reactions.

> *Phantastica*
> Lewis Lewin, 1931

One conclusion was forced upon my mind. . . . It is that our normal waking consciousness, rational consciousness as we call it, is but one special type of consciousness, whilst all about it, parted from it by the filmiest of screens, there lie potential forms of consciousness entirely different.

> *Varieties of Religious Experience*
> William James, 1904

...she went back to the table ... this time she found a little bottle on it ... and tied round the neck of the bottle was a paper label with the words "DRINK ME" beautifully printed on it in large letters.

It was all very well to say "Drink me," but the wise little Alice was not going to do *that* in a hurry. "No, I'll look first," she said, "and see whether it's marked *poison* or not" ... she had never forgotten that if you drink much from a bottle marked "poison," it is almost certain to disagree with you sooner or later. However, this bottle was *not* marked "poison," so Alice ventured to taste it, and finding it very nice (it had, in fact, a sort of mixed flavor of cherry-tart, custard, pineapple, roast turkey, toffy, and hot buttered toast), she very soon finished it off. "What a curious feeling!" said Alice; "I must be shutting up like a telescope." And so it was, indeed; she was now only ten inches high, and her face brightened up at the thought that she was now the right size for going through the little door into that lovely garden.

Alice in Wonderland, Lewis Carroll

Alice could play many roles in the world of drugs. She certainly should be named patron saint of the OTC compounds because she compulsively read the label and followed directions. As queen of the hallucinogens she reigns supreme. For thousands of years before Alice and increasingly recently, people have believed what Alice said:

I know something interesting is sure to happen whenever I eat or drink anything.

As a result, Alice is not the only one who has eaten or drunk some substance and experienced strange and unique body sensations, changes in perceptions, and alterations of consciousness. This chapter and the next will detail some of the substances and experiences.

INTRODUCTION

...man found it necessary to try to explain these extraordinary powers of some of the plants in his environment. In all primitive cultures, this explanation invariably ascribed to the plant some particular divinity or spirit which, in many instances, was thought to be efficacious as an intermediary between man's world of humdrum reality and the supernatural or spirit realm.*

*From Schultes, R. E.: Hallucinogenic plants of the New World, The Harvard Review **1**(4):18, 1963.

If God can be found through the medium of any drug, God is not worthy of being God.*

Over 4,500 years ago a South American tribe buried one of its members and included his snuff tube and snuffing tablets. Already there must have been some expectation of an existence beyond physical death, another reality. This chapter discusses some of the ways in which people have tried to explore other realities during life by using chemicals. Many groups in the past, and some of the so-called primitive tribes today, have looked at "the beyond within" in a religious or ceremonial context. Except in more advanced cultures people never take drugs, they use plants. This is an important distinction. Drugs and chemicals are derived from plants but chemicals aren't used by natives; they use plants, which they believe to have a life, a resident divinity. Eating the plant meant taking and acquiring the spiritual power of the plant.

The idea that plants had spirits meant that they were not used indiscriminately. Only in religious ceremonies did you use a plant that had power, and any plant with psychoactive properties had power. One writer comments:

This principle was true of even so mildly psychedelic a drug as tobacco. Aboriginally, tobacco was *always* used in a sacred magico-religious context, and never for mere secular-indulgent enjoyment.... And when ... Indian chiefs ... smoked the sacred calumet or peace pipe, the rite meant the invoking of the power of tobacco upon their sacred oath.†

As we know, some of the psychoactive plants with long histories in western civilization have been adopted for "mere secular-indulgent enjoyment." Those who use drugs today in the search for religious experiences have voiced a similar concern:

To turn on means to find a sacrament which returns you to the temple of God, your own body, to go out of your mind. To tune in means

*From Baba, M.: God speaks, New York, 1955, Dodd, Mead & Co.
†From LaBarre, W.: Old and New World narcotics: a statistical question and an ethnological reply, Botany **24**(1):77, 1970.

to be reborn; to drop back in, to start a new sequence of behavior that reflects your vision; in other words, to manifest in a behavioral way the religious experience you have had. . . .

Today, the sacrament is LSD. However, sacraments wear out. They become part of the social game. Treasure LSD while it still works. In fifteen years it will be a tame, socialized routine.*

Many plants have been found that have the property of being able to transport the individual to what he feels is a new reality. In the Americas, eighty to one hundred different plants have been used at different times and by different groups because of their psychoactive characteristics. The rest of the world never used more than seven species, and some feel that this is more a reflection of cultural differences than of botanical differences. Only a few of these agents can be commented on here. These plants and the psychoactive chemicals they contain are classed as hallucinogens because their distinguishing characteristic, to our society, is the ability to induce bizarre alterations in perception and states of consciousness. Most of the hallucinogens are agents that were included in Lewin's category, phantasticants. As usual the thrust will be to show the interrelationship of the drug and its effects on society as well as on the individual.[a]

CLASSIFICATION

Classification of the hallucinogens must be based on the same principles as the classification of other drugs (see Chapter 4). These agents could be meaningfully grouped as naturally occurring or synthetic compounds, or on whether they have a New World or Old World origin. Some authorities use other dimensions:

. . . a great number of drugs can induce psychotic reactions characterized by disorders in perception (including hallucinations), thinking, feeling (affect), and behavior. These can be roughly divided into two main drug classes: (1) drugs like lysergic acid diethylamide (LSD) and mescaline that produce states something like the functional psychoses such as schizophrenia and mania, and (2) drugs like atropine and diisopropylfluorophosphate

(DFP) that produce a syndrome more like a delirium or organic psychosis. We can further distinguish between drugs like LSD that, at adequate dosage, induce their psychotomimetic effect in most, if not all, people, and drugs like amphetamine that affect only a few particularly susceptible individuals. The distinction between the LSD group and the deliriants is not absolute but forms two ends of a continuum. Similarly, there has been a good deal of dispute as to whether the effects of LSD do or do not resemble schizophrenia.*

For some authorities there is no dispute; the drug-induced psychosis and schizophrenia are very different. A review summarized the work of one authority.

Withdrawal from interpersonal contacts is characteristic of schizophrenics; it is atypical of the drug-induced psychoses. Schizophrenics and drug subjects communicate poorly, but the former seem not to care; the latter are greatly concerned about it. The nature of the hallucinations is different. In schizophrenia they tend to be auditory and threatening; in the drug-induced states they are visual and pleasant or impersonal. Subjects under drugs tend to be highly suggestible; that is why the drug tends to be cultogenic. Schizophrenics are highly resistant to suggestion. In a blind study of tape-recorded mental status interviews of six schizophrenics and six subjects under drugs, a large group of professional raters had little difficulty in distinguishing between the two groups.†

For our purposes it seems most appropriate to group the hallucinogens according to the neurotransmitter through which they probably act. The three neurotransmitter substances named in Chapter 3—acetylcholine, noradrenaline, and serotonin—have very different chemical structures, each with a definite chemical nucleus. Serotonin is based on an indole nucleus:

*From Smith, D. E.: Symposium: psychedelic drugs and religion, Journal of Psychedelic Drugs **1**(2):48, 1967-68.

*From Smythies, J. R.: The mode of action of psychotomimetic drugs, Neurosciences Research Program Bulletin **8**(1):5, 1970.
†From Lipton, M. A.: The relevance of chemically-induced psychoses to schizophrenia. In Efron, D. H., editor: Psychotomimetic drugs, New York, 1970, Raven Press, p. 236. (The authority being referred to is Leo Hollister.)

The most notorious, most maligned, and most potent hallucinogen and the agent that made this a psychedelic society is the indole-based d-lysergic acid diethylamide, LSD. It is a synthetic compound closely related to naturally occurring hallucinogenic agents found in some morning glory seeds. The indole nucleus is also the basic structure in psilocybin, the active ingredient of the magic mushrooms of Mexico. The indole hallucinogens are discussed in Chapter 14.

Noradrenaline and the other adrenergic transmitters have a catechol nucleus:

The catechol nucleus is related to the phenethylamine structure of amphetamine, which could easily have been included in this section. The prototype catechol hallucinogen is mescaline, the primary active agent in the peyote cactus used in religious ceremonies by the Indians of southwestern United States. A synthetic hallucinogen with the catechol nucleus is DOM (STP).

Acetylcholine, easily the best-established neurotransmitter, has no chemical nucleus with a specific name, but the structure does have a unique characteristic that determines its activity. This is the existence of a positively charged atom a fixed distance from a carboxyl group.

Hallucinogens that act via the cholinergic system are unique, for only with these agents is there poor memory for the period of altered consciousness. There are three anticholinergic agents in this category that occur naturally in many plants, including henbane, the deadly nightshade plant, and Datura. Ditran is an example of a synthetic anticholinergic hallucinogenic drug.

THE CATECHOL HALLUCINOGENS
Peyote

Peyote is truly unique among the hallucinogenic agents since it is the only American plant used in sacred and religious ceremonies from before written history that has been retained as an integral part of a recognized religious group. Peyote (peyotl) is the cactus Lophophora williamsii, which is a synonym for an earlier designation, Anhalonium lewinii. It was so named to honor Lewin, who studied some of the plant that he acquired during his 1886 trip to the United States.

When Cortez moved into Mexico in the early 1500's, he took with him Christian missionaries whose goal was to drive out all remnants of the Aztec civilization and religion. They were also, and rather incidentally, to save the heathens. Before the ancient religious and ceremonial customs were forced underground, many reports were made of plants being used for sacred purposes.

One extensive report (and the most reliable since the author was not a professional missionary) on the pharmacopoeia and medicine of Mexico was compiled by Dr. Francisco Hernandez between 1570 to 1575. Hernandez was Court Physician to King Philip II of Spain, who named him Protomedico of the Indies. Philip told Hernandez to collect information about all aspects of the Mexican civilization but especially about its herbs and medicines. Mexican medicine in the sixteenth century must have been extensive, for Hernandez reported 1,200 remedies.

The peyote cactus was described by Hernandez: "The root is of nearly medium size, sending forth no branches or leaves above the ground. . . Both men and women are said to be harmed by it . . . it causes those devouring it to be able to foresee and predict things. . ." Earlier and later reports in the sixteenth century emphasized even more the psychoactive aspects of its use: ". . . those who eat or chew it see visions either frightful or laughable . . ." and ". . . see visions of terrifying sights like the devil. . . ." Briefly:

Peyote (from the Aztec peyotl) is a small, spineless, carrot-shaped cactus, Lophophora williamsii Lemaire, which grows wild in the Rio Grande Valley and southward. It is mostly subterranean, and only the grayish-green pincushion-like top appears above ground. . .*

*From LaBarre, W.: Twenty years of peyote studies, Current Anthropology 1(1):45, 1960.

In pre-Columbian times the Aztec, Huichol, and other Mexican Indians ate the plant ceremonially either in the dried or green state. This produces profound sensory and psychic derangements lasting twenty-four hours, a property which led the natives to value and use it religiously *

Only the part of the cactus that is above ground is easily edible, but the entire plant is psychoactive. This upper portion, or crown, is sliced into disks that dry and are known as "mescal buttons." These slices of the peyote cactus remain psychoactive indefinitely and are the source of the cactus between the yearly harvests. The journey by Indians in November and December to harvest the peyote is an elaborate ceremony, sometimes taking almost a month and a half. When the mescal buttons are to be used, they are soaked in the mouth until soft, then formed by hand into a bolus and swallowed.

Mescal buttons should not be confused with the mescal beans or with mescal liquor, which is distilled from the fermentation of the agave cactus. Mescal buttons are slices of the peyote cactus and contain mescaline as the primary active agent. Mescal beans, however, are dark red seeds from the shrub *Sophora secundiflora.* "These seeds, formerly the basis of a vision-seeking cult, contain a highly toxic alkaloid, cysticine, the effects of which somewhat resemble nicotine, causing nausea, convulsions, hallucinations and occasional death from respiratory failure."[1] The mescal bean has a long history, and there is some evidence that use of the bean diminished and ceased when the safer peyote became available in the southwestern United States. In the transition from a mescal bean to a mescal button cult there appeared, in some tribes, a period in which a mixture of peyote and mescal seeds was concocted and drunk. These factors contributed to considerable confusion in the early (and some recent) literature.

It would be a serious error if an anthropologist or ethnobotanist confused the two. In a legislative situation such a confusion could have a devastating impact. In a weighty report

to the House of Representatives in 1918 on "Prohibition of Use of Peyote," one of the supporting documents was a 1909 letter by an Indian agent who confused the two. (Compare his description with those of the mescal bean and mescal button effects noted previously.) In part, his report said:

... with reference to the effects of the peyote, commonly known as mescal ...

Several deaths have been reported to me which were clearly caused by the use of peyote; two, in particular, which resulted from an apparently healthy Indian dying while in the stupor from the use of peyote.

... the customary dose for beginners is eight peyote beans, taken in the form prescribed below, together with from two to five drinks of the water in which the beans have been steeped ...

... death is caused from malnutrition and by a violent disturbance of the digestive organs, and also by action on the respiratory centers.

The users of the peyote have described to me a feeling which they say they experience after using it a short time resembling that of suffocation. ... It is most commonly used among the Indians of this agency by first steeping the bean in hot water; then the bean is mashed and rolled in the fingers, and from 8 to 50 are taken at one time or during one meeting of the peyote users. In addition to eating the bean, they also drink the water in which the bean has been steeped ...*

Use in religion. Peyote played an important role in some of the religious groups in Mexico. The early missionaries attempted to stop its use. A Spanish missionary, Padre de Leon, had priests include the following questions in the confessional to be used with penitent Indians:

Art thou a sooth-sayer? Dost thou fortell events by reading omens, interpreting dreams, or by tracing circles and figures on water? ... Dost though suck the blood of others? Dost thou wander about at night, calling upon demons to help thee? Hast thou drunk peyotl, or given it to others to drink. ...†

Nothing succeeded in eliminating its use,

*From Thackery, F. A.: Prohibition of use of peyote, House Reports (Public) No. 560 **2**:18-19, 1917-1918.
†Quoted in LaBarre, W.: The peyote cult, op. cit., p. 23.

*From LaBarre, W.: The peyote cult, Hamden, Connecticut, 1964, The Shoe String Press, p. 7.

but peyote did go underground, along with the other magic plants of Mexico, only recently to reemerge. Although there was evidence that the use of peyote had moved north into the United States as early as 1760, it was not until the late nineteenth century that a peyote cult was widely established among the Indians of the plains.

From that time to the present, Indian missionaries have spread the peyote religion to almost a quarter of a million Indians, some as far north as Canada. The development of the present form of this sect has been summarized:

> . . . the independent groups of the Peyote Religion have federated into the Native American Church during the 20th century, like the independent congregations of the Jesus Cult federated into the Catholic Church during the 4th century. However, just as not all congregations accepting the basic doctrines of Christianity belonged to the Catholic Church, so not all groups accepting the basic doctrines of Peyotism belong to the Native American Church.*

In 1960 peyotism was ". . . the major religious cult of most Indians of the United States between the Rocky Mountains and the Mississippi. . . ."[2]

One version of how this variant of Christianity developed was told by a member of one tribe:

> A long time ago Indians were fighting: they killed each other and one woman was left from the tribes. She walked over the Desert—there was no food nor water: she was almost starved. Then a voice was heard from the sky. It was Jesus, and said, "Look down at this thing (pointing to Father Peyote, a large peyote disc) and you will get food and drink." She walked over a hill and on the other side she found water—it was her food from the skies, and the voice said this, peyote, was her food.†

The Native American Church of the United States was first chartered in Oklahoma in 1918 and is an amalgamation of Christianity and traditional beliefs and practices of the Indians. Its basic beliefs are simply stated in the articles of incorporation:

> The purpose for which this corporation is formed is to foster and promote religious believers in Almighty God and the customs of the several Tribes of Indians throughout the United States in the worship of a Heavenly Father and to promote morality, sobriety, industry, charity, and right living and cultivate a spirit of self-respect and brotherly love and union among the members of the several Tribes of Indians throughout the United States . . . with and through the sacramental use of peyote.*

As in all religions there has developed a whole series of rituals surrounding the use of peyote in religious ceremonies. Peyote is also used in other ways because the Indians attribute spiritual power to the peyote plant. As such, peyote is believed to be helpful, along with prayers and modern medicines, in curing illnesses. It is also worn as an amulet, much as some Christians wear a St. Christopher's medal, to protect the wearer from harm.

In the charter year, 1918, bills were introduced into the United States Congress, as they had been before, to restrict the use of peyote by the Indians. The entire report to the House of Representatives on "Prohibition of Use of Peyote" is interesting, but only a few of the more relevant issues can be mentioned here.

Reviewing some of the clear thinking presented by those advocating restricting the use of peyote, it is surprising that the bill was not enacted. For example, considering the question of whether alcohol or peyote is more harmful the report of a physician says:

> So far as its results upon the human economy are concerned from a pathological standpoint, alcohol is altogether the safest and least harmful. The alcoholic subject may, by careful system of dietetics, escape physical and mental weakness, but the mescal fiend travels to absolute incompetency. It is a vicious thing.†

Some testimony was solicited from scientific authorities, and Dr. H. W. Wiley, who spearheaded the enactment of the 1906 Pure Food

---

*From Slotkin, J. S.: Religious defenses (the Native American Church), Journal of Psychedelic Drugs 1(2):80, 1967-68.
†From Bromberg, W., and Tranter, C. L.: Peyote intoxication: some psychological aspects of the peyote rite, Journal of Nervous and Mental Disease 97:524, 1943.

*From LaBarre, W., and others: Statement on peyote, Science 114:582-583, 1951.
†From Prohibition of use of peyote, House Reports (Public) No. 560 2:17, 1917-1918.

and Drugs Act, sent a letter that said, in part:

> It is driving many of them to ruin. Its effects may be compared in some particulars to those of cocaine. It causes the victim, who becomes semiconscious, to have the most wonderful sensations of delight and pleasure, especially through the visions of flowers, sunshine, and verdure, which rise before him. The intoxication lasts from 24 to 48 hours and then gradually passes away. During its continuation the person is totally unfit for any useful purpose. It is a typically habit-forming drug, and to those who indulge in it the desire for its use becomes uncontrollable. The active principle is probably a resin or a glucoside. It probably is of the same nature of the poison in Indian hemp. Its use can no more be regarded in the light of a religious rite than that of alcohol, morphine, or cocaine. Its entire prohibition would conserve the financial, physical, mental, and spiritual welfare of the Indians.*

A petition to the Commissioner of Indian Affairs to prohibit peyote on Indian reservations was rejected by the Secretary of Interior who prohibited "absolutely any interference by the Indian Bureau with the religious practices of the Native American Church."[3] This proved to be a good decision.[3a]

Over 30 years later as "the-baby-with-the-bath-water" type of thinking reemerged in the drug world, five famous anthropologists felt it necessary to issue a statement on peyote which begins:

> ... there has been some propaganda to declare illegal the peyote used by many Indian tribes. ... our duty to protest against a campaign which only reveals the ignorance of the propagandists concerned.†

After a thousand well-chosen words this distinguished group concluded:

> ... the Native American Church of the United States is a legitimate religious organization deserving of the same right to religious freedom as other churches; also, that peyote is used sacramentally in a manner corresponding to the bread and wine of white Christians.‡

Hallucinogenic use. Near the end of the nineteenth century, Heffter isolated several alkaloids from peyote and showed that mescaline was the primary agent only for the

visual effects induced by peyote. Spath in 1919 finally synthesized mescaline and most experiments on the psychoactive and/or behavioral effects since then have used synthesized mescaline. There have now been over thirty psychoactive alkaloids identified in peyote, but mescaline does seem to be the agent responsible for the vivid colors and other visual effects. The fact that mescaline is not equivalent to peyote is not always made clear in the literature.

One of the early investigators of the effects of peyote was Dr. Weir Mitchell, who used an extract of peyote and who reported, in part:

> The display which for an enchanted two hours followed was such as I find it hopeless to describe in language which shall convey to others the beauty and splendor of what I saw. Stars, delicate floating films of color, then an abrupt rush of countless points of white light swept across the field of view, as if the unseen millions of the Milky Way were to flow in a sparkling river before my eyes ... zigzag lines of very bright colors ... the wonderful loveliness of swelling clouds of more vivid colors gone before I could name them.*

Another early experimenter was Havelock Ellis. Interestingly, he took his peyote on Good Friday in 1897, 65 years before the much noted Good Friday experiment with psilocybin. His experience is described in detail in a 1902 article entitled "Mescal: A Study of a Divine Plant" in *Popular Science Monthly,* but a brief quotation gives the essence of the experience:

> On the whole, if I had to describe the visions in one word, I should say that they were living arabesques. There was generally a certain incomplete tendency to symmetry, the effect being somewhat as if the underlying mechanism consisted of a large number of polished facets acting as mirrors. It constantly happened that the same image was repeated over a large part of the field, though this holds good mainly of the forms, for in the colors there would still remain all sorts of delicious varieties. Thus at a moment when uniformly jewelled flowers seemed to be springing up and extending all over the field of vision, the flowers still showed every variety of delicate tone and tint.†

---

*From Wiley, H. W. Quoted in Congressional Record-Senate **56**:4130, 1918.
†From LeBarre and others, op. cit., p. 582.
‡Ibid., p. 583.

*From De Ropp, R. S.: Drugs and the mind, New York, 1957, Grove Press, Inc., p. 34.
†From Ellis, H.: Mescal: a study of a divine plant, Popular Science Monthly **61**:59, 1902.

In reflecting on his experience Ellis comments:

> It should be added that a sense of well-being is not an essential part of these sensory manifestations. In this respect mescal is entirely unlike those drugs of which alcohol is the supreme type. Under the influence of a moderate dose of alcohol the specific senses are not obviously affected at all, but there is a vague and massive consciousness of emotional well-being, a sense of satisfaction tending to a conviction that 'all's well with the world.' Alcohol has a dulling influence on sensory activity and on the intellectual centers. . . . Mescal, on the other hand, is not mainly emotional in its effects but mainly sensory and it leaves the intellect almost unimpaired even in large doses. It is true that at one stage of mescal intoxication, and more especially in quite healthy persons, there is a feeling of well-being, and even of beatitude, accompanied by an illusory sense of quite unusual intellectual activity; but there is no stage of maudlin emotionality; on the whole there is a condition of fairly unimpaired and alert intellect, untiringly absorbed in the contemplation of the strange world of new sensory phenomena into which the subject has been introduced.*

In an earlier article (1897) entitled "Mescal: A New Artificial Paradise," Ellis concluded by stating:

> . . . unlike the other chief substances to which it may be compared, mescal does not wholly carry us away from the actual world, or plunge us into oblivion; a large part of its charm lies in the halo of beauty which it casts around the simplest and commonest things. . . .

> The few observations recorded in America and my own experiments in England do not enable us to say anything regarding the habitual consumption of mescal in large amounts. That such consumption would be gravely injurious I can not doubt. Its safeguard seems to lie in the fact that a certain degree of robust health is required to obtain any real enjoyment from its visionary gifts. It may at least be claimed that for a healthy person to be once or twice admitted to the rites of mescal is not only an unforgettable delight, but an educational influence of no mean value.†

It may well be that not every healthy individual wants every educational opportunity that is offered him. William James, surprisingly, was one who did not. He wrote to his brother Henry: "I ate one but three days ago, was violently sick for twenty-four hours, and had no other symptoms whatever except that and the Katzenjammer the following day. I will take the visions on trust." Even Dr. Weir Mitchell, who had the effect previously recorded, said: "These shows are expensive . . . The experience, however, was worth one such headache and indigestion but was not worth a second."

Even if you get by without too much nausea and physical discomfort, which the Indians also report, all may not go well. Huxley, whose 1954 *The Doors of Perception*[4] made him a guru in this area, admitted: "Along with the happily transfigured majority of mescaline takers there is a minority that finds in the drug only hell and purgatory." It is reported that natives sometimes wished for "bad trips" when taking this or other plants. By meeting their personal demons, much like Saint Anthony, they hoped to conquer them and remove problems from their lives.

Pharmacodynamics of mescaline. Mescaline is readily absorbed if taken orally. There is a maximal concentration of the drug in the brain after 30 to 120 minutes. About half of it is removed from the body in 6 hours, and there is evidence that some mescaline persists in the brain for up to 9 to 10 hours. Similar to the indole hallucinogens, the effects obtained with low doses, about 3 milligrams per kilogram, are primarily euphoric, while doses in the range of 5 milligrams per kilogram give rise to a full set of hallucinations. Most of the mescaline is excreted unchanged in the urine, and the metabolites identified thus far are not psychoactive.

A dose that is psychoeffective in man causes pupil dilation, pulse rate and blood pressure increases, and an elevation in body temperature. All of these effects are similar to those induced by LSD, psilocybin, and most other alkaloidal hallucinogens. There are other signs of central stimulation, such as EEG arousal, following mescaline intake. In rats the LD 50 is about 370 milligrams per kilogram, ten to thirty times the dose that causes behavioral

---

*Ibid., p. 65.
†From Ellis, H.: Mescal: a new artificial paradise, Annual Report of the Smithsonian Institution **52:**547-548, 1897.

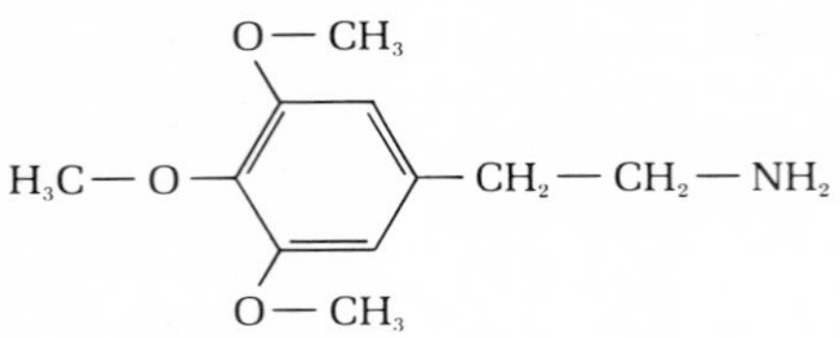

Mescaline
(3,4,5-trimethoxyphenethylamine)

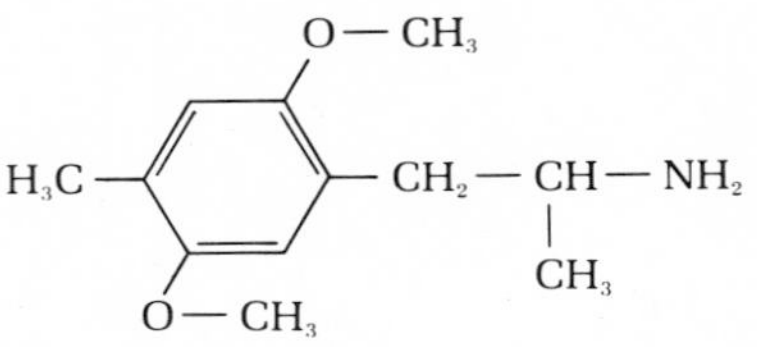

DOM (STP)
(2-amino-1-[2',5'-dimethoxy-4'-methyl]-
phenylpropane)

Fig. 13-1. Catechol hallucinogens.

effects. Death results from convulsions and respiratory arrest. Tolerance develops more slowly to mescaline than to LSD, and even though these drugs appear to act via different mechanisms, there is cross tolerance between them. As with LSD, the mescaline intoxication can be blocked with chlorpromazine.

Fig. 13-1 contains the chemical structure of both mescaline and DOM and clearly shows the relationship to the phenethylamine structure and the catechol nucleus.

DOM (STP)

DOM is 2,5-dimethoxy-4-methylamphetamine. According to most users, DOM is called STP, and street talk is that the initials stand for serenity, tranquility, and peace. Little human work has been done with this drug in controlled laboratory situations.[5, 6] Its actions and effects, however, are highly similar to mescaline and LSD, with a total dose of 1 to 3 milligrams yielding euphoria most often and 3 to 5 milligrams a 6- to 8-hour hallucinogenic period. This makes DOM about 100 times as potent as mescaline but only one-thirteenth as potent as LSD.

DOM has a reputation of inducing an extraordinarily long experience, but this seems to be caused by the very large amounts being used. Pills of DOM bought on the street contained about 10 milligrams—a very big dose. Reports by users had suggested that DOM was unlike other hallucinogens and that its effects were enhanced rather than blocked by chlorpromazine. Controlled laboratory work with normal volunteers, however, has clearly shown that the effects of DOM are similar to those of other hallucinogens and that chlorpromazine does attenuate the DOM experience.[7]

An early report[8] and an excellent review

from the Haight-Ashbury Clinic[9] contains most of the essential information about the rise and fall of DOM use. The latter paper concludes:

It appears then that DOM produces a higher incidence of acute and chronic toxic reactions than any of the other commonly used hallucinogens. . . . It appears that the effects of DOM are like a combination of amphetamine and LSD with the hallucinogenic effects of the drug very often putting the peripheral amphetamine like physiological effects out of perspective. . . .*

DOM may be taken more frequently than is known. It is often substituted for mescaline. In one study none of twenty-three "mescaline" purchases contained mescaline, but several were DOM.[9a] Analysis of 1800 street buys of different drugs found 7% to contain *no* drug and only 54% to contain the drug they were represented to be.[9b] If you can't trust your friendly neighborhood pusher, whom can you trust?

ANTICHOLINERGIC HALLUCINOGENS

It may be a bit discouraging to those whose ancestors came from Europe that so far not one of the hallucinogens has had its noble, or ignoble, history in traditional western culture. Unfortunately, now it is necessary to deal with the drugs that poisoned Hamlet's father as well as the Roman Emperor Claudius. Strange that they should be the same agents that probably made Cleopatra bright-eyed if not bushy-tailed and the same magic potions that gave witches liftoff power and put the kick in Vietnam marijuana.

*From Smith, D., and Meyers, F.: The psychotomimetic amphetamine with special reference to STP (DOM) toxicity. In Smith, D., editor: Drug abuse papers, 1969, Section 4, Berkley, 1969, University of California, p. 4.

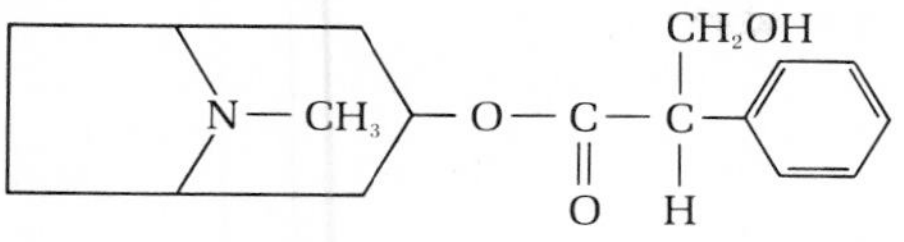

Atropine (*dl*-hyoscyamine)
(1αH,5αH-tropan-3α-ol, [+]-tropate [ester])

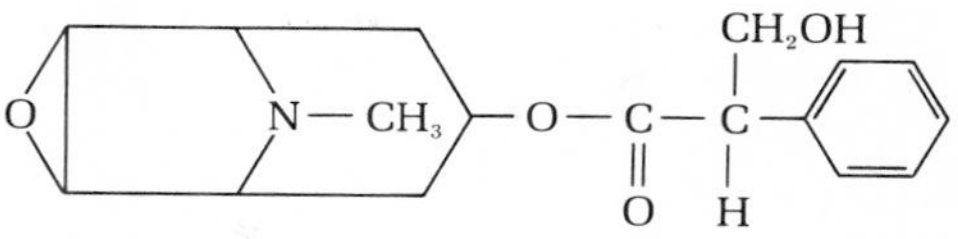

Scopolamine (*l*-hyoscine)
(6β,7β-epoxy-1αH,5αH-tropan-3α-ol,[−]-tropate [ester])

Fig. 13-2. Naturally occurring anticholinergic hallucinogens.

The potato family contains all the naturally occurring agents to be discussed here. Three of the genera—*Atropa, Hyoscyamus,* and *Mandragora*—have a single species of importance and were primarily restricted to Europe. The fourth genus, *Datura,* is worldwide and has many species containing the active agents.

The family of plants in which all these genera are found is *Solanaceae,* herbs of consolation, and three pharmacologically active alkaloids are responsible for the effects of these plants. Atropine, which is *dl*-hyoscyamine, scopolamine or *l*-hyoscine, and *l*-hyoscyamine are all potent central and peripheral cholinergic blocking agents. These drugs occupy the acetylcholine receptor site but do not activate it, and, thus, their effect is primarily to block the parasympathetic system. The relative potencies of atropine and scopolamine vary at different structures. In their central actions scopolamine may be as much as 100 times as potent as atropine. The *l* form of hyoscyamine is up to fifty times as potent centrally as atropine, which is a combination of the *d* and *l* forms of hyoscyamine. The structures of the two most widely studied anticholinergic agents, atropine and scopolamine, are shown in Fig. 13-2.

These agents have potent peripheral as well as central effects, and some of the psychological responses to these drugs are probably a reaction to peripheral changes. These alkaloids are frequently ingredients in cold symptom remedies because they block the production of mucus in the nose and throat. They also prevent salivation, so the mouth becomes uncommonly dry, and perspiration stops. Temperature may increase to fever levels (109° has been reported in infants with atropine poisoning) and heart rate may show a fifty beat per minute increase with atropine. Even at moderate doses these chemicals cause considerable dilation of the pupils of the eyes with a resulting inability to focus on nearby objects.

Centrally these drugs depress the reticular formation and cause a slowing of the EEG. With large enough doses, a behavioral pattern develops that resembles that of a toxic psychosis; there is delirium, mental confusion, loss of attention, drowsiness, and loss of memory for recent events. It was the loss of memory and confusion that was the basis for Lewin's classifying these agents as hypnotics rather than as phantasticants. These two characteristics—a clouding of consciousness and no memory for the period of intoxication—plus the absence of vivid sensory effects separate these drugs from the indole and catechol hallucinogens.

These agents are rapidly absorbed from the gastrointestinal tract and from the mucous membranes of the body. There are no definitive studies but it is probable that they are excreted unchanged in the urine. At high doses death results from paralysis of the respiratory muscles.

Atropa belladonna

The deadly nightshade, *Atropa belladonna,* has as its active ingredient atropine, which was isolated in 1831. The name of the plant reflects two of its major uses in the Middle Ages and before. The genus name reflects its use as a poison. Atropos was the oldest of the three Fates in Greek mythology and it was her duty to cut the thread of life when the time came. The deadly nightshade was one of the plants used extensively by both professional and amateur poisoners, since fourteen of its berries contain enough of the alkaloid to cause death.

Belladonna, the species name, refers to the "beautiful woman," a term that is a result of the use of an extract of this plant to dilate the pupils of the eyes. Interestingly, Roman and Egyptian women knew something that science did not learn until quite recently. In the 1950's it was demonstrated, by using pairs of photographs identical except for the amount of pupil dilation, that most people judge the girl with the most dilated eyes as the prettiest.

Of more interest here than pretty girls or poisoned men is the sensation of flying reported by witches. The first step toward completing this experiment is to make an ointment. Although there are many recipes, a good one seems to be: baby's fat, juice of water parsnip, aconite, cinquefoile, deadly nightshade, and soot. The soot makes the mixture black and, when rubbed on, serves to camouflage the body at night. The baby fat is added in amounts to suit the individual and makes the concoction adhere to the skin. The water parsnip is most likely not the kind used in salads but rather hemlock (yes, the same hemlock Socrates was forced to use), which is quite similar in appearance. Aconite is a pretty plant from the buttercup family and the deadly poison that killed Romeo. In very small doses the *Aconitum napellus* plant will cause a slowing and irregular heartbeat. The deadly nightshade containing atropine is the only other active ingredient in our flying recipe. With moderate doses there is some excitement and delirium along with impaired vision because of the pupillary dilation.

When the ointment is made it is rubbed on the body and especially liberally between the legs and on a stick that is to be straddled. This stick served as a phallic symbol during the ceremony of the Sabbat. The Sabbat, or Black Mass, worshipped Satan, and both males and females engaged in a nightlong orgy. Straddling the stick and hopping and shrieking around a circle they felt able "...to be carried in the aire, to feasting, singing, dansing, kissing, culling and other acts of venerie, with such youthes as they loue and desire most!"[10] The feeling of levitation perhaps comes from the irregular heartbeat in conjunction with drowsiness.

Some have reported that changes in heart rate coupled with falling asleep sometimes results in a sensation of falling (or flying?),[11] but a more likely explanation is simply the power of suggestion.

Other actions were important in causing the effects of the Sabbat. The pounding of the heart would certainly convey excitement and the excitement might cause sexual arousal. One of the reputations of belladonna was as an aphrodisiac, so it may all fit together. Perhaps the physiological effects of the agents coupled with a good placebo effect was enough for the witches who attended the Sabbat. It is to be noted that, unfortunately, the recipe will not work on the well-scrubbed American of today. Few agents are absorbed through unbroken skin, but in the typical individual of the Middle Ages—unwashed and with vermin bites, open sores, and the like—there is a good chance that the alkaloids would get into the bloodstream from the ointment.

Mandragora officinarum

The famous mandrake plant *(Mandragora officinarum)* contains all three alkaloids. One writer suggests that the root may contain up to 0.4% of the agents, a healthy dose. Although many drugs could be traced to the Bible, it is particularly important to do so with the mandrake because its close association with love and lovemaking has persisted from Genesis, Chapter 30, verses 14-16, to recent times.

> In the time of wheat-harvest Reuben went out and found some mandrakes in the open country and brought them to his mother Leah. Then Rachel asked Leah for some of her son's mandrakes, but Leah said, "Is it so small a thing to have taken away my husband, that you should take my son's mandrakes as well?" But Rachel said, "Very well, let him sleep with you tonight in exchange for your son's mandrakes." So when Jacob came in from the country in the evening, Leah went out to meet him and said, "You are to sleep with me tonight; I have hired you with my son's mandrakes." That night he slept with her....*

*From Genesis 30:14-16, The New English Bible, Oxford University Press and Cambridge University Press, 1970, p. 33.

The root of the mandrake is forked and, if you have a vivid imagination, resembles a human body. The root contains the psychoactive agents and was endowed with all sorts of magical and medical properties as a result of the "Doctrine of Signatures," which was phrased nicely by Mr. Stone in Chapter 9. It was the association with the human form that led Juliet in her farewell to use the phrase: "And shrieks like mandrakes torn out of the earth, That living mortals hearing them run mad."

One of the foremost experts in the field of psychoactive plants, in referring to the mandrake, states:

> Its intricate history as a magic plant has hardly been equalled by any other species. . . . Folk medicine regarded *Mandragora* as a panacea and recommended its use, notwithstanding its great toxicity, as a sedative and hypnotic agent in treating nervous conditions and pain. . . . It was employed further for many other illnesses and abnormal conditions, and, in many regions was considered to be an effective aphrodisiac.*

Hyoscyamus niger

Compared to the deadly nightshade and the mandrake, the *Hyoscyamus niger* has had a most uninteresting life. This is strange, since it is pharmacologically quite active and contains both scopolamine and *l*-hyoscyamine. There are other plants of this genus that contain effective levels of the alkaloids, but it is *Hyoscyamus niger* that appears throughout history as henbane, a highly poisonous substance and truly the bane of hens as well as other animals.

Pliny in 60 A.D. said: "For this is certainly known, that, if one takes it in drink more than four leaves, it will put him beside himself." Hamlet's father must have had more than four leaves, because it was henbane that was used to poison him.

Henbane may also have been used for socially popular purposes. This is brought home in the following quotation, in which a close relationship is suggested between the orgies of the ancients and the Sabbats of the Middle Ages:

> These plants were undoubtedly used in the ancient world in connection with orgiastic rites characterized by sexual excesses. Thus at the Bacchanalia, when the wild-eyed Bacchantes with their flowing locks flung themselves naked into the arms of the eager men, one can be reasonably certain that the wine which produced such sexual frenzy was not a plain fermented grape juice. Intoxication of this kind was almost certainly a result of doctoring the wine with leaves or berries of belladonna or henbane. The orgiastic rites were never totally suppressed by the Church and persisted in secret forms through the Middle Ages. Being under the shadow of the Church's displeasure, they were inevitably associated with the Devil, and those who took part in them were considered to be either witches or wizards.*

Datura

The distribution of the many *Datura* species is worldwide, but they all contain the three alkaloids under discussion—atropine, scopolamine, and hyoscyamine—in varying amounts. Almost as extensive as the distribution are its uses and its history. Some hint of the length of this history is seen in a quote from a 1970 article: "The Chinese valued this drug far back into ancient times. A comparatively recent Chinese medical text, published in 1590, reported that 'when Buddha preaches a sermon, the heavens bedew the petals of this plant with rain drops.' "[12] The text does suggest the importance of the plant, *Datura metel*, by associating it with Buddha much as tea and Daruma were related in legend.

Halfway around the world 2,500 years before the Chinese text, virgins sat at Delphi and, probably under the influence of *Datura*,[12] mumbled sounds that holy men phrased as predictions that always came true. The procedure was straightforward and:

> . . . preliminary to the divine possession, she appears to have chewed leaves of the sacred laurel . . . [prior to speaking] . . . she was supposed to be inspired by a mystic vapour that arose from a fissure in the ground.†

Probably either the plant material eaten

---

*From Schultes, R. E.: The plant kingdom and hallucinogens (part III), Bulletin on Narcotics **22**(1):43, 44, 46, 1970.

*From De Ropp, op. cit., p. 272.
†From Encyclopedia Brittanica, vol. 16, 1929, p. 831.

was one of the *Datura* species or the burning seeds and leaves of the *Datura* plant formed the mystic vapor she inhaled.

Datura was part of love potions in India and the practice of mixing the crushed seeds of *Datura metel* in tobacco and food in Asia persists even today. But, as one writer stated:

> The real centre of the hallucinogenic use of *Datura* lies in the New World, where many more species play major roles in magic, medicine and religion in sundry cultures.*

The ever-busy chronicler Hernandez mentioned the use of *Datura inoxia* by the Aztecs, and the use of various *Datura* species by Indians of the United States southwest for magical and religious purposes is well substantiated.[9] One of the interesting uses of *Datura stramonium*, which is native and grows wild in eastern United States, was devised by the Algonquin Indians. They used the plant to solve the problem of the adolescent search for identity.

> The youths are confined for long periods, given "...no other substance but the infusion or decoction of some poisonous, intoxicating roots..." and "they become stark, staring mad, in which raving condition they are kept eighteen or twenty days...". These poor creatures drink so much of that water of Lethe that they perfectly lose the remembrance of all former things, even of their parents, their treasure and their language. When the doctors find that they have drunk sufficiently of the wysoccan...they gradually restore them to their senses again...Thus they unlive their former lives and commence men by forgetting that they ever have been boys.†

This same plant is now called the Jamestown weed, or shortened to jimson weed, as a result of an incident that happened in the seventeenth century. This was fortunately recorded for history in the famous book *The History and Present State of Virginia*, published first in 1705 by Robert Beverly.

> The *James-Town* Weed (which resembles the Thorny Apple of *Peru*, and I take to be the Plant so call'd) is supposed to be one of the greatest Coolers in the World. This being an early Plant, was gather'd very young for a boil'd

Salad, by some of the Soldiers sent thither, to pacifie the Troubles of *Bacon*; and some of them eat plentifully of it, the Effect of which was a very pleasant Comedy; for they turn'd natural Fools upon it for several Days: One would blow up a Feather in the Air; another wou'd dart Straws at it with much Fury; and another stark naked was sitting up in a Corner, like a Monkey, grinning and making Mows at them; a Fourth would fondly kiss, and paw his Companions, and snear in their Faces, with a Countenance more antick, than any in a *Dutch* Droll. In this frantick Condition they were confined, lest they should in their Folly destroy themselves; though it was observed, that all their Actions were full of Innocence and good Nature. Indeed, they were not very cleanly; for they would have wallow'd in their own Excrements, if they had not been prevented. A thousand such simple Tricks they play'd, and after Eleven Days, return'd to themselves again, not remembring any thing that had pass'd.*

Some authorities[13] believe that some of the marijuana being used now in Southeast Asia is spiked with *Datura*. Reports of these marijuana users, and observation of their behavior, fit nicely into the type of syndrome discussed here. There may also be marijuana liberally laced with opium or hashish, but *Datura* probably is part of the mixture in some of the cigarettes.

Synthetics

Both atropine and scopolamine are found in many prescription drugs and preparations, but they are most easily available in some of the over-the-counter cold remedies and sleeping preparations.[14]

Ditran is a synthetic anticholinergic agent that causes a toxic psychosis much like that induced by atropine or scopolamine. Doses, orally, are in the range of:

> ...2-20 mg in adult males. The autonomic effects of Ditran exceed those of LSD. Mydriasis, flushing, nausea, vomiting, dryness of the mouth, tachycardia, hyperreflexia, and ataxia are encountered. More mental confusion, speech disturbances, and disorientation are seen than with other hallucinogens. Blocking, amnesias, thought disorganization, and feelings of strangeness

---

*From Schultes, The plant kingdom and hallucinogens (part III), op. cit., p. 44.
†Ibid.

*From Beverly, R.: The history and present state of Virginia, 1705, Chapel Hill, 1947, University of North Carolina Press, p. 139.

are often mentioned. All contact with reality and insight into the cause of the mental disruptions may be lost.*

To this time this agent has not been reported in use illegally.

CONCLUDING COMMENT

Before closing this section on the anticholinergic hallucinogenic plants, several points should be reemphasized. Clearly these plants have a much wider geographical distribution than any of the indole or phenethylamine hallucinogens. The effects are quite different from those of the other two groups and would seem to be much less desirable agents, since they cause a real clouding of consciousness and impair memory for the period of intoxication. The autonomic effects are also more severe with these plants and could easily be seen as adverse reactions in another context such as therapeutic use. Only the absence of memory for the event and the lack of a kinder substance seems to explain the willingness of some South American natives to use a drink resulting in the following effects:

Intoxication . . . is marked usually by initial effects so furious that the partaker must be restrained pending the onset of a deep, disturbed sleep during which hallucinations, interpreted as spirit visitations, enabling the witch-doctor to diagnose disease, discover thieves and prophesy the future of tribal affairs and aspirations, are experienced.†

*From Cohen, S.: The hallucinogens. In Clark, W. G., and del Giudice, J., editors: Principles of psychopharmacology, New York, 1970, Academic Press, Inc., p. 503.
†From Schultes, The plant kingdom and hallucinogens (part III), op. cit., p. 46.

PRECEDING QUOTES

1. Horne, C. H. W., and McCluskie, J. A. W.: The food of the gods, Scottish Medical Journal **8**:489, 1963.
2. Lewin, L.: Phantastica, narcotic and stimulating drugs: their use and abuse, New York, 1931, E. P. Dutton and Co., p. 1.
3. James, W.: The varieties of religious experience, New York, 1904, Longmans, Green, and Co., p. 388.

REFERENCES
a. Furst, P. T.: Flesh of the gods, the ritual use of hallucinogens, New York, 1972, Praeger Publishers, Inc.
1. Schultes, R. E.: The plant kingdom and hallucinogens (Part II), Bulletin on Narcotics 21(4): 26-27, 1969.
2. LaBarre, W.: Twenty years of peyote studies, Current Anthropology 1(1):45, 1960.
3. Collier, J.: The peyote cult, Science **115**:503, 1952.
3a. Bergman, R. L.: Navajo peyote use: its apparent safety, American Journal of Psychiatry **128**(6): 51-55, 1971.
4. Huxley, A.: The doors of perception, New York, 1954, Harper & Row, Publishers.
5. Synder, S. H., Faillace, L. A., and Weingartner, H.: DOM (STP), a new hallucinogenic drug, and DOET: effects in normal subjects, American Journal of Psychiatry **125**:357-363, 1968.
6. Hollister, L. E., Macnicol, M. F., and Gillispie, H. K.: An hallucinogenic amphetamine analog (DOM) in man, Psychopharmacologica **14**:62-73, 1969.
7. Snyder, S. H., Faillace, L., and Hollister, L.: 2,5-Dimethoxy-4-methyl-amphetamine (STP): a new hallucinogenic drug, Science **158**:669-670, 1967.
8. Meyers, F. H., Rose, A. J., and Smith, D. E.: Incidents involving the Haight-Ashbury population and some uncommonly used drugs, Journal of Psychedelic Drugs **1**(2):140-146, 1967-1968.
9. Smith, D., and Meyers, F.: The psychotomimetic amphetamine with special reference to STP (DOM) toxicity. In Smith, D., editor: Drug abuse papers, 1969, Section 4, Berkley, 1969, University of California, p. 4.
9a. 70% burns: street drugs analyzed, Rolling Stone, Feb. 17, 1972.
9b. Drug rip-offs cited by street analysis project, Drugs and Drug Abuse Education Newsletter **5**(3):3-4, March, 1974.
10. Briggs, K. M.: Pale Hecate's team, New York, 1962, The Humanities Press, p. 81.
11. Langdon-Brown, W.: From witchcraft to chemotherapy, Cambridge, 1941, Cambridge University Press, p. 30.
12. Schultes, R. E.: The plant kingdom and hallucinogens (part III), Bulletin on Narcotics **22**(1): 43-46, 1970.
13. Evans, W. O., and Kline, N. S., chairmen: Symposium and panel discussion on social patterns of drug use, historically and in nonwestern cultures, San Juan, Dec. 10, 1970, American College of Neuropsychopharmacology.
14. Long, R. E., and Penna, R.: Drugs of abuse. In Drug abuse education, ed. 2, Washington, D. C., 1969, American Pharmaceutical Association, pp. 6-15.

14 The major hallucinogens

The wish for instant paradise is as old as man himself. For ages, people have searched for artificial means to improve their condition, and drugs have played an important role in this quest.

    Jean Paul Smith, 1967

The LSD feeling would seem to have more fraternity with that tantalizing moment of total clarity, that complete understanding of what life is all about that illuminates a man in the midst of an evening's alcoholic revels. He can't explain the way he feels, and doesn't even remember very clearly the next day, but he tries again and again to recapture that counterfeit moment of truth. Goaded like the gold-hungry conquistadores, to whom El Dorado invisibly beckoned, he endures the "bad" trip or a "morning after" for the promise that is still there.

    Don McDonagh, 1967

The alchemists of the present day are the members of the drug cult. With LSD, or something else exotic from the chemical retort, they believe this leaden old world can be turned into instant gold. . . . What are the social consequences of several thousand young people regularly taking LSD, involving themselves with the psychedelic subculture . . . . It is quite important for the adult community in the dominant culture to be aware of the "psychedelic syndrome," primarily to shatter their stereotypes that "hippiness" is a fad, a passing phase similar to their adolescent rebellion of "swallowing goldfish." . . . The dominant attitudes of violence, competition, racism, and exploitation in virtually every aspect of American life have produced intolerable conflicts in many intellectual, passive, noncompetitive youth and the only solution the individual can accept is to "turn on, tune in, and drop out" into the antienvironment which may or may not resolve his own hate and disgust for "straight" society.

    David E. Smith, 1969

The hallucinogens that have attracted the most popular and scientific attention in recent years are those that most probably exert their effects by actions on the neurotransmitter serotonin. These indole-based agents span the continents and written history. They have been used in sanctuaries and on street corners, in ceremonies and in orgies. Only four of these phantasticants can be mentioned in any detail. Three are found in nature and have a rich history associated with their use, but the most famous of them all has only the heritage of a test tube beginning.

TEONANACATL

The magic mushrooms of Mexico have a long history of religious and ceremonial use in Central America. Large stone mushrooms dating from about 1000 B.C. have been found in Guatemala, and their importance is suggested by the figure of a god carved in the stem.

When Hernandez recorded the remedies of Mexico in the 1570's he included three hallucinogenic mushrooms and a "vision-producing flower." He drew a picture of this flower, which showed it to be a morning glory, the ololiuqui described in the next section. All of these plants, as well as peyote, dropped from western sight (but not from native use) for 300 years. The mushrooms were to be particularly suppressed. Their name "teonanacatl" can be translated as "God's flesh" or as "sacred mushroom," and either name was very offensive to the Spanish priests.

However, use was not limited to religious ceremonies. Already the secularization had begun. Summarizing some of these early reports:

Teonanacatl was not only ingested at social and festival occasions but also by witch doctors and soothsayers. The mushroom god—which the Christian missionaries called the devil—endowed them with clairvoyant properties, which enabled them, besides other things, to identify the causes of diseases and indicate the way in which they could be treated.*

*From Hofmann, A.: Psychotomimetic agents. In Burger, A., editor: Drugs affecting the central nervous system, vol. 2, New York, 1968, Marcel Dekker, Inc., p. 175.

It was not until the late 1930's that it was clearly shown that these mushrooms were still being used by natives in southern Mexico and that the first of many species was identified. The real breakthrough came in 1955. During that year a New York-banker-turned-ethnobotanist and his wife established rapport with a native group still using mushrooms in religious ceremonies. Gordon Wasson became the first outsider to participate in the ceremony and to eat of the magic mushroom. In language quite unlike a banker you can almost hear Wasson's soul cry out as he tries to describe the experience:

It permits you to travel backwards and forward in time, to enter other planes of existence, even (as the Indians say), to know God . . .
. . . What is happening to you seems freighted with significance, beside which the humdrum events of every day are trivial. All these things you see with an immediacy of vision that leads you to say to yourself, 'Now I am seeing for the first time, seeing direct, without the intervention of mortal eyes'. (Plato tells us that beyond this ephemeral and imperfect existence here below, there exists another ideal world of Archetypes, where the original, the true, the beautiful patterns of things, exist for evermore. Poets have pondered his words for millenia. It is clear to me where Plato found his ideas, it was clear to his contemporaries too. Plato had drunk of the potion in the Temple of Eleusis and had spent the night seeing the great vision) . . .

Your body lies in the darkness, heavy as lead, but your spirit seems to soar and leave the hut, and with the speed of thought, to travel where it listeth, in time and space, accompanied by the shaman's singing . . . at last you know what the ineffable is, and what ectasy means. Ecstasy! The mind harks back to the origin of that word. For the Greeks ekstasis meant the flight of the soul from the body. Can you find a better word to describe this state?*

The mushroom that seems to have the greatest psychoactive effect is *Psilocybe mexicana*. The primary active agent in this mushroom is psilocybin, which the discoverer of LSD, Albert Hofmann, isolated in 1958 and later synthesized. Before he did this, however,

*From Crahan, M. E.: God's flesh and other pre-Columbian phantastica, Bulletin of the Los Angeles County Medical Association **99**:17, 1969.

he ate thirty-two of the mushrooms (an average dose) to determine the potency of his mushroom supply. Hofmann's report of this experience is interesting because of the contrast with his experience with LSD, where he had had no prior expectations of the hallucinogenic effects. The comparison of Hofmann's experience with Wasson's account reemphasizes the importance of both the personality and the setting in trying to understand the effects of these drugs.

> Thirty minutes after taking the mushrooms the exterior world began to undergo a strange transformation. Everything assumed a Mexican character. As I was perfectly well aware that my knowledge of the Mexican origin of the mushroom would lead me to imagine only Mexican scenery, I tried deliberately to look on my environment as I knew it normally. But all voluntary efforts to look at things in their customary forms and colors proved ineffective. Whether my eyes were closed or open I saw only Mexican motifs and colors. When the doctor supervising the experiment bent over me to check my blood pressure, he was transformed into an Aztec priest and I would not have been astonished if he had drawn an obsidian knife. In spite of the seriousness of the situation it amused me to see how the Germanic face of my colleague had acquired a purely Indian expression. At the peak of the intoxication, about 1½ hours after ingestion of the mushrooms, the rush of interior pictures, mostly abstract motifs rapidly changing in shape and color, reached such an alarming degree that I feared that I would be torn into this whirlpool of form and color and would dissolve. After about six hours the dream came to an end. Subjectively, I had no idea how long this condition had lasted. I felt my return to everyday reality to be a happy return from a strange, fantastic but quite really experienced world into an old and familiar home.*

The dried mushrooms contain 0.2% to 0.5% of psilocybin. Psilocybin is unique (Fig. 14-1) because it is the only known naturally occurring indole to contain phosphorus. Even so the hallucinogenic effects of psilocybin are quite similar to those of LSD and the catechol hallucinogen mescaline, and cross tolerance exists among these three agents.

The psychoactive effects are clearly related to the amount used, with up to 4 milligrams

*From Hofmann, op. cit., p. 176.

yielding a pleasant experience, relaxation, and some body sensations. Higher doses cause considerable perceptual and body image changes with hallucinations in some individuals. Accompanying these psychic changes are dose-related sympathetic arousal symptoms. There is some evidence that psilocybin has its central nervous system effects only after it has been changed in the body to psilocin. Psilocin is present in the mushroom only in trace amounts but is about one and one-half times as potent as psilocybin. Perhaps the greater central nervous system effect of psilocin is the result of its higher lipid solubility.

OLOLIUQUI

Of the psychoactive agents used freely in Mexico in the sixteenth century ololiuqui, seeds of the morning glory plant *Rivea corymbosa*, perhaps had the greatest religious significance. In Hernandez's words: "... when the priests wanted to commune with their gods and to receive a message from them, they ate this plant to induce a delirium. A thousand visions and satanic hallucinations appeared to them...." When one has a good plant it should not be saved only for the priests; thus, ololiuqui was used medicinally "... to cure flatulence, to remedy venereal troubles, to deaden pain, and to remove tumors."[1]

These seeds tie America to Europe and today, for when Albert Hofmann analyzed the seeds of the morning glory he found several active alkaloids as well as d-lysergic acid amide. d-Lysergic acid amide is about one-tenth as active as LSD. The presence of d-lysergic acid amide is really quite amazing (to botany majors) because prior to this discovery in 1960, lysergic acid had been found only in much more primitive plants such as the ergot fungus.

A different species of morning glory, *Ipomoea violacea*, seems to be the primary source in the United States of most commercial morning glory seeds containing effective amounts of these alkaloids. Considering the psychoactivity of these seeds the commercial names seem quite appropriate: Pearly Gates, Flying Saucers, Heavenly Blue!

Morning glory seeds were something quite

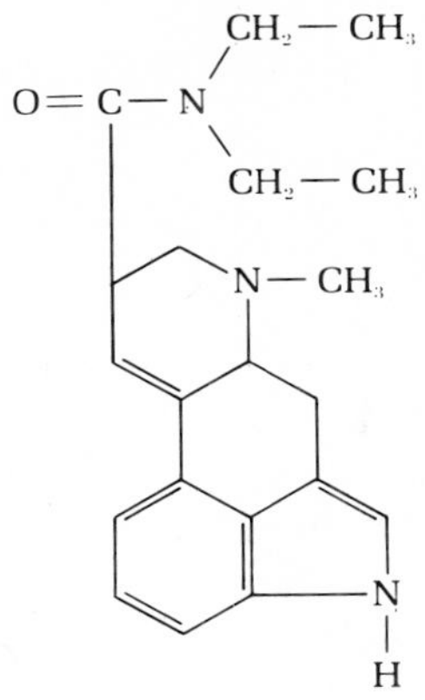

dl-lysergic acid diethylamide (LSD)
(9,10-didehydro-N,N-diethyl-6-methyl-ergoline-8β-carboxamide)

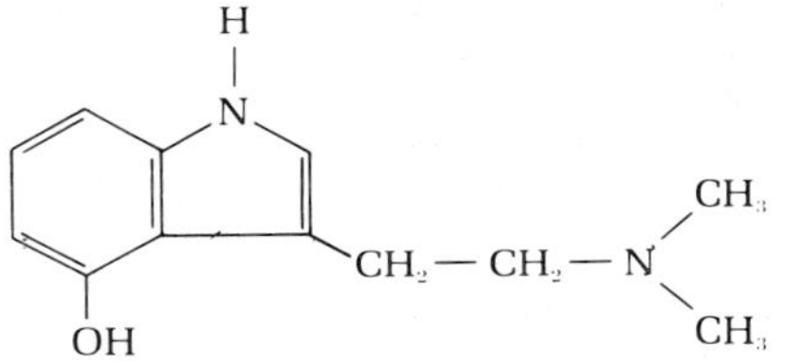

Psilocin
(3-[2-(dimethylamino)ethyl]-indol-4-ol)

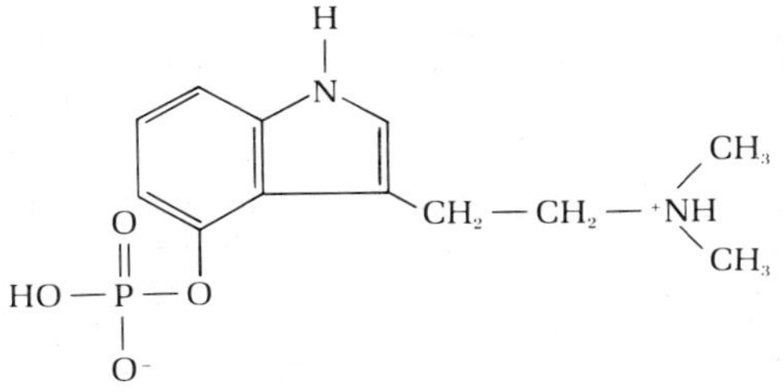

Psilocybin
(3-[2-(dimethylamino)ethyl]-indol-4-ol dihydrogen phosphate ester)

Fig. 14-1. Indole hallucinogens.

different from mushrooms. Seeds could be bought at your nearby-and-neighborly garden supply store, and were. When eaten, some of these commercial seeds produced psychoactive effects similar to LSD and psilocybin, according to reports in the literature, and there is at least one instance of an extract of the seeds being taken intravenously.[2, 3]

DMT

Only brief mention will be made of DMT, since it is not widely used in the United States although it has a long, if not noble, history. In fact, on a worldwide basis, DMT is probably the most important naturally occurring hallucinogenic compound, and it occurs in many plants. Dimethyltryptamine is the active agent in Cohoba snuff, which is used by some South American and Carribean Indians. It is ineffective when taken orally and must be inhaled, via snuff or smoking, or taken by injection.

The effective intramuscular dose (of the drug, not the snuff, which is not readily available) is about 1 milligram per kilogram of body weight. Since the effect only lasts about an hour, it can be used during lunch; the experience has been called a "businessman's trip."[4]

AMANITA MUSCARIA

...it got down off the mushroom, and crawled away into the grass, merely remarking as it went, "One side will make you grow taller, and other side will make you grow shorter."

"One side of *what*? The other side of *what*?" thought Alice to herself.

"Of the mushroom," said the Caterpillar, just as if she had asked it aloud: and in another moment it was out of sight.

Alice remained looking thoughtfully at the mushroom for a minute, trying to make out which were the two sides of it; and, as it was perfectly round, she found this a very difficult question. However, at last she stretched her arms round it as far as they would go, and broke off a bit of the edge with each hand.

"And now which is which?" she said to herself, and nibbled a little of the right hand bit to try the effect.

Alice in Wonderland

The mushrooms are personified as little men, one dwarf to a mushroom, and when under its influence one used to speak of these dwarfs as all-powerful.*

If Mexico has magic mushrooms, then Russia and the Scandinavian countries must lay claim to the mushroom that is reusable. The *Amanita muscaria* mushroom has been used for centuries, and Gordon Wasson suggests (even though there was no tobacco in Eurasia):

...It will be necessary for us all to make room in our own remote past for the part played by this mushroom, and the fly agaric will take its place by the side of alcohol, hashish, and tobacco as an outstanding

inebriant utilized by *Homo sapiens* living in Eurasia.*

This mushroom is also called "fly agaric," perhaps because it has insecticidal properties! It doesn't kill the flies but when they suck its juice it puts them into a stupor for 2 to 3 hours. Recently several authorities have suggested another explanation for the name:

...the association throughout the middle ages and earlier, of madness with the fly. People who were possessed were believed to be infested with flies. This was true throughout northern Eurasia...the fly spelled insanity. When you were treated, they waited for a fly to emerge from your nostril and you were cured....these flies in Fly Agaric are... symbols for the demonic power of Fly Agaric.†

The older literature suggests that eating five to ten *Amanita* mushrooms results in "severe effects of intoxication such as muscular twitching, leading to twitches of limbs; raving drunkenness with agitation and vivid hallucinations. Later partial paralysis with sleep and dreams follow for many hours."[5] A recent article summarizes the behavioral effects:

Effects of *Amanita muscaria* vary appreciably with individuals and at different times. An hour after the ingestion of the mushrooms, twitching and trembling of the limbs is noticeable with the onset of a period of good humor and light euphoria, characterized by macroscopia, visions of the supernatural and illusions of grandeur. Religious overtones—such as an urge to confess sins—frequently occur. Occasionally, the partaker becomes violent, dashing madly about until, exhausted, he drops into a deep sleep.‡

A 1963 report on a case of *Amanita* intoxication comments: "In these days of drugs, pep pills, and 'goof balls' it was almost refreshing recently to encounter a revival of addiction

*From Brekhman, I. I., and Sam, Y. A.: Ethnopharmacological investigation of some psychoactive drugs used by Siberian and Far-Eastern minor nationalities of USSR. In Efron, D. H., editor: Ethnopharmacologic search for psychoactive drugs, Washington, D. C., 1967, National Institute of Mental Health, p. 415.

*From Wasson, R. G.: Fly agaric and man. In Efron, D. H., editor: Ethnopharmacologic search for psychoactive drugs, Washington, D. C., 1967, National Institute of Mental Health, p. 405.
†From Wasson, R. G., and Eugster, C. H.: Discussion. In Efron, D. H.: Ethnopharmacologic search for psychoactive drugs, Washington, D. C., 1967, National Institute of Mental Health, p. 441.
‡From Schultes, R. E.: Hallucinogens of plant origin, Science **163**:246, 1969.

to the old ambrosia." The authors go on to speak of the reported effects of the mushroom: "They enjoyed the effects of eating the *A. muscaria*. The feeling of unreality and detachment was always pleasant. They felt an increase in power and a degree of invulnerability."[6]

Perhaps because the written history on the mushroom is not very old, going back only to about the seventeenth century, and in part because the active chemical constituent still eludes the biochemist, there are many speculations about the role in our history of this red-topped and white-spotted poisonous fungus.

First stop is the land of the midnight sun and the Icelandic legends that describe the phenomena of Berserksgang—going berserk. When this happened the warriors showed a shivering and chattering of teeth, and in battle they would fight with a tremendous rage. The rage was well known to the Christians of medieval times and is clearly reflected in one of their prayers, which has been oft-repeated in movies: "From the intolerable fury of the Norsemen Oh Lord deliver us!"

The intolerable fury has come down to us today in the word "beserk," which is derived from the uniform worn in battle by one of the heroes of a Norse legend, a bear (ber) skin (serk). In the eighteenth century and again in the nineteenth, Scandinavian botanists suggested that the fury of the Norsemen resulted from eating fly agaric prior to battle.[7] There is considerable doubt today over the validity of this interpretation.

The suggestion has also been made that the ambrosia food of the gods'—mentioned in the secret rites of the god Dionysius in Greece—was a solution of the *Amanita* mushroom.[8] Another proposal is that this fungus is the famous unidentified Soma of the Rig Veda poems written about 2000 B.C.,[9] and most scholars accept this interpretation. A last, really far-out, suggestion is that *Amanita muscaria* use formed the basis for the cult that originated about 2,000 years ago and today calls itself Christianity.[10]

There is no resolution of the role this magic mushroom of the North has played in our past, but its use continues today in Russia.

Use of the Amanita mushroom by Siberian tribes continues today largely free from social control of any sort. Use of the drug has a Shamanist aspect, and forms the basis for orgiastic communal indulgences. Since the drug can induce murderous rages in addition to more moderate hallucinogenic experiences, serious injuries frequently result.*

The mushrooms are expensive; sometimes several reindeer are exchanged for an effective number of the mushrooms. They do have the unique property of being reusable and during the long winter months they may be worth the price. The mushrooms themselves are not reusable—once eaten they're gone. But this is a hallucinogen that is excreted unchanged in the urine. When the effect begins to wear off, "midway in the orgy the cry of 'pass the pot' goes out."[11] The active ingredient can be reused four or five times in this way!

Until a few years ago the psychoactive agent in *Amanita muscaria* was thought to be bufotenin (N,N-dimethyl serotonin or 5-hydroxy-N,N-dimethyl-tryptamine). It has an indole structure and has been suspected of being a hallucinogen, but the evidence is far from clear. If bufotenin does prove to be psychoactive it may have been the important ingredient in the witches' brew discussed in *Macbeth*:

Round about the cauldron go;
In the poisoned entrails throw.
Toad that under cold stone,
Days and nights has thirty-one.

since the skin of toads have a fair amount of bufotenin. The fly agaric mushroom, however, has very little.

The total list of active ingredients of *Amanita muscaria* is not known, but two that have much importance at this time are ibotenic acid and muscimol.

Muscimol and ibotenic acid, two psychotomimetic principles of *Amanita muscaria*, have effects similar to those of LSD on norepinephrine, dopamine and serotonin concentrations in the brains of mice and rats. The increased serotonin concentration in the hypothalamus and midbrain is probably caused by a diminished turnover or liberation of serotonin,

*From Hallucinogens, Columbia Law Review **68**(3): 521, 1968.

perhaps resulting from a diminished pulse flow in serotonergic neurons.*

d-LYSERGIC ACID DIETHYLAMIDE

The historical background to d-lysergic acid diethylamide (LSD) presented in the literature has been confusing. LSD was originally synthesized from ergot alkaloids extracted from a fungus *Claviceps purpurea*. This mold occasionally grows on grain, especially rye, and eating infected grain results in an illness called ergotism. LSD is a synthetic chemical and does not occur in nature under any conditions.

St. Anthony's fire

Grain that has been infected with the ergot fungus is readily identified and is usually immediately destroyed. During periods of famine, however, the grain may be used in making bread. In France between 945 A.D. and 1600 A.D. there were at least twenty outbreaks of ergotism, the illness that results from eating infected bread. A brief description of the symptoms of the illness was recorded following an outbreak in 857 A.D.,[12] but a better picture of the condition under which gangrenous ergot intoxication occurred in this period was that in 993 A.D.:

> . . . a horrible plague raged among men, namely a hidden fire which, upon whatsoever limb it fastened, consumed it and severed it from the body. Many were consumed even in the space of a single night by these devouring flames. . . . Moreover, about the same time, a most mighty famine raged for five years throughout the Roman world, so that no region could be heard of which was not hungerstricken for lack of bread, and many of the people were starved to death. In those days also, in many regions, the horrible famine compelled men to make their food not only of unclean beasts and creeping things, but even of men's, women's, and children's flesh, without regard even of kindred: for so fierce waxed this hunger that grown-up sons devoured their mothers, and mothers, forgetting their maternal love, ate their babes.†

*From Waser, P. G., and Bersin, P.: Turnover of monoamines in brain under the influence of muscimol and ibotenic acid, two psychoactive principles of Amanita muscaria. In Efron, D. H., editor: Psychotomimetic drugs, New York, 1970, Raven Press, p. 161.

†From Coulton, G. G.: Life in the Middle Ages, vol. I, New York, 1910, pp. 2-3.

Although the cause of the illness was established before 1700, only symptomatic treatment exists even today. There are two forms of the disease. In one there are tingling sensations in the skin and muscle spasms that develop into convulsions, insomnia, and various disturbances of consciousness and thinking. In the other form, gangrenous ergotism, the limbs become swollen and inflamed, with the individual experiencing "violent burning pains" before the affected part became numb. Sometimes the disease moves rapidly, with less than 24 hours between the first sign and the development of gangrene. Gangrene develops because the ergot causes a contraction of the blood vessels, cutting off blood flow to the extremities, sometimes with dramatic results.

> The separation of the gangrenous part often took place spontaneously at a joint without pain or loss of blood. It is related that a woman was riding to the hospital on an ass, and was pushed against a shrub; her leg became detached at the knee, without any bleeding, and she carried it to the hospital in her arms.*

It was not until 1085 that the burning sensation, the fire, was called holy (*sacro igne*). Eight years later the Order of St. Anthony was founded and a hospital built in France near the church where the Saint's relics resided. During the twelfth century ergotism became associated with St. Anthony, although the reason for this is not completely clear. It may be that the hospital for the treatment of ergotism was built near the shrine of St. Anthony because he had suffered from a minor attack of ergotism. Some suggest that the demons he reported battling were the result of the disease.[13] Others believe the illness was called St. Anthony's Fire because those who made the pilgrimage to Egypt, where St. Anthony had lived, were cured. No matter, those who journeyed to Egypt as well as those who entered the hospital did lose their symptoms, probably as a result of a diet that did not include ergot-infected rye.

There have been no recent reports of the illness but special note must be made of a book[14] suggesting that there was an outbreak of ergotism in 1951 in a small French town.

*From Barger, G.: Ergot and ergotism, London, 1931, Gurney and Jackson, p. 30.

This suggestion has been frequently repeated in the popular literature with the symptoms of the illness attributed to ergot and/or LSD. In fact, the illness that spread rapidly through the inhabitants of the town was mercury poisoning resulting from eating bread made from mercury-treated wheat. The illness had nothing to do with the ergot alkaloids or LSD.

LSD

In the Sandoz Laboratories in Basle, Switzerland, in 1938 Dr. Albert Hofmann synthesized *lysergsaurediethylamid*, the German word from which LSD comes and the equivalent of the English *d*-lysergic acid diethylamide. (See Fig. 14-1.) Hofmann was working on a series of compounds derived from ergot alkaloids that had as their basic structure lysergic acid. LSD was synthesized because of its chemical similarity to a known stimulant, nikethamide. It was not until 1943, however, that LSD entered the world of biochemical psychiatry when Hofmann recorded in his laboratory notebook:

> Last Friday, April 16, 1943, I was forced to stop my work in the laboratory in the middle of the afternoon and to go home, as I was seized by a peculiar restlessness associated with a sensation of mild dizziness. Having reached home, I lay down and sank in a kind of drunkeness which was not unpleasant and which was characterized by extreme activity of imagination. As I lay in a dazed condition with my eyes closed (I experienced daylight as disagreeably bright) there surged upon me an uninterrupted stream of fantastic images of extraordinary plasticity and vividness and accompanied by an intense, kaledioscope-like play of colors. This condition gradually passed off after about two hours.*

Hofmann was sure that the experience he had had resulted from the accidental ingestion of the compounds with which he was working. The next Monday morning he prepared what he thought was a very small amount of LSD, 0.25 milligrams, and made the following record in his notebook:

> April 19, 1943: Preparation of an 0.5% aqueous solution of *d*-lysergic acid diethylamide tartrate.

*From Hofmann, op. cit., pp. 184-185.

4:20 P.M.: 0.5 cc (0.25 mg LSD) ingested orally, The solution is tasteless.

4:50 P.M.: no trace of any effect.

5:00 P.M.: slight dizziness, unrest, difficulty in concentration, visual disturbances, marked desire to laugh . . . At this point the laboratory notes are discontinued:

> The last words could only be written with great difficulty. I asked my laboratory assistant to accompany me home as I believed that my condition would be a repetition of the disturbance of the previous Friday. While we were still cycling home, however, it became clear that the symptoms were much stronger than the first time. I had great difficulty in speaking coherently, my field of vision swayed before me, and objects appeared distorted like images in curved mirrors. I had the impression of being unable to move from the spot, although my assistant told me afterwards that we had cycled at a good pace. . . .

> By the time the doctor arrived, the peak of the crisis had already passed. As far as I remember, the following were the most outstanding symptoms: vertigo, visual disturbances; the faces of those around me appeared as grotesque, colored masks; marked motor unrest, alternating with paresis; an intermittent heavy feeling in the head, limbs and the entire body, as if they were filled with metal; cramps in the legs, coldness and loss of feeling in the hands; a metallic taste on the tongue; dry, constricted sensation in the throat; feeling of choking; confusion alternating between clear recognition of my condition, in which state I sometimes observed, in the manner of an independent, neutral observer, that I shouted half insanely or babbled incoherent words. Occasionally I felt as if I were out of my body.

> The doctor found a rather weak pulse but an otherwise normal circulation.

> . . . Six hours after ingestion of the LSD-25 my condition had already improved considerably. Only the visual disturbances were still pronounced. Everything seemed to sway and the proportions were distorted like the reflections in the surface of moving water. Moreover, all objects appeared in unpleasant, constantly changing colors, the predominant shades being sickly green and blue. When I closed my eyes, an unending series of colorful, very realistic and fantastic images surged in upon me. A remarkable feature was the manner in which all acoustic perceptions (e.g., the noise of a passing car) were transformed into optical effects, every sound causing a corresponding colored hallucination constantly changing in shape and color like pictures

in a kaleidoscope. At about 1 o'clock I fell asleep and awakened next morning somewhat tired but otherwise feeling perfectly well.*

The amount Albert Hofmann took orally is five to eight times the normal effective dose, and it was the potency of the drug that attracted attention to it. Mescaline had been long known to cause strange experiences, alter consciousness, and lead to a particularly vivid kaleidoscope of colors, but it took 4,000 times as much mescaline as LSD. LSD is usually active when only 0.05 milligram is taken, and in some people a dose of 0.03 milligram is effective. At this dose level it seemed possible that a physiological action was taking place, that is, an action that might occur normally in the body. Early reports suggested that LSD caused a reversible psychosis. Since LSD was active in such small quantities, it seemed possible that it was mimicking the biochemical process that might normally cause schizophrenia!

The search began in earnest for the endogenous chemical that caused schizophrenia. The task still continues, and though many chemicals have been suggested, no agreement has been reached. Perhaps the major lasting impact of the psychedelics will prove to be increased study of nondrug highs and investigation of altered states of consciousness.[14a-d]

Only an overview of the history of legal LSD is mentioned here. The developing illegal use of LSD and other hallucinogens will be detailed in the following section. The first report on LSD in the scientific literature came from Zurich in 1947, but it was 1949 before the first North American study on its use in humans appeared. In 1953 Sandoz applied to the Food and Drug Administration to study LSD as a new investigational drug. Between 1953 and 1966 Sandoz distributed large quantities of LSD to qualified scientists throughout the world. Most of this legal LSD was used in biochemical and animal behavior research.

In April of 1966 the Sandoz Pharmaceutical Company recalled the LSD it had distributed and withdrew its sponsorship of work with LSD. Large quantities of illegally manufactured

LSD of uncertain purity were being used in the street, and Sandoz decided to give the responsibility for the legal distribution of LSD to the federal government. Sandoz still manufactures LSD and research continues under the combined sponsorship of the National Institute of Mental Health and the Food and Drug Administration, but from June of 1967 through 1970 there were fewer than 500 requests from scientists for LSD and/or other hallucinogens for research purposes. It will be repeatedly emphasized that the pharmacodynamic actions of LSD and the other hallucinogens reported here are based on results obtained with legally manufactured and pure drugs. Reports from street use of these drugs— behavioral effects, adverse effects, and the like—are almost always based on an illegal product of unknown purity that may contain other chemical agents as well.

The bootleg hallucinogen story

The illegal LSD story starts with legal psilocybin, or perhaps at West Point, where Timothy Leary discovered Oriental mysticism. The eponym for the "Psychedelic Era" will certainly be Timothy Leary. More than any other single person Leary made the mind-altering drugs newsworthy, and the media spread his gospel.

The story proper starts in the summer of 1960 in Mexico, where for the first time Leary used the magic mushrooms containing psilocybin. As he later said, he realized then that the old Timothy Leary was dead; the "Timothy Leary game" was over. Working at Harvard University, he collaborated with Dr. Richard Alpert and discussed the meaning and implication of this new world with Aldous Huxley.

During the 1960-1961 school year Leary and Alpert began a series of experiments on Harvard graduate students using pure psilocybin, which they had obtained through a physician. Leary's original work was apparently done under proper scientific controls and with a physician in attendance because drugs were used. The use of a physician was later eliminated, against state requirements, and then other controls were dropped. That is, Leary believed strongly that not only the

*Ibid., pp. 185-186.

subject should use the drug but also the experimenter, so that he could communicate with the subject. This practice removes the experimenter from the role of an objective observer and can hardly be classified as seriously scientific.

Leary's drug taking in the role of an experimenter and the apparent abandonment of any possible former semblance of a scientific approach was definitely questioned by the Harvard authorities and other scientists and was the beginning of the end. As early as the fall of 1961 there was open question about the "research" being carried out by Leary and Alpert. There were many legitimate complaints, as noted, but attitudes were not completely unbiased. This is suggested by a memorandum by the psychologist in charge of the Center for Research in Personality, which had hired Leary. The memorandum said, in part:

> It is probably no accident that the society which consistently encourages the use of these substances, India, produced one of the sickest social orders ever created by mankind, in which thinking men spent their time lost in the Buddha position . . . while poverty, disease, social discrimination and superstition reached their highest and most organized form in all history.*

Leary continued his work and in 1963 he founded the International Federation for Internal Freedom (IFIF). IFIF was an organization to encourage research on psychedelic substances. His own research in this field was not viewed as very rigorous, and the Federation died for lack of outside interest or support. In this same year, however, one of Leary's followers completed the now classic Good Friday study.[15]

The Good Friday study was designed to investigate the ability of psilocybin to induce meaningful religious experiences in individuals when the drug was used in a religious setting. Twenty seminarians participated in a double-blind study, with half receiving 30 milligrams of psilocybin and half placebos 90 minutes before attending a religious service. Tape

recordings of the subjects' experiences were made immediately after the 2½-hour service, which was held in a chapel. Within a week a questionnaire was completed, followed by a similar one 6 months later. The first was directed at determining the magnitude and type of change that occurred during the experiment, and the later one at assessing the durability of the change. Leary later summarized the outcome of the Good Friday study by saying:

> . . . the results clearly support the hypothesis that, with adequate preparation and in an environment which is supportive and religiously meaningful, subjects report mystical experiences significantly more than placebo controls.*

He then commented on the results of some other studies that looked at the relationship between hallucinogens and religious experience and concluded:

> . . . data . . . indicate that (1) if the setting is supportive but not spiritual, between 40 to 75 per cent of psychedelic subjects will report intense and life-changing religious experiences; and that (2) if the set and setting are supportive and spiritual, then from 40 to 90 per cent of the experiences will be revelatory and mystico-religious.†

Another experiment compared the effects of LSD and methylphenidate (Ritalin).[16] It reported that LSD produced more sensations of a religious or mystical nature, but methylphenidate (a stimulant) was more effective in eliciting reports of increased self-understanding.

All did not go well at Harvard for Leary. A combination of things not acceptable to the University gradually developed in 1962 and 1963. Some of the major issues were that no doctor was present when drugs were administered, undergraduates were used in drug experiments, and drug sessions were conducted outside the laboratory in Leary's home as well as at other places off the campus.

---

*From Caldwell, W. V.: LSD psychotherapy, New York, 1968, Grove Press, Inc., p. 54-55.

*From Leary, T.: The religious experience: its production and interpretation, Journal of Psychedelic Drugs 1(2):5, 1967-1968.
†Ibid., p. 6.

As a result, Alpert and Leary were dismissed from their academic positions in the spring of 1963. The University's reason for Leary's dismissal was his failure to meet his classes, which Leary admits he did not do since he understood he was on leave from the school.

1963 was the year that the White House Conference on Narcotics and Drug Abuse stated: "As yet these drugs (hallucinogens) are of minor importance in the general picture of drug abuse, in part because of their limited availability and inordinate high cost."[17] Already, though, the illegal production of the hallucinogens had begun, and the effects of pure LSD were to be confounded with the effects of impurities and other drugs.

All was reasonably quiet in 1964 and 1965. Alpert separated from Leary and lectured on the West Coast while Leary settled in at an estate in Millbrook, New York, which was owned by a wealthy supporter of Leary's beliefs. In 1964 Leary announced that drugs were not necessary to rise above and go beyond one's ego. He reiterated this again in 1966 after he was arrested for possession of marijuana at the Millbrook estate. He has repeatedly held since then that drugs are not necessary; they are only a help, a key to open consciousness to the inner experience he believes everyone should have.

1966 was a busy year for Leary. He appeared at three Congressional hearings; one interchange with Senator Edward Kennedy about LSD is particularly interesting. Interesting first because Leary so clearly predicted what was to come, and second because Senator Kennedy and Dr. Leary didn't seem to be touching the same bases.

> Kennedy: You said you do not know about the quality. What is it about the quality that you are frightened about?
>
> Leary: We do not want amateur or black-market sale or distribution of LSD.
>
> Kennedy: Why not?
>
> Leary: Or the barbiturates or liquor. When you buy a bottle of liquor—
>
> Kennedy: This is not responsive. As to LSD, why do you not want it?
>
> Leary: On possession?
>
> Kennedy: Why do you not want the indiscriminate manufacture and distribution? Why not? Is it because it is dangerous?

> Leary: Because you do not know what you are getting.
>
> Kennedy: Is it because it is dangerous? Are you interested only in the consumer and whether, like truth in packaging, whether there are too many strawberries or not enough strawberries in the pie, or is it something more dangerous than that, Dr. Leary?
>
> Leary: No sir; I think LSD is much less dangerous than the amphetamines and barbiturates.
>
> Kennedy: I am not asking that. The reason, as I would gather it, is because this is a dangerous drug; is that right?
>
> Leary: No, sir; LSD is not a dangerous drug.*

Also in 1966 Leary started his religion, the League of Spiritual Discovery, with LSD as the sacrament. The League got off to a slow start and Leary's home base at Millbrook was under attack around the same time. Concern was that Leary would attract ". . . drug addicts to Millbrook. When their money runs out, they will murder, rob, and steal, to secure funds with which to satisfy their craving."[18]

The world moves too quickly for new prophets today. Although the guru of the age, Leary's sacrament was already being secularized. Increasing numbers of young people were responding to the motto of the League for Spiritual Discovery, "Turn On, Tune In, and Drop Out." Leary phrased it meaningfully:

> Turning on correctly means to understand the many levels that are brought into focus; it takes years of discipline, training and discipleship. To turn on on a street corner is a waste. To tune in means you must harness rigorously what you are learning . . . To drop out is the oldest message that spiritual teachers have passed on. You can get only by giving up.†

Noble words, perhaps, but street corner turn-ons were becoming more frequent. A combination of many things increased the use of hallucinogens, and especially LSD, during the early and mid-1960's. LSD's promise of new sensations (which were delivered), of potent aphrodisiac effects (which were not

*From Hearings before a Special Subcommittee of the Committee on the Judiciary, U. S. Senate, Eighty-ninth Congress, Second Session, May 13, 1966, p. 253.
†From Celebration #1, New Yorker **42**:43, 1966.

forthcoming), of kinship with a friendly peer group (which occurred) spread the drug rapidly.

Users and potential users were reported to be more suggestible on a hypnotic suggestibility test and to be less concerned about loss of self-control than those who rejected the opportunity to use hallucinogens. However, by the mid-1960's, several studies had been carried out in an attempt to characterize the personality and background of the hallucinogen drug user. Some studies suggested there were differences between users, or those who said they were willing to use these drugs, and those who said they would not and also did not.[19, 20] A 1967 report rejected the idea that any common psychological or sociological characteristics would identify the moderate LSD user.

There is considerable support now for that attitude. Three obvious concerns in this type research will be mentioned. Most investigators search out only the chronic, heavy user of hallucinogens (much as alcoholics are studied and not just those who use alcohol). This gives a very different picture from that which would be obtained if a random selection were made from the 5% of Americans who report having tried hallucinogens as of 1972.[20a] One 1968 study[21] compared male college students who were regular users to nonusers matched for age, education, and social class. In contrast to the nonuser, the hallucinogen user came from:

> . . . a generally cold and rejecting family background which fails to develop adequate super-ego strength or socialization in the user who then, despite a middle class background and regular college attendance, resembles at least in some respects, the psychological test picture of the juvenile delinquent.*

This picture of a middle-class youth who has "slipped the traces" and became an acidhead appears also in other reports.[22] Prior to heavy use of LSD, these individuals are reported to be predominantly middle class in economics and beliefs. Usually they are nonathletic, above average in intelligence, and

*From Kleckner, J. H.: An investigation into the personal characteristics and family backgrounds of psychedelic drug users, Dissertation Abstracts 29B:4380-B, 1969.

poor in competitive situations. Frustrated with life and angry at their parents, these youths responded with passivity. They denied their hate in the easiest way possible, by turning it to love. True flower children.

Another problem is possible regional differences in the characteristics of heavy LSD users. Is the heavy user who trips in southern California the same type as the acidhead in Minneapolis? Probably not. But there are no real data. Out of the West in the late 1960's came multiple reports of a close interaction between chronic LSD use and the supernatural. It was not enough to reject technology; a positive belief in magic, extrasensory perception, and astrology was usually acquired. Still unknown is whether rising interest in the supernatural in the mid-1970's will increase or decrease hallucinogen use.

The final problem is the poor quality of most research in this area. An excellent 1973 review of research on psychosocial correlates concluded: "The foregoing suggests a multitude of preproblem use correlates of adolescent psychodelic use. At the same time, there is very little consensual validation and there are many contradictory findings."[22a, p. 102]

While chronic users of LSD and similar drugs were being identified and studied, a decline began in the use of these drugs. LSD use reached a peak during the winter of 1967-1968 and fell thereafter. Three factors seem to be primarily responsible. One was the increasing incidence of bad trips, bummers. These bad trips probably resulted in part from the spread of LSD use into less stable and more anxious individuals. As the capacity of the individual to deal with problems decreases, or as his anxiety level increases, the probability of a bad drug experience becomes greater. Another item still contributing its share of bad trips is impure LSD. Leary's forecast was right. Not only poorly synthesized LSD but also addition of other drugs to the LSD made street acid a risky buy (see p. 220).

Methamphetamine was and is one of the additives. A 1967-1968 report commented that methamphetamine combined with LSD "increases the likelihood of a 'bad trip', primarily due to the intense sympathomimetic effects of the amphetamines . . . [which are] often magnified by the LSD-sensitized mind into a panic reaction."[23]

A second factor that may have contributed to the decrease in the use of LSD was the report in 1967 that LSD damages chromosomes (see p. 247). A third reason for the decline of LSD use after 1968 was the availability of other drugs. Mescaline and/or peyote became the hallucinogens of choice for many previous LSD users. Most users are not looking to find themselves or God through their drug experience so mescaline is probably the drug of choice. It seems to offer less of an inner experience but an even better sensory show than LSD (see p. 220, however).

The final chapter in the Timothy Leary story, but not the LSD story, is probably already written. Even as the guru announced his League for Spiritual Discovery in 1966, his position as anything more than a symbol for an era was washing away. A series of arrests on drug charges and finally sentence to a minimum security prison in 1969 helped maintain interest in the symbol of the turned-on decade. When he escaped by walking away from the prison in September of 1970, he turned off the flame he ignited 10 years earlier in 1960. A real cop-out. In January, 1973, he was rearrested in Afghanistan and returned to a California prison.[23a]

Pharmacodynamics

LSD is an extremely potent, odorless, colorless, and tasteless compound. One ounce contains about 300,000 human adult doses. There are no data on the lethal dose in man, but in monkeys the LD 100 is about 5 milligrams per kilogram. In the laboratory rat the LD 50 is 16.0 milligrams per kilogram, while easily reproducible behavioral effects are obtained with 0.1 milligram per kilogram.

Absorption from the gastrointestinal tract is rapid, and most human laboratory experiments administer LSD via the mouth. (Although street users primarily take the drug orally, some feel it is necessary to inject LSD intravenously.)[24] At all postingestion times, the brain contains less LSD than any of the other organs in the body, so it is not selectively taken up by the brain. Within the brain, however, the levels of the drug are highest in visual areas, parts of the limbic system, and areas of the reticular system. Half of the LSD in the blood is metabolized every 3 hours, so blood levels decrease fairly rapidly. LSD is metabolized in the liver and excreted as 2-oxy-lysergic acid diethylamide, which is inactive.

Tolerance develops rapidly, repeated daily doses becoming completely ineffective in 3 to 4 days. Recovery is equally rapid, so weekly use of the same dose of LSD is possible. Cross tolerance has been shown between LSD, mescaline, and psilocybin, and the effects of each can be blocked or reversed with chlorpromazine. Physical dependence or addiction has not been shown to LSD or to any of the hallucinogens.

LSD is a sympathomimetic agent and the autonomic signs are some of the first to appear after LSD is taken. Typical symptoms are dilated pupils, elevated temperature and blood pressure, and an increase in salivation.

The basic pharmacological mechanism through which the LSD experience is generated is not known. There is some evidence that LSD actions on both the adrenergic and the serotonergic systems are necessary for its hallucinogenic properties.

There are suggestions that LSD has some effects via its interaction with the neurotransmitter serotonin. There is considerable evidence to support this idea. LSD probably occupies the receptor site for serotonin since it is a potent inhibitor of serotonin uptake by cells and inhibits the central nervous system actions of serotonin. LSD probably competes with serotonin for the receptor site, since if serotonin levels are lowered, there is usually an increase in the effects of LSD. An increase in serotonin levels (as occurs following a monoamine oxidase inhibitor) decreases the LSD effect.

Until recently a powerful argument against the idea that LSD produces its hallucinogenic effects by antagonizing serotonin was the finding that 2-brom-lysergic acid diethylamide was more potent than LSD as a serotonin antagonist but had no hallucinogenic effects. Recent work has demonstrated, however, that LSD is a more potent serotonin inhibitor than brom-LSD on some central nervous system serotonergic neurons. It could be the serotonin-antagonist properties of LSD in these neurons that are important for the drug's hallucinogenic properties; therefore, the serotonin hypothesis for LSD action is again very much alive.

Electrophysiological effects have been most frequently (though perhaps not correctly) associated with the hallucinogenic actions of LSD. One of its major effects is to increase the sensitivity of the sensory collaterals that feed into and activate the reticular formation. LSD is not like amphetamine. LSD lowers the threshold for reticular arousal via sensory input but does not directly increase the sensitivity of the reticular formation. By sensitizing the sensory collaterals, LSD administration makes possible activation of the central nervous system following sensory input below the normally effective level.

Although LSD apparently does not act on the sensory pathways themselves (except perhaps in the visual system), it does increase the effect of sensory input by increasing the size of the signal delivered to the cortex. This increase in the size of the signal and the increased activation of the cortex via reticular arousal could, of course, be a partial basis for the vividness of sensory experiences regularly reported following LSD ingestion. As might be anticipated from the effects on the reticular system, LSD also causes an activation of the EEG.

The reticular system is sometimes viewed as having two major functions with respect to the other areas of the brain. One is to control the activation or arousal level, and the second is to monitor and regulate the flow of sensory inputs. The reticular system can operate to increase or decrease the effect on the cortex of a given sensory signal. Thus it has a major role in determining the impact of sensory stimulation on an individual's awareness.

One of the workers in this area suggested that LSD has its effects by influencing "the processes concerned with the filtration and integration of sensory information."[25] If one recognizes that a large part of the LSD experience may be the reaction to changes in external and internal sensory inputs and to the way these inputs are integrated, then the actions

of the reticular system would seem to be basic to the hallucinogenic experience.

A summary[26] of a conference that included many of those doing research on the mechanisms of action of the hallucinogens states:

> The psychotomimetic drugs, particularly LSD, may produce their complex psychic effects by the inhibition of a basic brain stem mechanism . . . the function of which is to integrate the sensory inflow and the emotional and ideational state of the organism, and in particular to suppress irrelevant information. This system may depend on a complex interaction of serotonin and noradrenaline mechanisms. The basic requirements of a hallucinogen seem to be that it should (in specific doses) inhibit serotonin systems and potentiate noradrenaline systems. If these systems are normally mutually inhibitory, normal homeostasis might survive interruption of one of these mechanisms but would not survive simultaneous interruption of both in opposite senses. . . . LSD may also affect serotonin and noradrenaline mechanisms in the retina and other visual systems.*

Support your local travel agent

The heading for this section is from a lapel button and clearly says, "Take a Trip!" Why is an LSD experience called a trip? An excellent article starts from the premise that, among serious psychedelic drug users, the experience is viewed as ". . . a process of self-discovery, of self-confrontation, of deep self encounter, hopefully leading to self-acceptance, a heightened capacity to love, and spiritual harmony."[27] The essay weaves its way through Christianity's *Pilgrim's Progress* and Oriental religion to successful television shows such as *The Fugitive* and *The Immortal* to suggest that the find-yourself-by-losing-yourself theme frequently involves physical as well as psychological movement. ". . . every real trip is also a trip of spiritual growth, and every spiritual trip brings a heightened awareness of the real world."[27]

Some authorities reject almost categorically the idea that a religious or personally meaningful experience can be reached via hallucinogens:

As of now the self-denial, contemplation, and

*From Action of hallucinogenic drugs, Nature **220**:961, 1968.

careful preparation that have characterized the lives of the great mystics of Eastern and Western civilizations are not likely to be replaced by the instant mysticism of a hallucinogenic trip; nor is it likely that a young college student or a beatnik in rebellion against society will discover divine truths or experience valid apocalyptical visions regarding himself, his society, or his world merely by ingesting a drug coated sugar cube that distorts perception and shatters reality.*

Others are believers and feel that:

> In our own work, the wealth of phenomena revealed in the psychedelic experience convinced us that chemicals of this type can be tools of great worth, providing the best access yet to the contents and processes of the human mind. Moreover, when a session is all that it can be, it liberates and sets in motion an entelechy, something that must reside in the depths of every self, a force and a process that not only can restore the sick to health, but can enable the normal individual to achieve a greater maturity, realize potentials, and even discover in large measure who he is and what his existence is about.

> It is because these possibilities are real, that I urge continuing, and greatly expanded, multidisciplinary research programs with the psychedelics. And I hope we will not persevere in the non sequitur of irrational attacks upon the psychedelics, and of prohibiting serious work with them, because, quite apart from such work, there is a problem of drug abuse in our society.†

As in reacting to the LSD experience itself, reactions to the use of LSD by others is influenced by the personality and history of the observer as well as his environment. The truth probably is somewhere between the two points of view just expressed, but the fact that most hallucinogen users also use many other drugs suggests that, primarily, users are seeking the experience, not using the experience to seek.

The experience of a trip is difficult, if not impossible, to describe. Coupled with the problem of adequately verbalizing a personal inner experience is the fact that it is never-before-experienced experiences that are to be related. Gordon Wasson, in speaking of the "psychic disturbance" from eating mushrooms, said:

> This disturbance is wholly different from the effects of alcohol, as different as night from day. We are entering upon a discussion where the vocabulary . . . is seriously deficient. We are all confined within the prison walls of our every-day vocabulary; with skill in our choice of words we may stretch accepted meanings to cover slightly new feelings and thoughts, but when a state of mind is utterly distinct, wholly novel, then all our old words fail. (How do you tell a man born blind what seeing is like?)*

One summary of the experience by a scientist stated:

> . . . the importance of mood, expectation, and setting on the subjective effects of LSD is well recognized. Therefore, the described effects can be quite variable from subject to subject and in the same subject at different times and under different conditions. The major effects are on sensory perception (especially visual) and emotions. Sensory changes vary with dose. At low doses mild distortions appear, with lights appearing brighter and sounds seeming clearer. Increasing the dose causes more severe distortions, often with extremely vivid coloration and the appearance of such phenomena as moving walls and moving staircases. With still larger doses pseudohallucinations appear; and, with very large doses, there is the occurrence of true hallucinations with loss of insight. Such effects as numbness, tingling, and nausea may occur. Emotionally the effects are quite variable. For some there is fear and even panic; for others there is diminution of panic; for others there is diminution of anxiety and feelings of a deep and transcendental experience . . .†

A journalist phrased it a little differently:

> Thirty minutes after the exploding ticket is swallowed, life is dramatically changed. Objects are luminescent, vibrating, 'more real.' Colors shift and split into the spectrum

---

*From Louria, D. B.: LSD—a medical overview, Saturday Review **50**:92, 1967, Copyright 1967 Saturday Review, Inc.
†From Houston, J.: Phenomenology of the psychedelic experience. In Hicks, R. E., and Fink, P. J., editors: Psychedelic drugs, New York, 1969, Grune & Stratton, Inc., pp. 6-7. By permission.

*From Wasson, R. G.: The mushroom rites of Mexico, The Harvard Review **1**(4):8, 1963.
†From Gorodetsky, C. W.: Marihuana, LSD, and amphetamines, Drug Dependence **5**:20, 1970.

of charged, electric color and light. Perceptions come as killing insights—true! true! who couldn't have seen it before! There is an oceanic sense of involvement in the mortal drama in a deeply emotional new way. Colors are heard as notes of music, ideas have substance and fire. A crystal vision comes: how full is the cosmos, how sweet the flowers!

The illusions beckoned to the surface by the drug are greatly influenced by expectation, atmosphere and the traveler's mental balance . . .*

It is not possible to say, "This is *the* description of the experience," since there are as many experiences as there are drug users. Part of the wonder of these agents is that they do not give repeat performances. However, although each trip differs, the general type of experience and the sequence of experiences are reasonably well delineated. When an effective dose is taken orally (0.5 to 1.5 micrograms per kilogram of body weight), the trip will last 6 to 9 hours. It can be greatly attenuated at any time through the administration of chlorpromazine intramuscularly.

The initial effects noticed are autonomic responses that develop gradually over the first 20 minutes. The individual may feel dizzy or hot and cold; his mouth may be dry. These effects diminish and, in addition, are less and less the focus of attention as alteration in sensations, perceptions, and mood begin to develop over the following 30 to 40 minutes. In one study,[28] after the initial autonomic effects, the sequence of events over the next 20 to 50 minutes was: mood changes, abnormal body sensation, decrease in sensory impression, abnormal color perception, space and time disorders, and visual hallucinations. One visual effect has been described beautifully:

The guide asked me how I felt, and I responded, "Good." As I uttered the word "Good," I could see it form visually in the air. It was pink and fluffly like a cloud. The word looked "Good" in its appearance and so it had to be "Good." The word and the thing I was trying

to express were one, and "Good" was floating around in the air.*

About 1 hour after taking LSD, the intoxication is in full bloom, but it is not until near the end of the second hour that major ego disruptions occur (if they are to occur).

Usually these changes center around a depersonalization. The individual may feel that the sensations he experiences are not from his body or that he has no body. Body distortions are common, the sort of thing suggested by the comment of one user: "I felt as if my left big toe were going to vomit!" Not unusual is a loss of self-awareness and loss of control of behavior.

In this personality disruption stage, the individual usually has the experiences that lead him, or an observer, to characterize the trip as "good" or "bad." Two frequent types of overall reactions in this stage have been characterized as "expansive" and "constricted." Some people show both. In the expansive reaction (a good trip) the individual may become hypomanic and grandiose and feel that he is uncovering secrets of the universe or profundities previously locked within himself. Feelings of creativity are not uncommon: "If I only had the time I could write the truly great American novel." The other end of the continuum is the constricted reaction in which the user shows little movement and frequently becomes paranoid and exhibits feelings of persecution. The prototype individual in this situation is huddled in a corner fearful that some harm will come to him or that he is being threatened by some aspect of his hallucinations. Few LSD users ever reach the stage where auditory hallucinations occur. If they do, the hallucinations are usually an outgrowth of experiences in earlier phases of the trip. As the drug effect diminishes, normal psychological controls of sensations, perceptions, and mood return. As discussed on p. 245, there may be problems on reentry into the nonaltered reality.

A trip can be viewed in ways other than the sequential manner just discussed. One expert

---

*From Farrell, B.: Scientists, theologians, mystics swept up in a psychic revolution, Life Magazine **60**:31, March 25, 1966, ©1966 Time Inc.

*From Krippner, S.: Psychedelic experience and the language process, Journal of Psychedelic Drugs **3**(1):48, 1970.

interpreter[29] of the hallucinogenic experience analyzes the total experience into four levels of consciousness: sensory, recollective-analytic, symbolic, integral. Each level is more difficult to attain than the one before it and is reached by fewer people. Similarly, with each succeeding level the potential of the experience increases, for good or bad.

At the sensory level, which is readily attained by all users, there are changes in the way the user perceives everything. The synesthesias, in which colors evoke musical rhythms or auditory patterns bring forth a cavalcade of forms and color, and time distortions combine with the attributing of new meanings to old sensations. These experiences have at least one major effect on many individuals that they carry back to the nondrug reality. As a result of the drug-altered perceptions, the individual frequently is forced to think and to categorize things, people, and experiences in a new way when in the nondrug condition. This new way of looking at old things is perhaps the single most important outcome of the experience at this level.

At the recollective-analytical level of consciousness, the same types of new perceptions are experienced, but now within one's own history and personality. Being forced to see yourself through LSD eyes may bring panic and anxiety or a new and fuller understanding of one's own potentials and hopes.

The symbolic and the integral levels of consciousness are further, to use a metaphor, descents and explorations into our true selves. At the symbolic level there is an appreciation of our oneness with the universal concepts expressed in myths and in the archetypes of jungian psychology. To experience the final level, the integral level, has been likened to a religious conversion, that is, the sudden awareness that we have been accepted by God and are saved. At this level the individual feels a unity with God and/or with the essence of the universe.[30] (See also references 16, 31, and 32.)

Some general characteristics of the entire experience that must be mentioned are: the setting, use of the guide, and the dose. As mentioned in the section on Pharmacody-namics (p. 239), LSD and the other hallucinogens seem primarily to disrupt sensory input and processing. The more unique and stimulating the environment, the greater the effect of the drug. In a typical laboratory setting the drug experience is much different from that which occurs in a crowded room surrounded by friends, flashing lights, and acid-rock music.

How are the new experiences, sensations, and feelings to be interpreted? What do they mean? This is the primary function of the guide, although he is also available to prevent the individual from hurting himself. (You are just as dead whether you go out an upper-story window to "escape" from something or to "fly to join the beautiful stars.") The guide usually functions as an interpreter of the experience to the novice. As it is necessary to learn what you are looking at when you look through a microscope, it is necessary to learn what the drug-induced experiences mean. The guide is usually a close acquaintance or friend who has used hallucinogens and thus experienced a trip, but, while acting as a guide, he will not be using drugs. He may suggest what is happening to the user and lead him through the trip. Or, in other cases, he may only interact with the user when negative reactions seem to be appearing.

The length and depth of the experience is governed in part by the amount of the drug. As the dose increases, the experience becomes more and more like the trip to which people usually refer. With LSD and other indole hallucinogens, there does not seem to be as much euphoria associated with low doses as there is in the case of the catechol hallucinogens. Low doses of the hallucinogens do not give a miniature trip but instead produce only the autonomic and perceptual effects. An approximation of the relationship between dose and experience is indicated in Fig. 14-2.

In closing this section attempting to describe what is impossible to describe, some points should be reemphasized. The sensations and other experiences following use of an hallucinogen are brand new to the user. As such they are very susceptible to influence by many factors; the same experience might be viewed as magnificent or horrendous, depending on

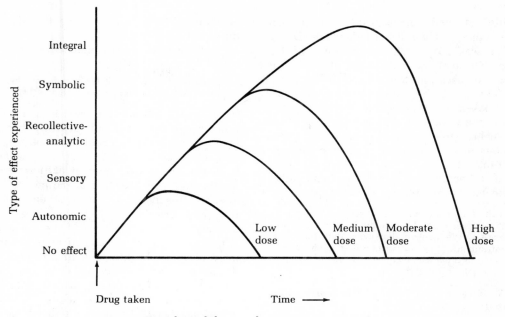

Fig. 14-2. Hypothetical dose- and time-response curve for LSD.

these factors. The feeling of depersonalization or of certain autonomic changes may be viewed as revealing—or only cause anxiety. Since there is memory for the period of altered consciousness, the experience may have considerable impact on how the individual reacts to the nondrug reality.

Adverse reactions

In the hands of experts these agents are relatively safe but they are potent mind-shakers which should not be lightly or frivolously consumed.*

The adverse reactions to LSD ingestion have been repeatedly emphasized in the popular as well as scientific literature. Since there is no way of knowing how much illegal LSD is being used or how pure the LSD is that people are taking, there is no possibility of determining the true incidence of adverse reactions to LSD. Adverse reactions to the street use of what is thought to be LSD may result from many factors. It is important to always remember that drugs obtained on the

*From Cohen, S.: A classification of LSD complications, Psychosomatics **7**:186, 1966.

Table 14-1. Estimated rates of major complications associated with LSD*

	Number per 1,000 persons		
	Attempted suicide	Completed suicide	Psychotic reaction over 48 hours
Experimental (control) subjects	0	0	0.8
Patients under-going psycho-therapy	1.2	0.4	1.8

*From Cohen, S.: Lysergic and diethylamide side effects and complications, Journal of Nervous and mental Diseases **130**:36, 1960.

street frequently are not what they are claimed to be—in purity or in chemical composition.

A 1960 study surveyed most of the legal United States investigators studying LSD and mescaline effects in humans. Data were collected on 25,000 administrations of the drug to about 5,000 individuals. Dosage range was 25 to 1,500 micrograms of LSD and 200 to 1,200 milligrams of mescaline. In some cases the drug was used in patients undergoing therapy; in other cases the drug was taken in an experimental situation to study the effects of the drug. Only LSD and mescaline used under professional supervision were surveyed. The results are noted in Table 14-1.

In reflecting on these data and others collected in the interim, a 1963 paper stated:

> The actual incidence of serious complications following LSD administration is not known. We believe, however, that they are infrequent. It is surprising that such a profound psychological experience leaves adverse residuals so rarely.*

A 1964 article, "The LSD Controversy," stated:

> It would seem that the incidence statistics better support a statement that the drug is *exceptionally safe* rather than dangerous. Although no statistics have been compiled for the dangers of psychological therapies, we would not be surprised if the incidence of adverse reactions, such as psychotic or depressive episodes and suicide attempts, were at least as high or higher in any comparable group of psychiatric patients exposed to any active form of therapy.

but then went on to say:

> It is also important to distinguish between the proper use of this drug in a therapeutic or experimental setting and its indiscriminate use and abuse by thrill seekers, "lunatic fringe," and drug addicts. More dangers seem likely for the unstable character who takes the drug for "kicks," curiosity, or to escape reality and responsibility than someone taking the drug for therapeutic reasons under strict medical aegis and supervision.†

It is also important to emphasize that a clear distinction must be made between the pure LSD used in the "therapeutic or experimental setting" and the impure drug or combination of drugs most frequently used in the street.

Finally, a 1967 report concluded:

> . . . it now appears that a variety of serious complications can result from both the therapeutic and non-therapeutic uses of LSD.*

The study of adverse reactions to LSD is an emotional area, and facts are hard to obtain. One survey[33] was taken in Los Angeles of professionals treating adverse reactions in illegal users. Sixty percent of those treating the users felt that half of the people with adverse reactions had been emotionally disturbed prior to taking the drug. This statement goes to the heart of the real question: can LSD elicit an adverse reaction in a mentally healthy individual? The evidence is divided, and no conclusion can honestly be drawn except to ask: "Are any of us without fears and anxieties, conscious or unconscious?" Given the right dose and the right conditions, probably anyone could have one of the adverse reactions noted in the following section. However, it is probably true that the more disturbed one is in the absence of the drug, the more likely it is that one will have a bad trip or other adverse reaction.

Some feel that novices have more serious reactions than habitual users, possibly because they have not learned how to handle the altered perceptions and states of consciousness. The same reason may be the basis for reports that individuals with more rigid and constricted personalities have more problems with the drug experience.[22] An overall factor that may be of great importance in minimizing the negative effects that do develop is the realization by the individual that the distortions and effects are time limited and drug related. This realization seems to be the key to "talking someone down" from a bad trip by continually emphasizing to the person that he has not changed and that it is the drug that is causing the effects, which will soon go away.

*From Cohen, S. and Ditman, K. S.: Prolonged adverse reactions to lysergic acid diethylamide, Archives of General Psychiatry 8:479, 1963.
†From Levine, J., and Ludwig, A. M.: The LSD controversy, Comprehensive Psychiatry 5(5):318-319, 1964.

*From Smart, R. G., and Bateman, K.: Unfavourable reactions to LSD: a review and analysis of the available case reports, The Canadian Medical Association Journal 97:1214, 1967.

Two of the types of adverse reactions that may develop during the drug-induced experience are the panic reaction and the overt psychosis. The panic reaction, which is an extreme anxiety attack, usually results from the individual's response to some particular aspects of the experience and is typified in the following case history:

A 21-year-old woman was admitted to the hospital along with her lover. He had had a number of LSD experiences and had convinced her to take it to make her less constrained sexually. About half an hour after ingestion of approximately 200 microgm., she noticed that the bricks in the wall began to go in and out and that light affected her strangely. She became frightened when she realized that she was unable to distinguish her body from the chair she was sitting on or from her lover's body. Her fear became more marked after she thought that she would not get back into herself. At the time of admission she was hyperactive and laughed inappropriately. Stream of talk was illogical and affect labile. Two days later, this reaction had ceased. However, she was still afraid of the drug and convinced that she would not take it again because of her frightening experience.*

When an overt psychosis develops, remedial treatment is not usually so rapid, and the next individual to be described was hospitalized for prolonged treatment. Usually such psychosis occurs in individuals with a precarious hold on reality in the nondrug condition. The flood of new experiences and feelings is too much for this type person to integrate.

A 23-year-old man was admitted to the hospital after he stood uncertain whether to plunge an upraised knife into his friend's back. His wife, an intelligent, nonpsychotic but masochistic woman, reported that he had been acting strangely since taking LSD approximately 3 weeks before admission. He was indecisive and often mute and shunned physical contact with her. On admission he was catatonic, mute and echopractic. He appeared to be preoccupied with auditory hallucinations of God's voice and thought he had achieved a condition of "all mind." On transfer to another hospital 1 month after admission, there was minimal improvement.

*From Frosch, W. A., Robbins, E. S., and Stern, M.: Untoward reactions to lysergic acid diethylamide (LSD) resulting in hospitalization, The New England Journal of Medicine **273**(23):1236, 1965.

During his adolescence the patient had alternated between acceptance of and rebellion against his mother's religiosity and warnings of the perils of sex and immorality. He had left college during his 1st year after excessive use of amphetamines. He attended, but did not complete, art school. His marriage of 3 years had been marked by conflict and concern about his masculinity. Increasing puzzlement about the meaning of life, his role in the universe and other cosmic problems led to his ingestion of LSD. Shortly after ingestion he was ecstatic and wrote to a friend, "We have found the peace, which is life's river which flows into the sea of Eternity." Soon afterward, in a brief essay, he showed some awareness of his developing psychosis, writing, "I am misunderstood, I cried, and was handed a complete list of my personality traits, habits, goals, and ideals, etc. I know myself now, I said in relief, and spent the rest of my life in happy cares asylum. AMEN."*

One of the frightening and interesting adverse reactions to LSD is the flashback. More than any other reaction, the recurrence of symptoms weeks or months after an individual has taken LSD brings up thoughts of brain damage and permanent biochemical changes. The next case history follows the usual pattern seen in flashback cases.

A man in his late twenties came to the admitting office in a state of panic. Although he had not taken any drug in approximately 2 months he was beginning to re-experience some of the illusory phenomena, perceptual distortions and the feeling of union with things around him that had previously occurred only under the influence of LSD. In addition, his wife had told him that he was beginning to "talk crazy," and he had become frightened. Despite a somewhat disturbed childhood and an interrupted college career he had carefully controlled his anxiety by a rigid obsessive-compulsive character structure, which had permitted him to work with reasonable success as a junior executive. Although for 6 years before admission he had felt the urge to seek help and self-understanding, he had never sought psychiatric care. He had tried marijuana, peyote and finally ground morning-glory seeds. Most of his 15 experiences with LSD had been pleasurable although he also had had 2 panic reactions, neither of which had led to hospital admission. On these occasions he thought that he was losing control and that his whole body was disappearing. At the time of admission he was concerned lest LSD have some perma-

*Ibid., p. 1237.

nent effect upon him. He wished reassurance so that he could take it again. His symptoms have subsided but tend to reappear in anxiety-provoking situations.*

Flashbacks consist of the recurrence of certain aspects of the drug experience after a period of normalcy and in the absence of any drug use. The frequency and duration of these flashbacks are quite variable and seem at this time to be unpredictable. One study[34] of flashbacks reported that they are most frequent just before going to sleep, while driving, and in periods of psychological stress. It was suggested that flashbacks may be attempts to resolve and master traumatic experiences. They seem to occur primarily in immature individuals and diminish in frequency and intensity with time if the individual stops using psychoactive drugs.

Where do all these reports leave us? Is LSD, or any of the better-known hallucinogens a dangerous drug? It is clear that some people do show immediate and/or long-lasting negative reactions to a hallucinogenic experience. The evidence strongly suggests that if the individual using the drug has a marginal adjustment in the nondrug condition, there is a higher probability of a bad reaction than if he is reasonably well adjusted.[22] However, considering the fact that even an apparently normal, mentally healthy person can have a bad trip or a prolonged adverse reaction, all of these drugs must be approached with extreme caution.

Beliefs about LSD

LSD is truly a legend in its own time. Although there are no data, probably more people have more ideas about what LSD does and does not do than they have about any other drug. Only a few of these beliefs can be mentioned. The reader should especially note that the conclusions drawn in this section may be altered in the future but as of now . . .

Creativity. One of the most widely occurring beliefs is that these hallucinogenic agents increase creativity or release the creativity that our inhibitions keep bottled

*Ibid., p. 1237.

inside us. Creativity is an ephemeral thing and not easily measured. Combining creativity with the use of a drug whose effects are very responsive to expectations and setting makes the problem very difficult to study. There have been several experiments that have attempted to study the effects of LSD on creativity, but there is no good evidence that the drug increases it. In one laboratory study using LSD at doses of 0.0025 or 0.01 milligram per kilogram body weight, "the authors concluded that the administration of LSD-25 to a relatively unselected group of people for the purpose of enhancing their creative ability is *not* likely to be successful."[35]

Therapy. Another common belief is that LSD has therapeutic usefulness, particularly in the treatment of alcoholics, even though in the literature: "Reports of results with LSD in alcoholism have gradually changed from glowing and enthusiastic to cautious and disappointing."[36] A recent well-controlled study compared the effectiveness of one dose of either 0.60 milligram of LSD or 60.0 milligrams of dextroamphetamine in reducing drinking by alcoholics. No additional therapy, physical or psychological, was used. The authors found ". . . LSD produced slightly better results early, but after six months the results were alike for both treatment groups."[37]

Some investigators[38] have reported considerable success with LSD in reducing the pain and depression of patients with terminal cancer. The LSD experiences were part of a several-day program involving extensive verbal interaction between the therapist and patient. Although not successful in every case, the LSD therapy was followed by a reduction in the use of narcotics, ". . . less worry about the future," and "the appearance of a positive mood state."[38] The authors concluded that they have a treatment "which may be highly promising for patients facing fatal illness if implemented in the context of brief, intensive, and highly specialized psychotherapy catalyzed by a psychedelic drug such as LSD."[38] The potential value of the hallucinogens in the treatment of many disorders is still very much discussed and studied, and, as with most issues, a final resolution has not yet been reached.[39]

Chromosomes. A credibility gap in the world of drugs developed in 1967 between the press and the public with the publication of a scientific report that LSD caused damage to chromosomes of white blood cells (leukocytes) in vitro. This report was quickly followed by a study showing a higher than normal incidence of chromosomal damage in the white blood cells of LSD users. These data received much attention in the mass media and are felt to be one of the reasons for the decrease in LSD use that has occurred since 1967. Not so widely publicized were the reports that did *not* show any relationship in vitro or in vivo between white blood cell chromosome damage and LSD use.

The popular reports also had a way of neglecting to emphasize (or mention) that the effects were on white blood cells and not on the germ cells, which are the only cells involved in reproduction. A poster distributed by the National Foundation—March of Dimes in this period showed a boy, in front of a possibly pregnant girl, making the statement: "Give me one good reason why I shouldn't use LSD." The poster replies "We can give you 46 . . . Broken chromosomes may cause birth defects. LSD can break chromosomes. Need we say more?"

A similar misemphasis showed up in a United Press International release in February of 1968 which used the headline, "Cancer Linked to LSD Use." In the story, however, LSD was only one of several agents:

> Evidence was building that LSD or any other agent that causes chromosomes to break—including caffeine additives in sufficient amounts—will shorten cell life in the user and "significantly increase the chance of cancer."*

Studies dealing with the effects of LSD on germ cells in animals have given both positive and negative results. Studies in mice show increased stillbirths and/or deformities when LSD is given during gestation. Data from humans are less clear since impure, street-obtained, LSD is ingested and malnutrition and inadequate prenatal care are common. Evidence is accumulating though that women who use LSD during pregnancy have a higher incidence of miscarriages and babies with congenital deformities. There is no way to identify the causative factors, and some investigators do not obtain similar results.[39a] It is true that:

> No one to date has conclusively proven that any birth defect is directly attributable to parental use of LSD.

And it is certainly true that:

> For the time being, it seems wiser to maintain a wait-and-see attitude.*

But it is most true of all that no drug used recreationally during pregnancy is good for the fetus, and some may be quite harmful (see p. 101).

Responsibility for acts committed in a drugged state. A question that occurs with reasonable frequency is whether an individual is legally responsible for his behavior while under the influence of a hallucinogen. It may be years before the nuances are resolved, but as of now the answer clearly is: it depends. In general the courts have used the precedents set in cases involving alcohol to judge hallucinogen cases. It seems probable that if ingestion of a hallucinogen is unknown to the individual, he will not be held responsible for his behavior while under its influence. In a 1969 Maryland case[40] a man broke into a house and confronted the owner's wife. The defendant pleaded not guilty because of temporary insanity and said that, unknown to him, he had been given LSD the night before the event. There was corroborating evidence and the defendant was acquitted on the grounds of temporary insanity.

It seems unlikely, however, that an individual will be allowed to voluntarily take a hallucinogen and then escape conviction on the grounds of drug-induced insanity. More probable will be the plea of drug intoxication, which does not preclude conviction for a crime. This plea may be the basis for a reduction in the charge though, such as from first

*From Doctor tells house of drug's dangers; cancer linked to LSD use, United Press International Release, February 19, 1968.

*From Egozcue, J., and Irwin, S.: LSD-25 effects on chromosomes: a review, Journal of Psychedelic Drugs 3(1):11, 1970.

degree murder to second degree or man-slaughter.[41] There have been innumerable precedents for this legal procedure when alcohol was the drug causing the intoxication, so its utilization with other drugs seems likely to increase.

CONCLUDING COMMENT

The hallucinogens are as fabulous in our time as coffee was a few hundred years ago in Europe. One big difference is that the hallucinogens have much more potential for personal good or harm than coffee ever had. Whether the secular and aperiodic use of hallucinogens will change the present world more than coffee and tea changed their world is a question only time can answer. The use of the hallucinogens for personal (and perhaps, therefore, social) good is an issue that is debated more and more.

A 1970 article in the *Minnesota Law Review* discussed the research done with LSD. The author concluded that a solution to the problem of LSD use:

> . . . is to be found, no doubt, where the answers to so many other social problems lie—in a general improvement of the quality of American society. If some such improvement came to pass, then either the need which LSD fills would disappear or its usage would become simply one very minor aspect of social life.*

*From Ford, S. D.: LSD and the law: a framework for policy making, Minnesota Law Review **54**:775-804, 1970.

PRECEDING QUOTES

1. Smith, J. P.: LSD: the false illusion, FDA Papers, vol. 1, July-August, 1967.
2. McDonagh, D.: Leary under the glass—some impressions by a turned-off observer, National Review **19**:377, 1967.
3. Smith, D. E.: LSD and the psychedelic syndrome, Clinical Toxicology **2**(1):69-73, 1969.

REFERENCES

1. Hofmann, A.: Psychotomimetic agents. In Burger, A., editor: Drugs affecting the central nervous system, vol. 2, New York, 1968, Marcel Dekker, Inc., pp. 169-235.
2. Fink, P. J., Goldman, M. J., and Lyons, I.: Morning glory seed psychosis, Archives of General Psychiatry **15**:210, 1966.
3. Cohen, S.: Suicide following morning glory seed ingestion, The American Journal of Psychiatry **120**(10):1024, 1964.
4. Szara, S.: DMT (N,N-Dimethyltryptamine) and

homologues: clinical and pharmacological considerations. In Efron, D. H., editor: Psychotomimetic drugs, New York, 1970, Raven Press, pp. 275-286.
5. Waser, P. G.: The pharmacology of Amanita muscaria. In Efron, D. H., editor: Ethnopharmacologic search for psychoactive drugs, Proceedings of a Symposium held in San Francisco, California, January 28-30, 1967, Washington, D. C., 1967, National Institute of Mental Health, p. 437.
6. Horne, C. H. W., and McCluskie, J. A. W.: The food of the gods, Scottish Medical Journal **8**:490, 1963.
7. Fabing, H. D.: On going berserk, The Prescriber **3**:30-31, 1956.
8. Graves, R.: Steps, London, 1958, Cassell & Co.
9. Wasson, R. G.: Fly agaric and man. In Efron, D. H., editor: Ethnopharmacologic search for psychoactive drugs, Proceedings of a Symposium held in San Francisco, California, January 28-30, 1967, Washington, D. C., 1967, National Institute of Mental Health, p. 405. (See also Wasson, R. G.: Soma, divine mushroom of immortality, New York, 1971, Harcourt, Brace, Jovanovich.)
10. Allegro, J. M.: The sacred mushroom and the cross, New York, 1970, Doubleday & Company, Inc.
11. Hallucinogens, Columbia Law Review **68**(3): 521, 1968.
12. Barger, G.: Ergot and ergotism, London, 1931, Gurney and Jackson, pp. 30, 43.
13. Hordern, A.: Psychopharmacology: some historical considerations. In Joyce, C. R. B., editor: Psychopharmacology: dimensions and perspectives, Philadelphia, 1968, J. B. Lippincott Co., p. 138.
14. Fuller, J. G.: The day of St. Anthony's fire, New York, 1968, The Macmillan Co., pp. 96,100.
14a. Fischer, R.: A cartography of the ecstatic and meditative states, Science **174**:897-904, 1971.
14b. Tart, C. T.: States of consciousness and state-specific sciences, Science **176**:1203-1210, 1972.
14c. Holden, C.: Altered states of consciousness: mind researchers meet to discuss exploration and mapping of "inner space," Science **179**: 982-983, 1973.
14d. Masters, R., and Houston, J.: The varieties of postpsychedelic experience, Intellectual Digest, pp. 16-18, March, 1973.
15. Clark, W. H.: Chemical ecstasy: psychedelic drugs and religion, New York, 1969, Sheed & Ward.
16. Ditman, K. S., and others: Dimensions of the LSD, methylphenidate and chlordiazepoxide experiences, Psychopharmacologia **14**:1-11, 1969.
17. White House Conference on Narcotics and Drug Abuse, Washington, D. C., 1963, U. S. Government Printing Office, p. 288.
18. Blumenthal, R.: Leary drug cult stirs Millbrook, New York Times, June 14, 1967, p. 49.

19. McGlothlin, W. H., and Cohen, S.: The use of hallucinogenic drugs among college students, The American Journal of Psychiatry 122(5): 572-574, 1965.

20. Brehm, M. L., and Back, K. W.: Self image and attitudes toward drugs, Journal of Personality 36:299-314, 1968.

20a. Drug use in America: problem in perspective, Second report of the National Commission on Marihuana and Drug Abuse, March, 1973.

21. Kleckner, J. H.: An investigation into the personal characteristics and family backgrounds of psychedelic drug users, Dissertation Abstracts 29B:4380-B, 1969.

22. Ungerleider, J. T., and Fisher, D. D.: The problems of LSD[25] and emotional disorder, California Medicine 106(1):49-55, 1967.

22a. Braucht, G. N., Brakarsh, D., Follingstad, D., and Berry, K. L.: Deviant drug use in adolescence: a review of psychosocial correlates, Psychological Bulletin 79(2):92-106, 1973.

23. Smith, D. E.: LSD: its use, abuse, and suggested treatment, Journal of Psychedelic Drugs 1(2): 120, 1967-1968.

23a. Cardoso, B.: Tim Leary and the long arm of the law, Rolling Stone, March 15, 1973.

24. Materson, B. J., and Barrett-Connor, E.: LSD "mainlining": a new hazard to health, Journal of the American Medical Association 200(12): 1126-1127, 1967.

25. Smythies, J. R.: The mode of action of psychotomimetic drugs. A report on an NRP work session held on November 17-19, 1968, Neurosciences Research Program Bulletin 8(1):63, 1970.

26. Action of hallucinogenic drugs, Nature 220:961, 1968.

27. Wallace, A. F. C.: The trip. In Hicks, R. E., and Fink, P. J., editors: Psychedelic drugs, Proceedings of a Hahnemann Medical College and Hospital Symposium sponsored by the Department of Psychiatry, New York, 1969, Grune & Stratton, Inc., p. 155. By permission.

28. Krippner, S.: Psychedelic experience and the language process, Journal of Psychedelic Drugs 3(1):48, 1970.

29. Houston, J.: Phenomenology of the psychedelic experience. In Hicks, R. E., and Fink, P. J., editors: Psychedelic drugs, Proceedings of a Hahnemann Medical College and Hospital Symposium sponsored by the Department of Psychiatry, New York, 1969, Grune & Stratton, Inc., pp. 1-7. By permission.

30. Moody, H.: Psychedelic drugs and religious experience. In Hicks, R. E., and Fink, P. J., editors: Psychedelic drugs, Proceedings of a Hahnemann Medical College and Hospital Symposium sponsored by the Department of Psychiatry, New York, 1969, Grune & Stratton, Inc., pp. 147-149. By permission.

31. Teenagers' logic slips from heavy LSD use, U.S. Medicine 4(9):24, 1968.

32. Katz, M. M., Waskow, I. E., and Olsson, J.: Characterizing the psychological state produced by LSD, Journal of Abnormal Psychology 73(1): 1-14, 1968.

33. Ungerleider, J. T., and others: A statistical survey of adverse reactions to LSD in Los Angeles County, American Journal of Psychiatry 125:352-357, 1968.

34. Shick, J. F. E., and Smith, D. E.: Analysis of the LSD flashback, Journal of Psychedelic Drugs 3(1):13-19, 1970.

35. Zegans, L. S., Pollard, J. C., and Brown, D.: The effects of LSD-25 on creativity and tolerance to regression, Archives of General Psychiatry 16:748, 1967.

36. Hayman, M., and del Giudice, J.: Psychotropic drugs in alcoholism. In Clark, W. G., and del Giudice, J., editors: Principles of psychopharmacology, New York, 1970, Academic Press, Inc., p. 520.

37. Hollister, L. E., Shelton, J., and Krieger, G.: A controlled comparison of lysergic acid diethylamide (LSD) and dextroamphetamine in alcoholics, American Journal of Psychiatry 125: 1352, 1969.

38. Pahnke, W. N., and others: Psychedelic therapy (utilizing LSD) with cancer patients, Journal of Psychedelic Drugs 3(1):74, 1970.

39. Abramson, H., editor: The use of LSD in psychotherapy and alcoholism, Indianapolis, 1967, The Bobbs-Merrill Co., Inc.

39a. Maugh, T. H., II: LSD and the drug culture: new evidence of hazard, Science 179:1973.

40. State v. Hannon, Howard County, Maryland, 1969.

41. Baumgartner, K. C.: The effect of drugs on criminal responsibility, specific intent, and mental competency, American Criminal Law Quarterly 8:118-127, 1970.

15 Marijuana and hashish

Continued use of the drug, for example, will lead to a delirious rage in which the addicts are temporarily irresponsible and inclined to commit the most horrible and violent crimes. Any increase in crime in a community usually is attributed by authorities to marijuana. Many murders are committed either by persons not responsible while under the influence of the drug, or by persons who deliberately smoke it to gain a false courage for the commission of a planned slaying. Prolonged use is said to lead to mental deterioration and eventual insanity.

Popular Science Monthly, 1936

With the possible exception of speeding on the highways, pot smoking is almost certainly the most widely committed crime in the
United States today.

Newsweek, September, 1970

October 17, 1967

Whether or not marijuana is a more dangerous drug than alcohol is debatable—I don't happen to think it is.

October 18, 1967

Some press reports allege that I see no difference between smoking marijuana and having a cocktail. This is false. The possession and use of marijuana carries a very severe legal penalty while the use of alcohol has no such severe legal penalties attached . . . .

Smoking marijuana and drinking both present dangers to the individual, and in this respect, as a physician, as well as a parent, I do not dismiss the subject as casually as reported.

James L. Goddard, Commissioner
Food and Drug Administration

We should not be hung up like some doctors who say on TV that marijuana is no worse than alcohol . . . . Alcohol can kill you. And if you look at all the problems that alcohol produces, with suggestions from Congress that hundreds of millions of dollars be spent on dealing with its problems, there is no reason to open the doors to marijuana and compound the problem.

John Mitchell, September, 1970
Attorney General

MARIJUANA

Marijuana perhaps more than any other drug is the NOW generation.[a] Not just the hippies or the dropouts or the alienated but the doctors, lawyers, and all kinds of chiefs of tomorrow say marijuana is it. It is better than booze, no hangover. It is a mind drug, not a body drug as is alcohol. It is a harmless drug while alcohol and nicotine are known to be responsible directly or indirectly for much illness and many deaths. It is a euphoriant in a world that needs joy, not the obliteration of sensation that accompanies alcohol. It is not addicting, whereas hard liquor is. No one dies when they stop using it; some have died when they stopped drinking. It represents and is part of a new attitude toward life while alcohol is regressive.

On the other hand . . .

Nonsense. Marijuana smoking is frequently the first step toward dropping out of life. It sometimes leads to the use of even more dangerous drugs. It has not been studied enough to say it is harmless. It is a symbol of an attitude that will destroy our country and lower everyone's standard of living. Alcohol does present problems but it is the drug of choice in all of the more technologically advanced countries, so it cannot be too bad. Marijuana, on the other hand, is used only in the backwater countries of the world.

These statements are but a few of the opinions that can be read or heard regarding marijuana. Be it good or bad, marijuana is here to stay. Just as coffee and tea came to dinner and stayed on, so too with marijuana. To appreciate our present attitudes toward marijuana, it may help to remember the type of attitude toward coffee and tea that was expressed only a hundred years ago. The French essayist Balzac contrasted the effects of wine and coffee by saying that coffee:

> . . . causes an admirable fever. It enters the brain like a bacchante. Upon its attack, imagination runs wild, bares itself, twists like a pythoness and in this paroxysm a poet enjoys the supreme possession of his faculties; but this is a drunkenness of thought as wine brings about a drunkenness of the body.*

*From Mickel, E. J.: The artificial paradises in French literature, Chapel Hill, 1969, University of North Carolina Press, p. 65. (Free translation from French.)

In the original French the description is even more stimulating and erotic. Unfortunately, it does not seem to refer to the effect most people have with their morning cup of coffee.

The plant Linnaeus named *Cannabis sativa* in 1753 is a single species genus that now grows worldwide but that originated in the Orient. It has been widely grown for its fibers, from which hemp rope is made. The psycho-active agent is concentrated in the resin of the plant, the concentration being greatest in the flowering tops and decreasing in the lower, more fibrous parts. The potency of this resin will vary with the conditions under which the plant is grown. The psychoactive potency of the *Cannabis* preparation depends on the amount as well as the strength of the resin present and therefore varies depending on the part of the plant used. Hash, or hashish in this country, is resin from the flowering tops and thus is highly potent. Much less potent is the preparation called marijuana, which consists chiefly of leafy material and fine stems and is used in smoking.

EARLY HISTORY

The history of the use of the plant *Cannabis sativa* is difficult to give because so little of it is known. *Cannabis* was never a staple in the doctor's black bag, so there are not extensive references to it in medical history. The earliest reference to *Cannabis* is in a pharmacy book written in 2737 B.C. by the Chinese Emporer Shen Nung. Referring to the euphoriant effects of *Cannabis*, he called it the "Liberator of Sin." There were some medical uses, however, and he recommended it for "female weakness, gout, rheumatism, malaria, beriberi, constipation and absent-mindedness"![1]

Since the earliest record is Chinese, a slight credibility gap exists in noting that the most popular story of marijuana's discovery is a legend from the Arabic world. The hero is Haider, a very stoic, seclusive monk, who built a monastery in the desert and made a point of never enjoying any pleasures. Things changed for Haider when:

> One burning summer's day when the fiery sun glared angrily upon Mother Earth as if he wished to wither up her breasts, Haider stepped out from his cloister and walked alone

to the fields. All around him lay the vegetation weary and without life, but one plant danced in the heat with joy. Haider plucked it, partook of it, and returned to the convent a happier man. The monks who saw him immediately noticed the change in their chief. He encouraged conversation, and acted boisterously. He then led his companions to the fields, and the holy men partook of the hasheesh, and were transformed from austere ascetics into jolly good fellows.*

The same characteristics of the plant to which Haider responded spread its use around the world. There are scattered references to *Cannabis* in India, China, and the Middle East between 2737 B.C. and recent years. One writer commented:

> Opium is mentioned in many medical texts because of its ability to relieve pain, references to hashish are confined to a more fanciful, vague world of religious and mystical experience. The drug's wondrous ability to set man's imagination free, to change the shape and color of his world, has caused it to be used quite differently from opium and for purposes more related to man's spiritual existence.†

Some of the early references were to the use of *Cannabis* as an inebriant. In 430 B.C. Herodotus reported that the Scythians burned hempseeds and inhaled the smoke to induce intoxication. Since the seeds contain little if any of the psychoactive agent, probably the entire top of the plant was used. The scattered reports of *Cannabis* as an intoxicant are of little importance here, but social use of the plant spread to the Moslem world and North Africa by 1000 A.D. Its social use increased to the point where it was considered epidemic in the twelfth century.[2]

In this period in the eastern Mediterranean area a legend developed around a religious cult that committed murder for political reasons. The cult was called "hashishiyya," from which our word "assassin" developed. In 1299 Marco Polo told the story he had heard of this group and their leader. It was a marvelous tale and had all the ingredients for surviving through the ages: intrigue, murder, sex, the use of drugs, mysterious lands. The story of this group and their

---

*From Robinson, V.: An essay on hasheesh, ed. 2, New York, 1925, E. H. Ringer, Publisher, pp. 29-30.
†From Mickel, op. cit., pp. 44-45.

activities was told in many ways over the years, and Boccaccios's *Decameron* contained one story based on it. Stories of this cult, combined with the frequent reference to the power and wonderment of hashish in *The Arabian Nights*, were widely circulated in Europe over the years.

MIDDLE HISTORY

At the turn of the nineteenth century, world commerce was expanding. New and exciting reports from the world travelers of the seventeenth and eighteenth centuries introduced new cultures and new ideas to Europe. The Orient and the Middle East had yielded exotic spices as well as the stimulants coffee and tea. Europe was ready for another new sensation, and she got it. The returning veteran, as usual, gets part of the blame for introducing what Europe was ready to receive.

> Napoleon's campaign to Egypt at the beginning of the nineteenth century increased the Romantic's acquaintance with hashish and caused them to associate it with the Near East. . . . Napoleon was forced to give an order forbidding all French soldiers to indulge in hashish. Some of the soldiers brought the habit to France, however, as did many other Frenchmen who worked for the government or traveled in the Near East.*

By the 1830's and 1840's, everyone who was anyone was using, thinking about using, or decrying the use of mind-tickling agents such as opium and hashish. One of the earliest (1844) popular accounts of the use of hashish is in *The Count of Monte Cristo* by Alexander Dumas. The story includes a reference to the Assassin story and contains statements about the characteristics of the drug that still sound contemporary.

Throughout the middle of the nineteenth century the great French writers of the period were in constant communication with each other. During the 1840's a group of artists and writers gathered monthly at the Hotel Pimodan in Paris' Latin Quarter to use drugs. This group became famous because one of the participants, Gautier, wrote a book, *Le Club des Hachischins*, which described their activities. From this group have come some of the best literary descriptions of hashish

---

*From Mickel, op. cit., p. 63.

intoxication. These French Romantics, as with the impressionistic painters of a later period, were searching for new experiences, new sources of creativity from within, new ways of seeing the world outside. A few of the regulars are well-known writers such as Baudelaire, Gautier, and Dumas. Balzac actually was pretty much of an antidrug man and even warned against the use of coffee, tea, alcohol, and sugar!

Baudelaire was addicted to opium, but at the time of his death, at an early age as a result of syphilis, he was opposed to the use of drugs. His writings, however, contain much of value for those who want to understand the use and attraction of *Cannabis*. The drug being used was hashish, the most potent form of the psychoactive material of *Cannabis*. Baudelaire repeatedly used this drug and was an astute observer of the effects in himself and in others. In his book *The Artificial Paradises* he echoes what Dumas had written about the kind of effect to expect from hashish.

> . . . the uninitiated . . . imagine hashish intoxication as a wondrous land, a vast theater of magic and juggling where everything is miraculous and unexpected. That is a preconceived notion, a total misconception. . . . the intoxication will be nothing but one immense dream, thanks to intensity of color and the rapidity of conceptions; but it will always preserve the particular tonality of the individual. . . . the dream will certainly reflect its dreamer. . . . he is only the same man grown larger . . . sophisticate and *ingénu* . . . will find nothing miraculous, absolutely nothing but the natural to an extreme. The mind and body upon which hashish operates will yield only their ordinary, personal phenomena, increased, it is true, in amount and vitality, but still faithful to their original. Man will not escape the fate of his physical and mental nature: to his impressions and intimate thoughts, hashish will be a magnifying mirror, but a *true* mirror, nonetheless.*

Baudelaire's actual experience with hashish is debatable, but he did identify (and exaggerate) three stages of intoxication following oral intake. These are still being rediscovered.

> At first, there is a certain absurd, irresistible hilarity that overcomes you. These unprovoked

paroxysms of mirth . . . recur frequently, interrupting periods of stupor during which you try in vain to collect yourself. The most ordinary words, the most trivial ideas, assume a new and bizarre aspect . . . endless puns, and comic sketches keep gushing from your brain. The demon has invaded you; it is useless to resist this hilarity, which racks you like a good tickling. Now and again you break out laughing at yourself, and at your own silliness and foolery . . . The mirth . . . generally last only a fairly short time. Soon, the relations between ideas become so vague . . . that only your fellows can understand you.

> . . . a new sharpness — a greater keenness — becomes apparent in all the senses. The senses of smell, sight, hearing and touch alike participate . . . One's eyes focus on infinity. One's ear perceives near-imperceptible sounds in the very midst of the loudest tumult. It is then that the hallucinations begin. One by one, external objects slowly assume strange appearances . . . Next . . . the shuffling and misunderstanding of ideas. Sounds are clad in color, and colors contain a certain music. This, you will say, is only quite natural, and any poetic mind, in its normal rational state, will easily comprehend such analogies. But I have *already* informed the reader that there is nothing exactly supernatural in hashish intoxication; it is only that now the analogies assume an unaccustomed vividness . . . It sometimes happens that your individual identity will disappear . . . the mere contemplation of external objects will cause you soon to forget your own existence, and become inextricably fused with theirs.*

As the end of the nineteenth century approached, the use of pain-reducing and anxiety-relieving drugs increased, but the hashish experience held little interest for the dweller in middle America. Just beginning, however, was the new science of psychology, whose interest was in the workings of the mind. The writings of William James and others introduced the possibility of using psychoactive agents in studying psychological processes. In 1899 one of the psychologists who had been using *Cannabis* in experiments said: "To the psychologist it [Cannabis] was as useful as the microscope to the naturalist; it magnifies psychological states and in this way is an aid to its study."[3]

This psychologist delivered a public lecture titled "Hashish and Its Effects" in January of 1899. He read from *The Count of Monte Cristo*

*Baudelaire, C.: Artificial paradises, on hashish and wine as means of expanding individuality, New York, 1971, Herder and Herder, pp. 41-43.

*Ibid., pp. 45, 54-55.

and commented that at least 5 grains of hashish was necessary to produce psychological effects. The newspaper report of his talk said in part:

> The outward symptoms noted after taking hashish were seen in the pulse, breathing and temperature. The pulse rose on one occasion from 70 to 156. Breathing is quickened and is superficial, while the muscular strength is diminished, although the one under the influence of the drug thinks his strength is vast, and feels as if he was making extraordinary muscular efforts. The steadiness of the hand is decreased, and there is also a tendency to move about and to make rhythmical movements. . . .
>
> An interesting thing which is found detailed in many of the accounts of hashish is the tendency to overestimate and to underestimate. This is true of heat, space, muscular efforts and of number of objects.
>
> Mentally the power of association is much increased. During the period of increase it is from 30 to 40 per cent larger. Along with the ease and rapidity of this action comes the richness of images—they are fuller of detail and thoughts. . . .
>
> Emotions, too, are very much intensified, both as to pleasure and pain. Apparently the drug had no effect on the memory; if anything it was decreased. Usually the accuracy of mental processes was the same as under normal condition. To sum up his observations, Prof. Delabarre stated that the effects noted were due to hyper-excitability of the nervous system. In the process from the normal to the maximum excitement there is a wave or rhythmical increase; it generally takes about seven hours for the full influence to be felt after the drug has been taken, and when its effect passes off there is no period of depression.
>
> He spoke of the symptoms, the thrills, glows, the increase in mental power and visions, which would vary with individuals. . . . The only danger attending its use is that of becoming an habitual user, aside from the danger to the health from this strain. One may think while under the influence of the drug that he is surely going to die, but on its effects passing off no harm has been incurred, so far as is known.
>
> In conclusion, a warning was given against danger attending the habitual use, although it was stated that none was apparent if a sufficient period elapsed in making tests with it.*

*From unpublished material in the Archives of the American Psychological Association, Department of Psychology, University of Akron, Akron, Ohio.

This is still a reasonable summary of the effects of a moderate amount of hashish or of a large amount of marijuana. In spite of the promised potential of the use of drugs to study the mind their use decreased in the early years of this century. In part this resulted from the passage of the 1906 Food and Drug Law.

THE COMING OF "MARIJUANA, ASSASSIN OF YOUTH"

During the beginning of the twentieth century, public interest in marijuana and its use were not very widespread. In the early 1920's there were a few references in the mass media to the use of marijuana by Mexican Americans, but public concern was not aroused. In 1926, however, a series of articles associating marijuana and crime appeared in a New Orleans newspaper. As a result, the public began to take an interest in the drug. Enough concern developed so that one news agency sought out a government authority on plants and interviewed him about the reported episodes involving the use of marijuana. This plant scientist commented:

> It made me smile a little when I saw the first reports that a young Mexican was "concealing" his patch of hemp plants in a New York park. The plant grows from six to ten feet tall and requires plenty of open sunlight; concealment would not have been easy.
>
> Recent reports of the smuggling and use in this country of the Mexican hemp derivative 'marijuana' or 'marihuana' were no news to us, . . . We have had correspondence with El Paso and other border cities in Texas for a good many years about this situation. The reported effects of the drug on Mexicans, making them want to "clean up the town," do not jibe very well with the effects of cannabis, which so far as we have reports, simply causes temporary elation, followed by depression and heavy sleep.*

The no-cause-for-alarm attitude expressed by this scientist seemed to be prevalent in government circles. The Commissioner of Narcotics, Harry Anslinger, said that in 1931, when only sixteen states had antimarijuana laws, that the Bureau of Narcotics' file on marijuana was less than 2 inches thick.[4]

*From Our home hasheesh crop, The Literary Digest, April 3, 1926, p. 64.

The same year, the Treasury Department stated:

A great deal of public interest has been aroused by the newspaper articles appearing from time to time on the evils of the abuse of marijuana, or Indian hemp. . . This publicity tends to magnify the extent of the evil and lends color to an inference that there is an alarming spread of the improper use of the drug, whereas the actual increase in such use may not have been inordinately large.*

Six years later, however, at Congressional hearings, Anslinger stated: ". . . traffic in marijuana is increasing to such an extent that it has come to be the cause for the greatest national concern."[5] In those 6 years it is true that the use of marijuana had spread throughout the country, but there is no evidence that there was wide use. The primary motivation for the Congressional hearings on marijuana came not because of the use of marijuana as an inebrient or a euphoriant but because of reports by police and in the popular literature stating: "Most crimes of violence . . . are laid to users of marihuana."[6]

When *Scientific American* reported in March of 1936 that:

Marihuana produces a wide variety of symptoms in the user, including hilarity, swooning, and sexual excitement. Combined with intoxicants, it often makes the smoker vicious, with a desire to fight and kill.†

and *Popular Science Monthly* in May of 1936 contained a lengthy article including such statements as:

. . . the chief of Philadelphia County detectives declared that whenever any particularly horrible crime was committed—and especially one pointing to perversion—his officers searched first in marijuana dens and questioned marijuana smokers for suspects.‡

it hardly seemed necessary for the readers to be told that marijuana had arrived as ". . . the foremost menace to life, health, and morals in the list of drugs used in America."[7]

The association was repeatedly made in this period between crime, particularly violent and/or perverted crime, and marijuana use. A typical report, cautiously phrased as were all of them, follows:

In Los Angeles, Calif., a youth was walking along a downtown street after inhaling a marijuana cigarette. For many addicts, merely a portion of a "reefer" is enough to induce intoxication. Suddenly, for no reason, he decided that someone had threatened to kill him and that his life at that very moment was in danger. Wildly he looked about him. The only person in sight was an aged bootblack. Drug-crazed nerve centers conjured the innocent old shoe-shiner into a destroying monster. Mad with fright, the addict hurried to his room and got a gun. He killed the old man, and then, later, babbled his grief over what had been wanton, uncontrolled murder.

"I thought someone was after me," he said. "That's the only reason I did it. I had never seen the old fellow before. Something just told me to kill him!"

That's marijuana!*

However, not all articles condemned marijuana as the precipitator of violent crimes. An article in *The Literary Digest* reported that the chief psychiatrist at Bellevue Hospital in New York City had reviewed the cases of over 2,200 criminals convicted of felonies. Referring to marijuana he said: "None of the assault cases could be said to have been committed under the drug's influence. Of the sexual crimes, there was none due to marihuana intoxication. . . . It is quite probable that alcohol is more responsible as an agent for crime than is marihuana."[8]

There was very poor documentation of the marijuana-crime relationship, which was stated as proved in the 1930's. A thorough review of Anslinger's writings, including the marijuana and vicious crime cases related throughout this period, concluded that:

In the works of Mr. Anslinger, there are either no references or references to volumes which my assistants and I have checked and which,

---

*From Snyder, S. H.: What we have forgotten about pot, The New York Times Magazine, December 13, 1970, p. 130.
†From Marihuana menaces youth, Scientific American **154:**151, 1936.
‡From Wolf, W.: Uncle Sam fights a new drug menace . . . marijuana, Popular Science Monthly **128:**14, 119, 1936.

*From Anslinger, H. J., and Cooper, C. R.: Marijuana: assassin of youth, The American Magazine **124:**19, 153, 1937.

in our checking, we find to be based upon much hearsay and little or no experimentation. We found a mythology in which later writers cite the authority of earlier writers, who also had little evidence. We have found, by and large, what can most charitably be described as a pyramid of prejudice, with each level of the structure built upon the shaky foundations of earlier distortions.*

With such poor evidence supporting the relationship between marijuana use and crime, it seems strange that the true story was never told. There are probably several reasons. One was the great depression, which made everyone acutely sensitive to, and wary of, any new and particularly foreign influences. The fact that it was the lower-class Mexican-Americans and Negroes that had initiated use of the drug made the drug doubly dangerous to the white middle class. These factors, combined with the broad cultural attitudes about marijuana use, further increased anxiety levels.

> Cannabis has been accepted for centuries in India and other eastern countries where cultural and religious teachings support introspection, mediation, and bodily passivity. On the other hand, the West, with its cultural emphasis on achievement, activity, and aggressiveness, has elected alcohol as its acceptable, almost semi-official euphoriant. These cultural differences are consonant with some of the important, pharmacological differences between the two drugs. Clearly the more introspective, meditative, non-aggressive stereotype associated with marihuana goes against our cultural mainstream. And while this contributes to its attractiveness to some, it makes it repellent, even threatening, to many others who identify with the active, aggressive, manly stereotype.†

There were other issues operating to build marijuana into a national menace. Perhaps some of the feelings against marijuana stemmed from the opinion that it offered pleasure without penalty.

> In the years which preceded the passage of the Marijuana Tax Act, the specter of "demon rum" was still quite clear in the minds of the moral entrepreneurs of this nation, when a

new menace, the "killer weed" raised its ugly head. Like alcohol, it was an intoxicant which was sought after primarily because of the pleasure it gave the user, but unlike alcohol, it did not provide for the spiritually-redeeming morning-after hangover. Its use, like alcohol, is a pleasurable, hedonistic, non-productive, and above all, a sinful practice.*

Another contributing factor probably was the regular reference in associating marijuana and crime to the murdering cult of Assassins as suggestive of the characteristics of the drug.[9] The 1936 *Popular Science Monthly* reference to the Assassins is the most concise.

> The origin of the word "assassin" has two explanations, but either demonstrates the menace of Indian hemp. According to one version, members of a band of Persian terrorists committed their worst atrocities while under the influence of hashish. In the other version, Saracens who opposed the Crusaders were said to employ the services of hashish addicts to secure secret murderers of the leaders of the Crusades. In both versions, the murders were known as "haschischin," "hashshash" or "hashishi" and from those terms comes the modern and ominous "assassin."†

In none of the actual stories and legends were the murders committed by individuals under the influence of hashish; rather, it was part of the reward for carrying out the murders.

Because of the fear aroused by the reports on marijuana users, many states in the early 1930's passed marijuana control laws with the blessing of the Federal Bureau of Narcotics headed by Mr. Harry Anslinger. In the mid-1930's the Narcotics Bureau acted to support federal legislation, and in the spring of 1937 Congressional hearings were held.

Passage of the Marijuana Tax Act was a foregone conclusion. There were few witnesses to testify other than law enforcement officers. The birdseed people had the act modified so they could import sterilized *Cannabis* seed for use in their product. An official of the American Medical Association testified on his own behalf, not representing the American Medical Association, against the

---

*From Whitlock, L.: Review: marijuana, Crime and Delinquency Literature 2(3):367, 1970.
†From Grinspoon, L.: Marihuana, International Journal of Psychiatry 9:510-511, 1970-1971.

*From Smith, R.: U. S. marijuana legislation and the creation of a social problem, Journal of Psychedelic Drugs 2(1):93, 99, 1968.
†From Wolf, op. cit., p. 119.

bill. His reasons for opposing the bill were multiple. Primarily, though, he thought the antimarijuana laws that already existed in 46 states were adequate enough and, also, that the social menace case against marijuana had not been proved at all. The bill was passed in August and became effective on October 1, 1937.

The general characteristics of the law followed the regulation-by-taxation theme of the Harrison Act of 1914. The federal law did not outlaw *Cannabis* or its preparations, it just taxed the grower, distributor, seller and buyer and made it, administratively, almost impossible to have anything to do with *Cannabis!* In addition, the Bureau of Narcotics prepared a uniform law that many states adopted. These laws made possession and use of marijuana illegal per se. Thirty-two years later, in May of 1969, the United States Supreme Court declared the Marijuana Tax Act unconstitutional because there was:

> . . . in the Federal anti-marijuana law—a section that requires the suspect to pay a tax on the drug, thus incriminating himself, in violation of the Fifth Amendment; and a section that assumes (rather than requiring proof) that a person with foreign-grown marijuana in his possession knows it is smuggled.*

AFTER THE ACT

Passage of the Marijuana Tax Act had an amazing effect. Almost immediately there was a sharp reduction in the reports of heinous crimes committed under the influence of marijuana! The price of the merchandise increased rapidly (the war came along, too), so that 5 years after the act the cost of a marijuana cigarette—a reefer—had increased six to twelve times and cost about $1.00.

The year after the law was enacted, 1938, Mayor Fiorillo LaGuardia of New York City, remembered what no one else wanted to recall. What he recalled were two army studies on marijuana use by soldiers in the Panama Canal Zone around 1930. Both reports found marijuana to be innocuous and that its reputation as a troublemaker "was due to its association with alcohol which . . . was always found the prime agent."[10]

*From Fort, J.: Pot: a rational approach, Playboy, October, 1969, pp. 131 and 154.

Mayor LaGuardia asked the New York Academy of Medicine to study marijuana, its use, its effects, and the necessity for control. The report, issued in 1944, was intensive and extensive and a very good study for its time. A 1966 pro-marijuana book called it: ". . . the most impressive collection of factual finding in the whole body of scientific literature on marihuana. . ."[11]

The complete report is available[11] and widely discussed, so only a part of the summary is quoted. (See also references 12 and 13.)

> It was found that marihuana in an effective dose impairs intellectual functioning in general. . . . Marihuana does not change the basic personality structure of the individual. It lessens inhibition and this brings out what is latent in his thoughts and emotions but it does not evoke responses which would otherwise be totally alien to him. It induces a feeling of self-confidence, but this expressed in thought rather than in performance. There is, in fact, evidence of a diminution in physical activity. . . . those who have been smoking marihuana for a period of years showed no mental or physical deterioration which may be attributed to the drug.*

This 1944 report, which was completed by a very reputable committee of the New York Academy of Medicine, brought a violent reaction. The American Medical Association stated in a 1945 editorial:

> For many years medical scientists have considered cannabis a dangerous drug. Nevertheless, a book called "Marihuana Problems" by New York City Mayor's Committee on Marihuana submits an analysis by seventeen doctors of tests on 77 prisoners and, on this narrow and thoroughly unscientific foundation, draws sweeping and inadequate conclusions which minimize the harmfulness of marihuana. Already the book has done harm. One investigator has described some tearful parents who brought their 16 year old son to a physician after he had been detected in the act of smoking marihuana. A noticeable mental deterioration had been evident for some time even to their lay minds. The boy said he had read an account of the La Guardia Committee report and that this was his justification for using marihuana. He read in *Down Beat,* a musical journal, an analysis of this report under the caption "Light Up Gates, Report

*Mayor LaGuardia's Committee on Marihuana. In Solomon, D., editor: The marihuana papers, New York, 1966, The New American Library, p. 408.

Finds 'Tea' a Good Kick." ... Public officials will do well to disregard this unscientific, uncritical study, and continue to regard marihuana as a menace wherever it is purveyed.*

As in all such reports and reactions to reports, there is little dispute over the facts, only over the interpretation. Since the La-Guardia Report is in substantial agreement with the Indian Hemp Commission Report of the 1890's,[14] the Panama Canal Zone reports of the 1930's,[15] and the recent comprehensive reports by the governments of New Zealand,[16] Canada,[17] Great Britain,[18] and the United States,[19, 19a] it is likely that the conclusions of the LaGuardia Report were and are for the most part valid.

The conflict between the LaGuardia Report and its opponents was debated in the mass media, and usually the LaGuardia Report lost. A 1945 article in a popular monthly, *Magazine Digest*, asks "How 'Mild' is Marihuana?" and, to its credit, adds some new horror stories to the list of those possibly completed by individuals perhaps under the influence of marijuana. Place particular attention on the wording of the story; nowhere does it even say the man used marijuana!

> That there is a certain anesthetic effect from marihuana cannot be denied. In medical records there is the case of a man in Texas who, out on bail pending appeal from a conviction for raping a 12-year-old girl, slashed to death two respectable women, and then turned the knife on himself, slashing his own body so severly and repeatedly that a doctor who examined him before he died declared that marihuana was the only thing which could have desensitized his nerves sufficiently to allow him to carry out such self-mutilation without fainting from pain after the first cut. Opiates in a sufficient dose for this anesthetic effect would have rendered the man unconscious.†

This post–Marijuana Tax Act period is best closed with the realization that in 1945: "The narcotic law enforcement officials are also faced with the problem of returned servicemen bringing home with them the 'hemp habit' from other countries."[20] C'est la vie, Napoleon!

*From Marijuana problems, Journal of the American Medical Association **127**(17):1129, 1945.
†From Esrati, A. E.: How "mild" is marihuana? Magazine Digest, June, 1945, pp. 85-86.

The 1950's and 1960's form a unique period in the history of marijuana. There was a hiatus in scientific research on marijuana and *Cannabis*, but experimentation in the streets increased continually. There were some rational reports in the mass media,[21] but they were easy to ignore. With the arrival of the "psychedelic sixties," the popular press could and did emphasize the more sensational hallucinogens. Marijuana, however, was everywhere the action was in the youth culture, but for the most part the major concern was on the more potent agents.

Toward the end of the 1960's, LSD use declined, heroin use increased rapidly in and out of the ghetto, and marijuana use was becoming the initiation rite of the turned-on generation.[22, 23] Discussion of the drug, however, no longer had the one-sidedness of the 1930's. Advocates of the legalization of marijuana, if not of marijuana, spoke out clearly, even at Senate hearings.[24]

MEDICAL USES OF CANNABIS

Cannabis has never attained the medical status of opium, so its medical record is spotted. The first report of medical uses was by Shen Nung in 2737 B.C. (see p. 251). Some 2,900 years after the Shen Nung report, another Chinese physician, Hoa-tho (200 A.D.) recommended *Cannabis* resin mixed with wine as a surgical anesthetic. Although *Cannabis* preparations were used extensively in medicine in India and after about 900 A.D. in the Near East, there was almost nothing about it in European medicine until the 1800's.

Early reports in European medical journals—such as de Sacy's 1809 article entitled "Intoxicating Preparations made with Cannabis"—awakened more interest in the writers and artists of the period than in medical men. In 1839, however, a lengthy article, "On the preparations of the Indian hemp, or gunjah," was published by a British physician working in India.[25] He reviewed the use of *Cannabis* in Indian medicine and reported on his own work with animals, which suggested that *Cannabis* preparations were quite safe. Having shown *Cannabis* to be nontoxic, he used it clinically and found it to be an effective anticonvulsant and muscle relaxant, as well as a valuable drug for the relief of the pain of rheumatism.

This article by W. B. O'Shaughnessy started the up-and-down history of the medical use of *Cannabis* in Europe and the United States. In 1860 the Ohio State Medical Society's Committee on *Cannabis indica* reported its successful use in the treatment of stomach pain, chronic cough, and gonorrhea. One physician felt he had to ". . . assign to the Indian hemp a place among the so-called hypnotic medicines next to opium. . . ."[26] By the 1890's a medical text included the statement: "Cannabis is very valuable for the relief of pain, particularly that depending on nerve disturbances. . . ."[1]

In 1938 a book-size review of the literature entitled *Marijuana, America's New Drug Problem* attributed the rapid increase in the medical use of *Cannabis* drugs in the last half of the nineteenth century to several causes.

> This popularity of the hemp drugs can be attributed partly to the fact that they were introduced before the synthetic hypnotics and analgesics. Chloral hydrate was not introduced until 1869 and was followed in the next 30 years by paraldehyde, sulfonal and the barbitals. Antipyrine and acetanilide, the first of their particular group of analgesics, were introduced about 1884. For general sedative and analgesic purposes, the only drugs commonly used at this time were the morphine derivatives and their disadvantages were very well known. In fact, the most attractive feature of the hemp narcotics was probably the fact that they did not exhibit certain of the notorious disadvantages of the opiates.*

Interestingly, although used widely, therapeutic doses of *Cannabis* were seldom reported to have intoxicating properties. One recent writer comments that the patients receiving *Cannabis* never "were 'stoned,' changed their attitudes about work, love, their fellow men or patriotism."[1]

One of the difficulties that has always plagued the scientific, medical, and social use of *Cannabis* is the variability of the product. A 1902 article reviewed the assay and standardization techniques used with many of the common plant drugs and stated: "In Cannabis Indica we have a drug of great importance and one which of all materia medica is undoubtedly the most variable."[27] In that same year Parke, Davis & Company, using new standardization procedures, claimed that "each lot sent out upon the market by us is of full potency and to be relied upon."[28] They listed a variety of *Cannabis* products available for medical use, including "a Chocolate Coated Tablet Extract Indian Cannabis 1/4 grain"!

In spite of improved standardization of potency and an increased number of preparations, the use of *Cannabis* declined.

> In 1885 there were 5 prescriptions out of every 10,000 as fluid extract; in 1895, 11.6; in 1907, 8 out of every 10,000; in 1926, 2.3, and in 1933, the last figures we have 0.4 out of every 10,000.*

Passage of the 1937 law resulted in all twenty-eight of the legal *Cannabis* preparations being withdrawn from the market, and in 1941 *Cannabis* was dropped from the National Formulary and the U. S. Pharmacopeia. Note well that the decline in the medical use of *Cannabis* occurred long before 1937 and that the law did not eliminate an actively used therapeutic agent. Four factors, however, certainly contributed to the declining prescription rate of this plant. One was the development of new and better drugs for most illnesses. Second was the variability of the available medicinal preparations of *Cannabis,* which was repeatedly mentioned in the 1937 hearings.[29] Third, *Cannabis* is very insoluble in water and thus not amenable to injectable preparations. Last, taken orally it has an unusually long (1- to 2-hour) latency to onset of action.

With the recent renewed interest in marijuana as a social drug has come some reevaluation and rethinking of the implications of some of the older therapeutic reports. Scientists are looking again at some of the more interesting reported therapeutic effects of *Cannabis.* One is its anticonvulsant activity.

*From Walton, R. P.: Marihuana: America's new drug problem, Philadelphia, 1938, J. B. Lippincott Co., p. 152.

*From Taxation of marijuana, House of Representatives, Committee on Ways and Means, Seventy-fifth Congress, First Session, Washington, D. C., May 4, 1937, p. 114.

A 1949 report[30] found it effective in some cases where Dilantin, the anticonvulsant of choice both then and now, was ineffective. Another area being explored is the bactericidal characteristics of *Cannabis*; maybe it is effective against gonorrhea! The fact that both Queen Victoria's physician and Sir William Osler, as well as others, found *Cannabis* to be very effective against tension headaches and/or migraine will probably be investigated in the future.[1, 31] Similarly, old and new reports that *Cannabis* can be used in the treatment of narcotic withdrawal[32] and recent reports that it may be beneficial with terminal cancer patients[33] are also sure to be further investigated.

EFFECTS OF CANNABIS SATIVA ON MAN

The *Cannabis sativa* plant has separate male and female plants, and both manufacture the psychoactive material in usable amounts. The psychoactive material is most concentrated in the resin of the plant, and this resin is secreted in highest quantity by the unfertilized flowers of the female. It is this highly resinous mixture of female flowering tops that is called hashish in the United States and charas in India.

The term "marijuana" comes from a Spanish or Portugese word meaning intoxicant and refers to a smoking preparation containing chopped leaves, flowers, and stems of either the male or the female plant or both. The leaves contain between 10% and 20% as much of the psychoactive material as is found in the resin. Most marijuana smoked is one-third to one-seventh as psychoactive as hash.

Even though there is a single species that grows worldwide—and thus older terms such as *Cannabis indica* and *Cannabis americanes* are botanically meaningless—there appears to be two genotypes. One has been cultivated for use as a fiber source and produces little of the psychoactive material. (This is the predominant form found growing wild in the Unites States.) The second genotype is cultivated as a source of the resin and contains 1% to 5% of the active ingredient. The actual amount of the psychoactive substance in the final preparation will vary with the conditions of growth, harvesting, and curing as well as the genetic variation of the plant.

Much of the basis for the difficulty of early workers (and users) to obtain a constant potency preparation may now be understood. In the plant there are regular cycles of variations in the amount of psychoactive material present. It seems probable, from the available data, that the active material is synthesized by the plant but because of its sensitivity to light, air, and temperature is then metabolized to inactive substances. This deactivation is accompanied by an increase in the precursor, which then decreases in amount as the active ingredient is again synthesized. There is thus a regular alternation of the precursor and the active ingredient in the plant, with one being high while the other is low.

Pharmacodynamics

The chemistry of *Cannabis* is quite complex, and isolation and extraction of the active ingredient are difficult even today. *Cannabis* is unique among psychoactive plant materials in that it contains no nitrogen and thus is not an alkaloid. This fact was established over 100 years ago by two chemists, the Smith brothers (yes, it's those Smith brothers). Because of its nonnitrogen content, the nineteenth century chemists who had been so successful in isolating the active agents from other plants were unable to identify the active component of *Cannabis*.

Before the turn of the century, a portion of the resin believed to be the active component was isolated and named cannabinol. Close examination 30 years later showed that the isolated material, cannabinol, was not the psychoactive portion of hashish![34] A second substance, cannabidiol, which is similar in chemical structure to cannabinol, was isolated around 1940 by one of the primary figures in the LaGuardia investigations. This isolation was the key to the chemistry of *Cannabis*.

Although cannabidiol, like cannabinol, is physiologically inactive, the study of its structure and its reactions was most revealing. The results served to determine completely the structure of cannabinol and led to the formation of tetrahydrocannabinols, products of high marihuana potency which are probably active principles in the red oil of hemp.*

*From Adams, R.: Marihuana, Bulletin of the New York Academy of Medicine **18**:709, 1942.

The 1971 Health, Education and Welfare report on *Marijuana and Health* stated:

> At present, four major cannabinoids have been found in the plant: the two isomers: (-)-trans-Delta-9 and Delta-8-tetrahydrocannabinols (Delta-9-THC and Delta-8-THC), cannabidiol (CBD) and cannabinol (CBN).... The major tetrahydrocannabinol believed to be responsible for the psychoactive properties of marihuana is the Delta-9-THC.*

The structures of these chemicals are shown in Fig. 15-1.

The synthesis of Delta-9-THC has been carried out and research quantities have been available from the test tube since the late 1960's. In the body Delta-9-THC is metabolized in the liver to 11-hydroxy-THC, and it is this substance that seems responsible for the physiological and psychological effects, although, to date, there are no accepted theories of the mechanism of action producing these effects.[34a]

Thus far the study of the effects of Delta-9-THC on the physiology of the body have done little more than quantify earlier reports in which resin extracts were used. The established physiological effects of *Cannabis* are dose related, for the most part minor, of indeterminate importance for the psychological effects, and of unknown toxicological significance. The 1971 federal government summary of physiological effects is not much different from a 1942 summary.[12] For 30 years there has been substantial agreement on the short-term physiological effects of *Cannabis*.

> Physiological changes accompanying marihuana use at typical levels of American social usage are relatively few. One of the most consistent is an increase in pulse rate. Another is reddening of the eyes at the time of use. Dryness of the mouth and throat are uniformly reported. Although enlargement of the pupils was an earlier impression, more careful study has indicated that this does not occur. Blood pressure effects have been inconsistent. Some have reported slightly lowered blood pressure while others have reported small increases. Basal metabolic rate, temperature, respiration rate, lung vital capacity and a wide range of other physiological measures are generally

unchanged over a relatively wide dosage range of both marihuana and the synthetic form of the principal psychoactive agent, delta-9-THC....

> There is evidence that the drug in large amounts can slow gastrointestinal passage of an experimental meal and relax an isolated intestine although it is not constipating. The sometimes reported enormous increase in appetite following marihuana smoking may also be related to effects in the gastrointestinal tract....

> Because smoking is the typical mode of use of marihuana in America, studies of its effects on lung function are of considerable potential importance ... even though preliminary experiments have not shown this form of smoking to be as damaging as tobacco smoking....

> ...[Regarding] blood sugar level ... recent studies have found no change.*

Some additional information, however, has been accumulated since 1942. The lethal dose of Delta-9-THC has not been extensively studied, and no human deaths have been reported from the use of *Cannabis*. The consensus now, however, is that death occurs only at a dose about 40,000 times as large as a psychologically effective dose. This number has more meaning, perhaps, when compared to the LD/ED ratio for alcohol, which is about 10. *Cannabis* also is not addicting and no withdrawal signs occur when use of the drug stops.

Tolerance is an issue still much debated since it has clearly been demonstrated in several animal experiments but not in human studies.[33] Some authorities feel that tolerance must develop in man. "How else could people take the huge doses of hashish that are taken in other countries without some of the 'zonked' effects that we see when somebody takes a lot of hash here?"[35]

There are reports of reverse tolerance or sensitization occurring, that is, less drug being necessary with each succeeding use of the drug. These results are difficult to evaluate since, in some cases, regular users have reported psychological effects when using placebos. Some biochemical work may provide

*From Marihuana and health, Department of Health, Education and Welfare, Washington, D. C., 1971, U. S. Government Printing Office, pp. 22-23.

*From Marihuana and health, op. cit., pp. 9-10, 94, 173-174.

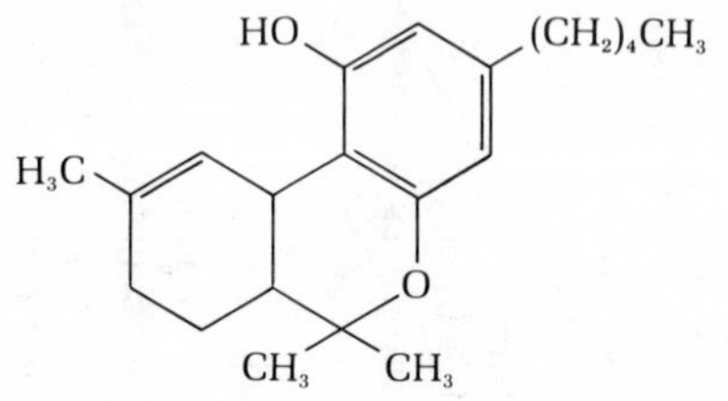

Δ⁹–Trans-tetrahydrocannabinol
Δ⁹–THC
(6a,7,8,10a-tetrahydro-6,6,9-trimethyl-3-pentyl-6H-dibenzo [b,d] pyran-l-ol)

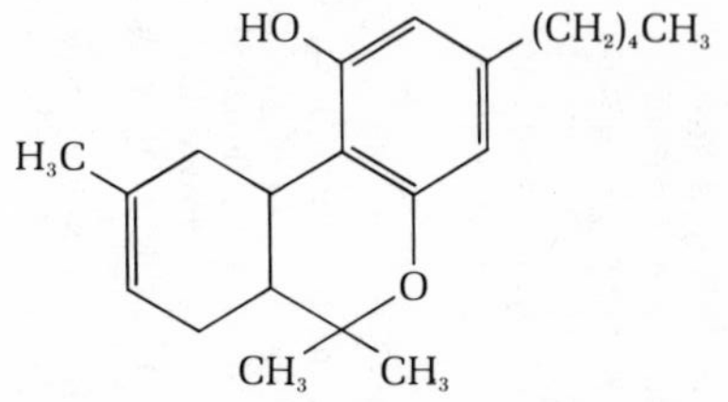

Δ⁸-Trans-tetrahydrocannabinol
Δ⁸-THC
(6,7,10a-tetrahydro-6,6,9-trimethyl-3-pentyl-6H-dibenzo [b,d] pyran-l-ol)

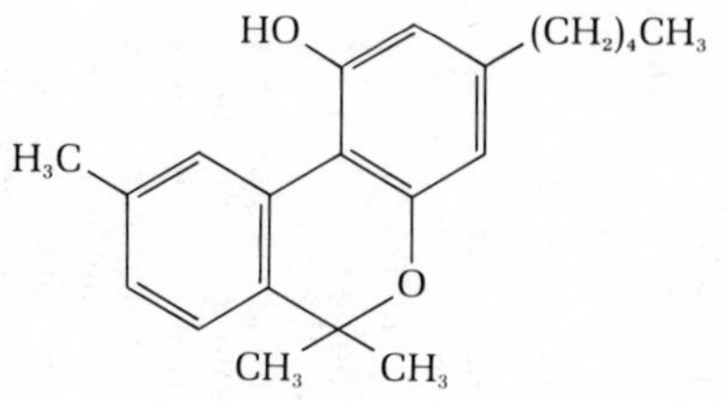

Cannabinol
CBN
(6,6,9-trimethyl-3-pentyl-6H-dibenzo [b,d] pyran-l-ol)

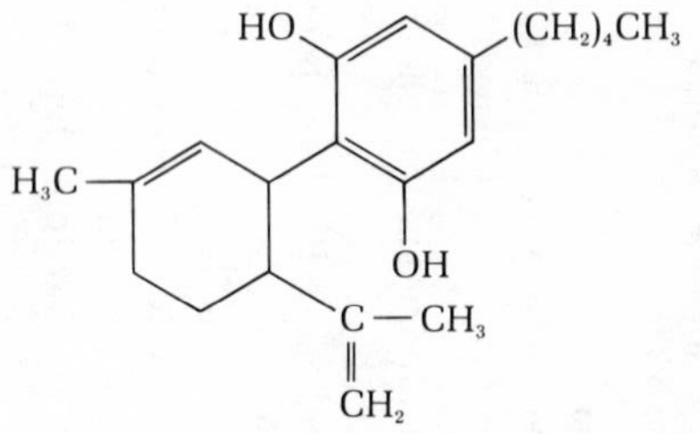

Cannabidiol
CBD
(2-p-mentha-1,8-dien-3-yl-5-pentyl-resorcinol)

Fig. 15-1. Delta-9-THC and related compounds found in *Cannabis sativa.*

a rationale for the sensitization, however. Radioactively labeled Delta-9-THC was found to persist in the body as an active metabolite as long as 8 days after use. With an accumulation of the active agent in the body, less and less new drug would be needed to reach a threshold level.[36] Because of the elaborate procedures involved in smoking marijuana, conceivably the placebo and sensitization effects could be the result of simply learning "when I do these things, and it tastes and smells this way, then these feelings and effects always follow." Still another basis for the reported sensitization may simply be that in the initial stages of marijuana use the smokers are learning to smoke more efficiently. Perhaps all three factors are operating, but the clear evidence supporting an accumulation of THC or its metabolites in the body make a biochemical basis for sensitization most probable.

With the advent of isolated Delta-9-THC, dose-response relationships could be determined and the differential response to oral and inhalation modes of intake evaluated.

> Threshold doses of 2 mg. smoked and 5 mg. orally produced mild euphoria; 7 mg. smoked and 17 mg. orally, some perceptual and time sense changes occurred; and at 15 mg. smoked and 25 mg. orally, subjects reported marked changes in body image, perceptual distortions, delusions and hallucinations.*

Oral intake is more frequently followed by nausea, physical discomfort, and hangover and the dose level cannot be titrated as accurately as is possible when smoking. There may be other differences in effects between comparable oral and smoking intake, although this has not been studied.

One of the major problems in communicating about Cannabis is that it is not readily placed in any of the usual pharmacological categories. It is not possible to summarize the effects of the drug with a single word, such as depressant or hallucinogen.

> ...the pharmacological action of marihuana has some similarities to properties of the stimulant, sedative, analgesic and psychotomimetic classes of drugs. In large doses, cannabis drugs bear many similarities to the psychotomimetics. Isbell described marked

*From Marijuana and health, op. cit., p. 88.

distortion of auditory and visual perception, hallucinations and depersonalization. He found LSD was 160 times more potent as a psychotomimetic than Delta-9-THC. . . . In low doses, the effects of marihuana and alcohol are similar. Both produce an early excitant and later sedated phase, and are commonly used as euphoriants, relaxants and intoxicants. At low doses, subjects experience difficulty differentiating the effects of alcohol from marihuana and placebo.*

Some users disagree very much with the implication that the marijuana and alcohol experiences are difficult to distinguish. One user has said:

> A pot high is quite different from a liquor high. Alcohol dulls the senses whereas pot sets them on edge. If a child were screaming in the next room, I'd take a drink, not a joint. If I were sitting with an arm around Jane Fonda and she had just told me I had beautiful eyes, I'd light up. Drink is for tuning out. Pot is for tuning in.†

A reminder. Cannabis is a drug that has primarily been used in two dosage forms of very different potency. Hashish and Cannabis extracts that gave rise to the experiences reported by Baudelaire and others are potent hallucinogenic agents. The drug delivery system that spread through the country in the 1920's and 1930's was a much less potent form, marijuana. The active ingredient is the same; the amount differs. Both marijuana and hashish are available and used in the United States today, although the great majority of users restrict themselves to marijuana.

Behavioral effects

Almost all of the recent writers emphasize that a new user has to learn how to smoke marijuana. They elaborate on three stages in the learning process.[37] The first step involves deeply inhaling the smoke and holding it in the lungs for 20 to 40 seconds. Then the user has to learn to identify and control the effects, and, finally, he has to learn to label the effects as pleasant. Because of this learning

*Ibid., pp. 105-106.
†From Pop drugs: the high as a way of life, Time, September 26, 1969, p. 39, 73. Reprinted by permission from TIME, The Weekly Newsmagazine; copyright Time, Inc., 1969.

process, most first-time users do not achieve the euphoric "stoned" or "high" condition of the repeater.

The effects accompanying marijuana smoking by the experienced user are relatively well established.

> A cannabis "high" typically involves several phases. The initial effects are often somewhat stimulating and, in some individuals, may elicit mild tension or anxiety which usually is replaced by a pleasant feeling of well-being. The later effects usually tend to make the user introspective and tranquil. Rapid mood changes often occur. A period of enormous hilarity may be followed by a contemplative silence.*

One investigator had experienced marijuana smokers indicate how frequently their marijuana intoxication included each of 206 effects listed on a sheet. Although there are great difficulties in looking for generalizations among idiosyncratic responses, the investigator was able to summarize 124 common subjective effects.

> Sense perception is often improved, both in intensity and in scope. Imagery is usually stronger but well controlled, although people often care less about controlling their actions. Great changes in perception of space and time are common, as are changes in psychological processes such as understanding, memory, emotion, and sense of identify. . . . To the extent that the described effects are delusory or inaccurate, the delusions and inaccuracy are widely shared. It is interesting, too, that nearly all the common effects seem either emotionally pleasing or cognitively interesting, and it is easy to see why marijuana users find the effects desirable regardless of what happens to their external behaviour.†

At the level of social intoxication there is a dose-related impairment in scores on psychomotor and cognitive tests with "moderate impairment . . . during the period of peak intoxication."[33, 37a] In laboratory studies naive users report fewer subjective effects but show greater decrement in test performance.

One of the consistent alterations in function is that on short-term memory. While intoxicated, the marijuana user is unable to easily recall information he just learned seconds or minutes before. This memory lapse not only affects the general thread of conversation among a group of users but also is probably the basis for the changes in time sense frequently reported. The user feels that more time has passed than actually has. Such overestimation of the passage of time is the most commonly reported psychological effect of marijuana smoking and has been validated in many experiments.

One group of researchers[38] has suggested that the impairment of immediate memory is the basic effect of marijuana intoxication and that many other effects, not just changes in time sense, result from it.

> . . . we have shown that impaired immediate memory may account, in part, for temporal disintegration. To make comparisons between *now* and *then*, a person must hold in mind and juxtapose diverse events, each embedded in a particular temporal series. . . . Moreover, if a person forgets what came before or after an experience, he will have difficulty locating that event in time. When an experience appears to have no before or after, it is isolated from time and, hence, may seem timeless. The sense of timelessness, emerging during THC intoxication, can be likened to the progressive fragmentation of a movie film.
>
> . . . The fragmentation of temporal experience co-varies with strange and unfamiliar feelings about the self, perhaps because the person during marihuana intoxication feels less familiar with himself as he loses the perspective of continuity of the self through time. Depending on personality factors, THC-induced temporal disintegration and depersonalization, so long as they are believed to be time-limited, are euphorigenic processes, perhaps because the person—with an altered sense of time and sense of self—is less concerned about what will happen to himself.*

These scientists also reported that, in individuals concerned with loss of control and individuality, these same temporal disruptions

---

*From Interim report of the Commission of Inquiry into the Non-medical Use of Drugs, Ottawa, 1970, Queen's Printer for Canada, p. 174. (Also called the LeDain Report.)
†From Tart, C. T.: Marijuana intoxication: common experiences, Nature **226**:704, 1970.

*From Melges, F. T., and others: Temporal disintegration and depersonalization during marijuana intoxication, Archives of General Psychiatry **23**:208-209, 1970.

and depersonalizations caused anxiety and sometimes panic reactions.

Many users report increased sensory awareness and sensitivity. For the most part changes in the sensory system have not been shown in laboratory experiments; probably it is the response to sensory input, not the input per se, that is altered.

In summary, there are a few statements concerning the behavioral effects of marijuana use for which relatively widespread consensus of opinion exists. First, a marijuana "high" requires learning on the part of the user. Second, the drug does impair short-term memory. Third, the user experiences an overestimation of the passage of time. However, each of these effects must be viewed in light of the conclusions of one reviewer who stated:

> The most consistently striking finding in all of these studies is that marijuana produced no striking findings. Indeed, one is impressed with how easily subjects could suppress the marijuana "high."*

Adverse reactions

A whole host of adverse reactions to normal marijuana use can be mentioned rapidly to show that there are no completely safe drugs. Flashbacks have been reported by several investigators and apparently occur under the same conditions as do LSD flashbacks.[39] Marijuana-precipitated psychosis has been long known. Psychotic reactions occurred in some of the prisoners studied for the LaGuardia Report, but the comment in that report is still true: ". . . (A) characteristic marihuana psychosis does not exist. Marihuana will not produce a psychosis de novo in a well-integrated, stable person."[13]

Some research into the relationship between marijuana use and chromosomal damage and birth defects has reported that marijuana does have such effects, but the case is far from proved. Much concern is voiced over the fact that long-term heavy marijuana users in parts of North Africa and India exhibit an amotivational syndrome; that is, they show a loss of motivation for the usually accepted personal or social accomplishments. One preliminary report on group therapy with apprehended marijuana smokers suggested a similar type of behavior. There were two general characteristics. These individuals were "strongly addicted to nonachievement" and "actually worked at getting caught for illegal drug usage."[40] The difficulties in assessing which came first, the marijuana or the absence of motivation, prevent any conclusions from being formed.

The marijuana equivalent of the alcoholic, the pothead, has been the subject of some direct research in this country. As with alcohol, heavy use of marijuana results from many factors. The pothead is perhaps as different from the social smoker as the alcoholic is from the social drinker. Although only the individuals at the ends of the continuum are usually studied, it should be clear that users need not be either only occasional smokers (or drinkers) or potheads (or alcoholics). Once heavy use is started, of either alcohol or marijuana, the circle continues, with the use of the drug reducing discomfort, but setting things up to cause more discomfort so that more drug is needed. . . . One study found that heavy marijuana use was correlated with:

> . . . psychological dependence, search for insight or meaningful experience, multiple-drug use, poor work adjustment, diminished goal directed activity and ability to master new problems, poor social adjustment and poor heterosexual relationships.*

It is the absence of an answer to the question of whether there is a physiological basis to the development of an amotivational syndrome that arouses the most concern in many scientists and clinicians. It is readily admitted by most researchers that the known acute physiological and psychological effects of marijuana use are minimal. The question really is: does long-term use at a moderate to high level necessarily lead to the amotivational syndrome: The federal government has funded several studies to investigate the phenomenon, but no clear answer has evolved.[40a]

---

*From Brill, N. Q.: The marijuana problem (UCLA Interdepartmental Conference), Annals of Internal Medicine 73(3):454, 1970.

*From Marihuana and health, op. cit., p. 112.

MARIJUANA USE TODAY

Virtually all of the American data indicate that use of marihuana has rapidly increased over the past several years. While the number of those who have tried the substance at some point in their lives remains a minority of the population it is continuing to increase rapidly. In some high school or college settings it is virtually certain that a majority have at least tried marihuana. By the end of 1970 about one college student in seven was using it on a weekly or more frequent basis. High school use has generally lagged behind that of colleges and universities, although in areas of high use as many as a third to a half have experimented with it. While comparable data are not available for non-school attending youth there is reason to believe that levels of use are at least comparable and for school drop outs are probably higher. In some west coast high schools which have had relatively high levels of use there is evidence that the increase in use may be decelerating and even declining. The likelihood of continuing, persistent use over an extended period of time by large numbers is not known at the present time.

Middle class users have tended to be individuals from higher income families attending larger, non-religiously affiliated urban universities rather than small, denominational colleges. However, as the number of users increases they become less clearly distinguishable from the more general youthful population. As use becomes more widespread there is reason to believe still younger as well as older populations are becoming involved.*

The world does move swiftly. Only 15 years ago a major textbook in pharmacology could reasonably state that the marijuana user was

> . . . usually 20 to 30 years of age, idle and lacking in initiative, with a history of repeated frustrations and deprivations, sexually maladjusted (often homosexual) who seeks distraction, escape and sometimes conviviality by smoking the drug. He almost uniformly has major personality defects and is often psychopathic.†

In the 1960's, however, things changed and use increased rapidly, even though the drug was illegal and severe penalties were man-

dated. In part the increased use in recent years may result from:

> . . . a contagion effect. The more users the less viable the official line on marihuana and to a lesser extent other drugs. The less respected rationale for such sanctions, the greater the experimentation. Greater experimentation increases the number of those who use and makes it easier for novices to obtain drugs. The more varied the user groups the less any potential user has to change his identity to begin using. The more users the more jobs open for drug traffickers and the more sellers will operate among their own kind; the more they blend with their clientele the more difficult it becomes to catch them. This leads to the perception of less risk and greater desirability of dealing. Over time the contagion effect reaches a point where serious doubt about official positions is replaced by contemptuous disregard.*

Marijuana use is definitely widespread today. Evidence for the relative lack of acute harmful physiological and/or psychological effects is convincing. This is not to say that it is a safe drug. At social use levels the overt behavioral effects of alcohol and marijuana seem comparable and a "high" from either drug impairs performance.[37a] There is, however, no basis for believing that marijuana smoking leads directly to the use of other drugs such as the opiates or the hallucinogens.[33] On the campuses today with more potent hallucinogens, as in the ghettos in the 1950's with heroin, the association of marijuana with other drugs and the acceptance of other drugs by the group using marijuana may result in some individuals who start with marijuana moving on to other agents. Some do, most don't.

In spite of the increased data available concerning the effects of marijuana, some ideas are slow to change. In 1967, a handbook written primarily for law enforcement officials stated:

> Marijuana, unlike opium, is an excitant drug. It disrupts and destroys the brain and distorts the mind, resulting in crime and degeneracy. It attacks the central nervous system, and violently affects the mentality and five physical

*From Marihuana and health, op. cit., pp. 6-7.
†From Goodman, L. S., and Gilman, A.: The pharmacological basis of therapeutics, ed. 2, New York, 1955, The Macmillan Co., p. 174.

*From Carey, J. T.: Marihuana use among the new bohemians, Journal of Psychedelic Drugs **2**(1):80-81, 1968.

senses. Time, space and distance are obliterated, and hallucinations occur. Marijuana, like cocaine, is the immediate and direct cause of the crime committed. This drug used with whiskey intensifies its violent properties. It gives a feeling of exaltation and physical power but, if continued, the drug develops a delirious rage.*

CONCLUDING COMMENT

Has the world gone to pot? It sure has! More and more frequently in the 1970's individuals[41, 42] and organizations,[43, 43a,b] as well as the National Commission on Marihuana and Drug Abuse,[43c] are arguing cogently that marijuana should, at least, be decriminalized. That is, *criminal* penalties for possession for private use should be abolished. The argument usually is that the damage done to society by the present stand on marijuana is far greater than the harm that might occur if legalization were accomplished with appropriate controls. Perhaps . . . perhaps . . .[44]

Marijuana is symbolic of a more passive, contemplative, and less competitive attitude toward life than has been traditional in the United States. It is usually denounced by people who like things the way they are. Whether society accepts or rejects the drug will undoubtedly have some influence on the evolution of our national character.†

True, true.

*From Williams, J. B., editor: Narcotics and hallucinogenics: a handbook, Beverly Hills, California, 1967, Glencoe Press, p. 141. By permission of the publisher.
†From Synder, S. H.: Uses of marijuana, New York, 1972, Oxford University Press, p. x, 128 pp.

PRECEDING QUOTES

1. Wolf, W.: Uncle Sam fights a new drug menace . . . marijuana, Popular Science Monthly **128**:119, 1936.
2. Newsweek, September 7, 1970, p. 20.
3 and 4. Goddard, J. L.: Drug chief equates peril of marijuana and that of alcohol, New York Times, October 19, 1967, p. 1.
5. Mitchell, J.: On marijuana, Newsweek, September 7, 1970, p. 22.

REFERENCES

a. Grass grows more acceptable, Time, Sept. 10, 1973.
1. Snyder, S. H.: What we have forgotten about pot, The New York Times Magazine, December 13, 1970, pp. 27, 121, 124, and 130.
2. Cannabis Study Group (Chairman: Alfred Freedman): The Ninth Annual Meeting American College of Neuropsychopharmacology, San Juan, Puerto Rico, December 8-11, 1970.
3. From unpublished material in the Archives of the American Psychological Association, Department of Psychology, University of Akron, Akron, Ohio.
4. Anslinger, H. J., and Cooper, C. R.: Marijuana: assassin of youth, The American Magazine **124**: 19, 153, 1937.
5. Taxation of marihuana, hearings before the Committee on Ways and Means, House of Representatives, 75th Congress, 1st Session, on H. R. 6385, April 27-30 and May 4, 1937, Washington, D. C., U. S. Government Printing Office.
6. Parry, A.: The menace of marihuana, American Mercury **36**:487-488, 1935.
7. Wolf, W.: Uncle Sam fights a new drug menace . . . marijuana, Popular Science Monthly **128**: 14, 119, 1936.
8. Facts and fancies about marihuana, The Literary Digest **122**:7-8, 1936.
9. Mandel, J.: Hashish, assassins, and the love of God, Issues in Criminology **2**(2):149-156, 1966.
10. The marihuana bugaboo, The Military Surgeon **93**:95, 1943.
11. Mayor LaGuardia's Committee on Marijuana. In Solomon, D., editor: The marihuana papers, New York, 1966, The New American Library, pp. 278 and 408.
12. Adams, R.: Marihuana, Bulletin of the New York Academy of Medicine **18**:709, 723, 1942.
13. Allentuck, S., and Bowman, K. M.: The psychiatric aspects of marihuana intoxication, American Journal of Psychiatry **99**:249, 1942.
14. Marijuana. Report of the Indian Hemp Drugs Commission 1893-1894, Baltimore, 1969, Waverly Press. (Originally published in 1894.)
15. Editorial: The marihuana bugaboo, The Military Surgeon **93**:94, 1943.
16. Drug dependency and drug abuse in New Zealand, first report, Board of Health, Report Series No. 14, Wellington, New Zealand, 1970, A. R. Shearer, Government Printer.
17. Interim report of the Commission of Inquiry into the Non-medical Use of Drugs, Ottawa, 1970, Queen's Printer for Canada, p. 174. (Also called the LeDain Report.)
18. Cannabis, Report by the Advisory Committee on Drug Dependence, London, 1968, Her Majesty's Stationery Office. (Also known as the Wooton Committee Report.)
19. Task force report: narcotics and drug abuse, President's Commission on Law Enforcement and Administration of Justice, Washington, D. C., 1967, U. S. Government Printing Office.
20. Esrati, A. E.: How "mild" is marijuana? Magazine Digest, June, 1945, pp. 81, 85-86.
21. Kolb, L.: Let's stop this narcotics hysteria! Saturday Evening Post **229**:19, 1956.
22. McGlothlin, W. H., and West, L. J.: The mari-

huana problem: an overview, American Journal of Psychiatry **125**:370-378, 1968.

23. Kaufman, J., Allen, J. R., and West, L. J.: Runaways, hippies, and marihuana, American Journal of Psychiatry **126**(5):717, 1969.

24. Competitive problems in the drug industry, hearings before the Subcommittee on Monopoly of the Select Committee on Small Business, United States Senate, Ninety-first Congress, First Session (July 16, 29, 30 and October 27, 1969), Part 13, Psychotropic Drugs, Washington, D. C., 1969, U. S. Government Printing Office, p. 5460.

25. O'Shaughnessy, W. B.: On the preparations of the Indian hemp, or gunja, Trans. Med. m. Phys. Soc., Bengal, pp. 71-102, 1838-1840; pp. 421-461, 1842.

26. Mikuriya, T. H.: Marijuana in medicine: past, present, and future, California Medicine **110**(1):35 1969.

27. Standardization of drug extracts, promotional brochure, Parke, Davis & Co., Detroit, 1898, p. 7.

28. Letter to E. P. Delabarre, 9 Arlington Avenue, Providence, R. I., from Parke, Davis & Company, Manufacturing Department, Main Laboratories, Detroit, Superintendent's Office, Control Department, March 10, 1902.

29. Taxation of marijuana, House of Representatives, Committee on Ways and Means, Washington, D. C., 1937, pp. 1, 114.

30. Davis, J. P., and Ramsey, H. H.: Antiepileptic action of marihuana-active substances, Federation Proceedings **8**:284-285, 1949.

31. Lieberman, C. M., and Lieberman, B. W.: Marihuana—a medical review, The New England Journal of Medicine **284**(2):88-91, 1971.

32. Walton, R. P.: Marihuana: America's new drug problem, Philadelphia, 1938, J. B. Lippincott Co., pp. 35 and 37.

33. Marihuana and health, Department of Health, Education and Welfare, Washington, D. C., 1971, U. S. Government Printing Office.

34. Todd, A. R.: The hemp drugs, Endeavor **2**:69-72, 1943.

34a. Lemberger, L., Crabtree, R. E., and Rowe, H. M.: 11-Hydroxy-$\triangle^9$-tetrahydrocannabinol: pharmacology, disposition, and metabolism of a major metabolite of marihuana in man, Science **177**:62-64, 1972.

35. Faltermayer, E. K.: What we know about marijuana—so far, Fortune **83**(3):130, 1971.

36. Lemberger, L., and others: Marihuana: studies on the disposition and metabolism of delta-9-tetrahydrocannabinol in man, Science **170**:1320-1322, 1970.

37. Becker, H. S.: Outsiders, studies in the sociology of deviance, New York, 1963, The Free Press.

37a. Rafaelsen, Bech, P., Christiansen, J., Christrup, H., Nyboe, J., and Rafaelsen, L.: Cannabis and alcohol: effects on simulated car driving, Science **179**:March 2, 1973.

38. Melges, F. T., and others: Temporal disintegration and depersonalization during marihuana intoxication, Archives of General Psychiatry **23**:208-209, 1970.

39. Keeler, M. H., Reifler, C. B., and Liptzin, M. B.: Spontaneous recurrence of marihuana effect, American Journal of Psychiatry **125**:384-386, 1968.

40. Cappannari, S. C., Griffith, J. D., and Shriver, T. H.: Achievers and non-achievers among marijuana users, paper read October 3, 1969, at the Central Neuropsychiatric Association, Nashville, Tennessee.

40a. Behavioral and biological concomitants of chronic marihuana smoking by heavy and casual users, Marihuana: a signal of misunderstanding **1**:68-246, March, 1972.

41. Kaplan, J.: Marihuana—the new prohibition. New York, 1970, World Publishing Company.

42. Grinspoon, L.: Marihuana reconsidered, Cambridge, 1971, Harvard University Press.

43. Pot and the law, Christian Century, October 28, 1970.

43a. Anderson, P.: The pot lobby, New York Times Magazine, January 21, 1973.

43b. Cahill, T.: The new pot advocates, Rolling Stone, January 3, 1974.

43c. Drug use in America: problem in perspective, Second report of the National Commission on Marihuana and Drug Abuse, March, 1973.

44. Hollister, L. E.: Marihuana in man: three years later, Science **172**:21-29, 1971.

UNIT

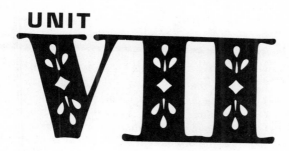

Conclusion

16 A rational look at drug use

It can come as a surprise to find that the longer a bad habit's history, the closer it has moved to being a good habit. Tradition alone seems to be able to brainwash whole societies, making their members ignorant of the fact that they have developed psychic dependence at least as deleterious as any arising from the officially recognized drugs of abuse.

All About Drugs
N. F. Bergel and D. Davies, 1970

... we have at our disposal hallucinogens and tranquilizers whose physiological price is amazingly low, and there seems to be every reason to believe that the consciousness-changers and tension-relievers of the future will do their work even more efficiently and at even lower cost to the individual. Human beings will be able to achieve effortlessly what in the past could be only achieved with difficulty, by means of self-control and spiritual exercises. Will this be a good thing for individuals and for societies? Or will it be a bad thing? ... all that one can predict with any degree of certainty is that it will be necessary to reconsider and re-evaluate many of our traditional notions about ethics and religion, and many of our current views about the nature of the mind, in the context of the pharmacological revolution. It will be extremely disturbing; but it will also be enormous fun.

The History of Tension
Aldous Huxley, 1957

I don't look with any favor ... on a society where everybody just floats around in his own tub of butter. A certain amount of tension and alertness is essential to keep things straight in life.

Dr. James H. Wall, 1956

Obviously, the question of whether to prohibit the drugs is one about which reasonable men could differ. But the answer preferred here is that the law should not prohibit them except to the extent necessary to protect the physical and mental health of the users. This sort of choice can be dangerous to the stability and health of our society; but a free society must often run risks as great or greater. It may be that the young people who are now using hallucinogens need guidance and restraint. But the law is not the only way, or the best way, to meet this kind of need.

Columbia Law Review
Robert M. Cover, 1968

One of the bright things about a book is that the concluding chapter does not have to be the end. Some readers will remember some of the facts, the stories, and the ideas and use them in looking at the drug scene now and tomorrow. A concluding chapter should offer a beginning, a new view as well as an overview of the problem.

This chapter will serve several purposes. First, it will summarize the themes and principles that have been everywhere evident. And we've been about everywhere—from the Andes to Vienna, from Turkey to the suburbs, from the laboratory to the streets of every city. To what end; why? Why not just the here-and-now? For one reason, to know that the drug situation is not new; we have been where we are now many times before. At the same time, we have never been where we are now—never in 4,000 years. That is what this chapter is about. How are we the same and how are we different from earlier periods of high drug use? What general principles can be derived about the use of psychoactive drugs? Not concepts about specific drugs in specific societies, but broad principles about the interactions that occur repeatedly among drugs, individuals, and society.

Another purpose of this chapter is to consider these general principles and to draw some conclusions. Of particular importance are the implications of these principles for the present culture. Finally, after reviewing the major themes and considering their implications, a rational view of drug use today in our society seems possible.

THEMES AND PRINCIPLES
Dimensions and determinants of drug effects

What are the determinants of the behavioral effects of a psychoactive drug? They are multiple and range from pharmacological and biochemical factors to the cultural history and social setting of the user. There is no simple answer to the general question: what is *the* behavioral effect of *this* drug? Nevertheless, at the most fundamental level, all drugs used recreationally on a regular basis directly or indirectly either increase pleasure or decrease discomfort. However, individuals and cultures may differ greatly in whether a particular

effect is experienced as pleasant or unpleasant.

To find the common physiological threads weaving through the psychoactive drug experiences, only two broad dimensions of brain activity need be considered for our purposes: level of arousal and information processing. The activity level of the brain is increased by stimulants, such as caffeine, amphetamine, and cocaine, and decreased by the depressants, including alcohol and the barbiturates. The action of these drugs seems primarily to be via their effect on the reticular formation. Some agents, such as LSD, have an alteration of activation level as a secondary rather than a primary effect.

Most of the drugs that have been adopted by western culture are those primarily affecting arousal level. Perhaps stimulation or depression, and thus a loss of inhibitions, has been compatible with our aggressively achieving but tightly moral society. Whether speeded up or slowed down, the user is still focused on the outside "real world."

The distortion-of-information-processing dimension results from one of two types of actions on the nervous system. The distortion can result from alterations of the primary or secondary sensory input pathways, or it can result from impaired retrieval and processing of memories. The hallucinogens, LSD, mescaline, and hashish have their primary effect on the information-processing systems. Images, colors, all experiences are partly unreal when hallucinogenic drugs are employed. Only at the extremes of the arousal dimension—high activation or extreme depression—does distortion of information processing become an important feature of those drugs that primarily influence level of arousal.

Drugs that alter information processing have been foreign to western civilization. There are probably many reasons for this fact, but one of them certainly has to be that by providing "multiple realities," hallucinogens would have impaired the single focus that is essential for rapid scientific and technological progress. It may be that the present movement away from such a single cultural focus will be coupled with an increase in the use of this class of agents.

Throughout the book it has been demonstrated that to meaningfully discuss drug use it is essential to specify dosage range, mode of administration, frequency of drug use, and setting in which the use occurs. The low oral dose of amphetamine that helps bored blimps make it through the day is a far cry from shooting speed, even though some people simply categorize both as drug misuse. The mild temporal and spatial distortions and the euphoria accompanying marijuana smoking have only a tenuous behavioral connection with the very personal hallucinations of hashish. Use of LSD and other hallucinogens in a laboratory setting certainly alters their effects from those obtained when they are used in a social situation surrounded by friends and containing pulsating lights and music.

Expectations are of great importance in determining the effects of an agent, as seen most vividly in work done with placebos. The belief that an authority, the physician, is giving a medicine that will have a specific effect is frequently enough to in fact produce the effect, even though an inert agent has been used. The expectations an individual has about various drugs obviously develop from his personal history of experiences and needs that occur in a social context. For that reason it is important that the social context present accurate and credible information about what a drug can and cannot do.

It cannot be emphasized too much that the greater the role played by mechanisms of consciousness and the integration of information in producing a drug's effects, the more variable can be these effects. A drug may have very specific biochemical actions and still have quite variable behavioral effects. Such variability results because drugs do not create new patterns of nervous system activity. Rather, they only serve to modify already existing patterns, most of which are the result of an individual's unique personal experiences. That is, these psychoactive drugs act by altering *ongoing information processing* and retrieval of *already stored memories.*

Psychoactive drugs, then, do not add new components to experience, or awareness, or consciousness. They may shape the existing components differently, distort them, mute or intensify them, but the drugs do not take the user beyond himself and his environment. If, in fact, each of us carries some of his own personal heaven or hell, then these agents may make it easier to experience each of these.

In spite of the uniqueness of the drug experience resulting from an interplay of all these factors, generalizations about the effects of these chemicals can be made because of three facts. First, the drugs do have specific biochemical actions (even if they are in part unknown) on areas, functions, or processes of the brain. This means that the range of effects an agent can produce is somewhat restricted. Second, the general culture, as well as the small subgroups in which each of us lives, presents a narrow range of experiences, hopes, and fears. It is from this set of possible experiences that drug effects must be selected. Last, one is taught which drug effects should be sought and emphasized and which are to be minimized. We learn, to some extent, whether the drug-induced effects are to be labeled as desirable or undesirable.

How safe are drugs?

There are at least three ways in which the harmfulness of a drug can be considered. One is the common medical usage referring to the toxic effects and lethality resulting from the use of the drug. Both short-term and long-term toxic effects need to be identified (these may be different). Furthermore, all statements refer only to what is now known. Toxic effects that may appear tomorrow cannot be predicted today. Therefore, medically speaking, the basic rule is to approach all drugs with respect and with caution.

From a medical point of view no drug is safe. With some doses, modes of administration, and frequency of use, all drugs cause toxic effects and even death. It is equally true that at some doses, modes of administration, and frequency of use all drugs are safe. The concern here is whether a drug, *used the way most people use it today,* is physically harmful. From this position, alcohol and marijuana are relatively safe drugs the way most people use them. Nicotine, in contrast, is a very harmful drug since the usual amount of cigarette smoking does increase mortality rate. (Appreciate, however, that when cigarette smoking began, the lethal effects were much less; people smoked fewer cigarettes and also did not live long enough for much of the cigarette-induced mortality to appear! If cigarettes appeared today for the first time, it would probably be no more than 5 to 10 years before their contribution to mortality would be identified.)

The regular, nonseptic use of intravenous injections makes any drug dangerous. The possibility of hepatitis, general infection, or an overdose clearly labels the usual form of heroin or injectable stimulant as medically dangerous. The fact that the users of these drugs frequently are also malnourished, with all that implies, only contributes to making the usual use of these agents clearly medically harmful.

Not so easy to categorize as medically safe or dangerous are the hallucinogens. In the normal, illegal, street use of these agents there is no way of knowing what drug is actually being used, or the purity of the agent, or the dosage, or whether one or more drugs are contained in the dose as taken. Under these conditions it is not surprising that bad trips, deaths, and long-term psychiatric hospitalizations do occur. Perhaps this situation parallels that seen in the realm of the over-the-counter drugs—safe if used as directed. When purity, dose, and the other factors are controlled, the hallucinogens have not resulted in a high incidence of adverse effects. Aspirin is a reasonably safe drug even though over 100 youngsters a year die because of misuse. Oral use of pure hallucinogens is medically more dangerous than oral use of aspirin but not as physically dangerous as regular, moderate cigarette smoking.

An increasing number of individuals is beginning to emphasize other implications of the word "harmful." This position considers the personal-social aspect of a drug's use to be of paramount importance. The question here is: to what extent does use of the drug lead to, or contribute to, a major disruption of the individual's relationship to his society? That is, does the use of the drug impair the interaction of the user and the existing culture?

When concern is directed to the degree of drug-induced impairment of the relationship between a user and society, different pictures appear. Nicotine is used regularly without greatly impairing the user's interaction with his world (up to the point where cigarette smoking causes hospitalization or death). Alcohol, however, is not harmless since at least 10% of those who use it at all use it to an extent that they are unable to function in society. The data are not as well established with respect to marijuana, but many feel that the incidence and extent of social impairment are about the same for users of alcohol and marijuana.

The injected agents also score high as dangerous drugs when impairment of social functioning is considered. Few heroin or intravenous stimulant users manage to maintain a useful relationship with society. It is not so easy to categorize the use of the hallucinogens since the data are fragmentary. Those users who center their life, for one reason or another, around the use of these drugs become dropouts and certainly fail to make any contribution to the present society. However, there must also be many occasional and irregular users who do maintain their positions in society, but a percentage division is not possible.

A third possibility is that the use of a drug may also have important interrelations with social trends in the culture. Concern is not with the medical effects of the drug or with the possible personal consequences of drug use but with the implications that extensive use of the drug may have for the society. Drug consumption by a large number of individuals may be important to the extent that a drug's effects support or oppose certain themes in the culture. That is, does the use of certain drugs fit more compatibly with certain philosophies of life?

It is suggested that two of the main threads of the American culture are aggressive achievement and tight inhibition of impulses. As a result of these closely knit threads, American society is at a standard of technology unmatched anywhere. All of our social institutions have reflected and supported these threads. For example, the schools supported these themes with the emphasis on grades (learn facts, you are not here to think) and winning sports teams (it is not how you play, it is whether you win or lose that counts) and a fairly rigid lock-step method of advancement through the system. The churches have reflected the national ethos by actively proselytizing and sending missionaries to foreign lands. Occasionally a sermon on Christian capitalism would be punctuated by a few verses of "Onward Christian Soldiers," which reaffirms the central themes of society. The emphasis on impulse control, from "nice boys don't fight" and "don't show your emotions" to the series of "thou shalt not's" that formed the basis of yesterday's religion, made it necessary to attack the environment and the problems of science and technology.

Even the drugs have contributed. All of the drugs that have become widespread through western societies have been those that alter arousal level. Not one drug whose primary action is to distort information processing has been part of the developing American scene. Within the class of drugs affecting arousal level, there have been some restrictions on their use, depending on their potency, but those of mild to moderate potency are generally attainable. Caffeine, amphetamines, alcohol, and barbiturates are clearly the drugs of choice for an outwardly oriented, achieving, inhibited society. Even oral opiates did not detract from the onmoving thrust of this society.

The hallucinogens, drugs that alter information processing, seem to be more supportive and more compatible with a different set of values. Drugs offering multiple realities and suggesting internal rewards far beyond those in the outside world seem hard to fit into a focused, accomplish-it-because-it's-there orientation. Instead of outward achievements and activation, these drugs would seem to offer inner exploration and passivity. Rather than a communion of individuals joining together to fight the infidels out there, these agents promise a personal, solitary adventure inside the soul. The hallucinogens are potent drugs. Their danger, though, seems primarily to be

to the achievement themes of our society. However, the point must be reemphasized that when any aspect of drug use is considered, all of the pharmacological and social variables must be specified if the total range of implications is to be detailed.

Perspective of history

Drug use has affected society, but social changes also affect the use of drugs. One overriding theme has certainly been that the perspective of history and of other cultures is needed to properly view drug use in America today. Drug use, as with other behaviors, takes place and has meaning only in a context, and the context for all social phenomena must be historical. For example, an important part of the context in which drug use occurs consists of the attitudes held about the drug and the user of the drug. Only by knowing how drugs have been used and viewed in the past can present attitudes toward the use of any drug be fully appreciated.

Lewin's sentiment, which is quoted in the frontispiece, seems almost axiomatic. Throughout history, when a psychoactive drug has been introduced to a culture its use has spread without stopping. However, until recently, most drugs started in the medicine man's bag of tricks and took years or centuries to disperse. From the chemist's test tube to the hamlets in the hills is now only a matter of weeks or months. Everything moves faster.

The transition from a select group of users of a drug to its acceptance as a critical component of the culture has been seen already with caffeine, nicotine, and distilled spirits. The recent flow of antipsychotic, antianxiety, and antidepressant drugs from the hospital pharmacy to the home medicine cabinet is but a modern version of the spread of a drug. The question still to be answered, of course, is which, if any, of the present illicit drugs will move into the homes of America.

In our society, the spread of a greater and greater number of drugs has been seen. From coffee in the morning through an aspirin during the day to the final nightcap—liquid or pill—we use drugs. Drugs are seen as problem solvers, and for some people they are. They make us feel good, forget the bad;

they lift us from the rat race of life to the ecstasy of eternity and remove the boredom of the banal and replace it with the excitement of the evernew. Drugs are also viewed as causing problems, and for some they do this. They make us ill, kill us, take a bad world and make it worse, and take a bright future and turn it into a dull haze. For most drug users, no matter what drug they use, none of this will happen. Whether legal or illegal, most of us use drugs in amounts and frequencies such that our lives are not seriously altered by our use of drugs. We are, however, becoming much more casual about our use of drugs.

Another principle abstracted from history is that if a psychoactive drug is to be widely used in a society, it must be integrated into and fill some need in that society. Once the agent occupies a niche, it cannot be dislodged except by changing the culture or offering a substitute to meet the same need. For example, in primitive groups the use of psychoactive plants was almost exclusively in a religious or spiritual setting. The active ingredient provided many of the experiences necessary for the participant to maintain the faith that sustained the group structure.

When a particular drug is widely used and used in a particular way, it seems to be a part of the glue that holds a culture together. Whether it is *Datura* in initiation rites or martinis at a business lunch, the drug is a part of and a supporter of that society's prevailing world view. When the drug no longer contributes to and supports the culture, the drug is dropped. More likely, however, the form of the drug use will shift to adjust to the changing culture. In some cases the culture shifts so as to incorporate the use of the drug.

The failure of the Eighteenth Amendment to dislodge alcohol from our society shows clearly that alcohol is firmly entrenched in our culture. It will not be eliminated without an acceptable substitute being offered or a major change occurring in our attitudes about life. The shifting pattern of caffeine use, from the formal and generally less convenient use of coffee to the casual and everywhere available colas, both reflects and supports our changing concepts of work and play. Therefore, the psychoactive drugs a culture selects for regular use and the form of that use can tell much about the culture. Each drug widely used in a particular way is as much of a supporting institution of the society as is its form of government, its churches, and its schools.

There are a number of reasons for the increase in the number of drugs used in our society. Only a few of the more obvious and important will be sketched here. In our generally affluent society each individual learns early that science and technology will supply answers to problems once the problems are identified. Because of the present rate of social and technological change and the great publicity given to even minor discoveries, the expectation of quick solutions to problems is now well ingrained in our culture. Drugs provide these quick solutions. The priming in the medical area was carried out over the first half of this century so that, by the post–World War II period, it was easy to believe that drugs would take care of everything, from a cold to cancer.

Throughout the 1950's and 1960's the United States was flooded with drugs that promised to solve most personal problems. Sniffles— take a pill; bad day at school or office— take two pills; trouble relating to those around you—take a tablet. The pressures for increased use of legal drugs to solve problems have been well identified throughout the book and their effectiveness is clear. The marketplace is replete with exhortations to use this or that drug to remedy a variety of uncomfortable situations. Such advertisements are not false, just misleading. The pill does not cure the cold; it just removes some symptoms! The tablet does not solve the problems you are having with other people, but it does make you less concerned about them.

However, the drugs that were being rapidly developed and marketed did temporarily solve some major problems for one group of individuals, the physicians. Physicians were confronted with increasing demands on their time, and over half of their patients presented symptoms resulting in large part from nonphysical problems. The drugs of the 1950's and 1960's made it possible for the physician to process a lot of patients and make most of them feel at least temporarily better. Cure, no. Resolution of problems, no. Relief for both the patient and the physician, yes. Little wonder that physicians dispense medication in large amounts.

Another factor that contributes to the increased drug use is simply the availability of more drugs. Not only are there more things to try, but each of the agents offers, and partially delivers, a different effect and thus different needs of more individuals may be met. Also, an affluent society such as this one may be conducive to increasing drug use. In an economically wealthy society it is possible to drop out and be a reasonably heavy drug user and still survive. This fact may be an important determinant of some individuals' behavior.

Another general cultural trend that seems to importantly interact with the increase in the use of illegal psychoactive drugs is the diminishing importance of the traditional arbiters of public and private behavior. Accepted patterns of behavior are shifting rapidly in many areas of society. The old black-and-white guidelines have been breeched and the social institutions—church, school, family—have not yet found their way out of the gray area where many behaviors "sound wrong, but I guess they are all right."

Closely intertwined with the fact that these groups no longer speak with authority on matters of individual behavior is the increase in personal freedom and rights that has accompanied the civil rights and woman's liberation movements. Such an emphasis on personal freedom has already had a major impact on what is moral, legal, and acceptable in the areas of sex and censorship. It seems probable that the expansion of individual rights—that is, the absence of restrictions on behavior that does not immediately and directly harm another person—might soon come to include drug-taking behavior. This thesis has already been repeatedly presented by those advocating reform of the current drug laws. It does appear difficult to justify expanding each individual's personal freedom in every area except that of drug use.

In addition to the dissolving traditional moral standards, which in the past have partially countered increased drug use by labeling it as *bad, immoral,* or *sinful,* the shifting patterns of drug use today make it difficult to combine opposition to drug use with already existing prejudices. Identifying the use of alcohol and saloons with the lower class, immigrant Catholic made it easy for the middle class, second generation Protestant to vote for prohibition in the early part of the century. Marijuana prohibition was easy in the 1930's; the drug had an obviously foreign name, it was primarily introduced into this country by Mexicans, and its usage was spread by lower-class Negroes. There was little conflict when the heroin problem of the 1950's was considered. The high incidence of use was in the black ghettos and the drugs were smuggled and sold by a foreign-dominated group, the Mafia. One could nicely compartmentalize the drug, the user, and the seller and be against all three with no problem.

One of the conflicts about drug use today, in contrast to previous times, is that patterns of use are changing and things are not so easily compartmentalized. Marijuana, a bad drug, is being used by white middle-class students and workers—good groups. The heroin—bad drug—problem has partly moved to the country club in the suburbs—nice people. All sorts of psychoactive drugs are being used by more and more people. No longer is it possible to categorically label those who experiment with drug use as bad, or degenerate, or sick.

Increased pressure for drug use may reflect the fact that the era of instant communication is upon us. The mass media has done an excellent job of spreading the word about the use of drugs, perhaps too good. Perhaps most stories about the use of drugs serve only to increase curiosity about the drugs and thus increase experimentation. Rarely reaching the level of news is the occasional user of any drug or the socially impaired user whose life *is* drugs. What makes the news is the exciting, the adventurous, the dramatic drug episode. Perhaps, as some have said, this is the time to cool it, to stop reporting the pot raids and the drug use by celebrities.

Similar comment could be made about the

exploding number of ill-conceived, rapidly established, and poorly aimed drug education programs in this country. By emphasizing drug use only in a moral and legal context (which is not accepted by many people today), it seems probable that drug education programs will increase the amount of drug experimentation. If these programs only emphasize the dramatic and then say *"don't!"* it is difficult to see how they can do more than support the confusion and interest already started by the news media.

A final aspect of our present society that must be briefly mentioned is the federal government. The national government is playing a pivotal and conflicting role in the expansion of illegal drug use in several ways. It is clear that there is now no consensus at the national level on the medical, personal, or societal meaning of drug use and abuse. Several issues are of concern. First, some of the antidrug material the federal government sponsors does no more than convince the younger generation that the older generation lies, is naive, or is stupid. Second, many pronouncements still insist on considering the drug problem as primarily one of law enforcement when it clearly goes beyond that to become a matter of social philosophy. Last, the decrease in penalties for marijuana possession and the developing emphasis on education and rehabilitation has not been paralleled by a shift in the thinking of those responsible for implementing the laws. As with the Marijuana Tax Act of 1937, the implementation of the law may greatly change the final meaning of the 1970 law.

A RATIONAL VIEW OF DRUG USE

One of the first steps that must be taken to rationally look at drug use is to clarify terms. The legal aspects of drug usage must be kept separate from the concept of abuse. Only by identifying the different patterns of drug usage do the problems stand out and make it possible to develop solutions.

Moderate drug use is almost straightforward. Most of us are drug users from coffee in the morning to martinis at lunch to an afternoon Coke. We use these drugs because they stimulate us a little and make us feel good or because they depress our anxieties and agitations and make us feel better. It is meaningful to restrict the term "drug abuse" to patterns of drug use that impair the individual's ability to function optimally in his personal, social, and vocational life. It complicates rather than clarifies the issues to label a 17-year-old moderate alcohol drinker as a drug abuser when in fact he is only an illegal drug user. Use of an illegal drug should not automatically be considered drug abuse. Similarly, misuse of a drug, as by overweight, bored, frustrated, depressed suburban housewives who continue to function as adequate wives and mothers, should not be labeled as drug abuse.

There is then the one problem of legal-illegal drug usage and the separate and distinct problem of drug use and drug abuse. The legal-illegal question is a dichotomy, but use-abuse is clearly a continuum. The major immediate problem for society is the drug abuser, whether he abuses a legal drug, such as alcohol, or an illegal drug, such as heroin. These abusers are the individuals whose life style is most disruptive and expensive to society.

With terminology clarified, some basic premises should be enunciated. These are not facts. They are, I believe, reasonable conclusions drawn from the available facts. Being conclusions they are debatable. Some people may feel that the conclusions do not follow from the facts, or that relevant facts were not considered, or that the assumptions made in moving from the facts to the conclusions were wrong. However, I believe these conclusions to be valid and justifiable. The basis for these premises will not be elaborated in detail. Either they appear reasonable enough from the material already presented so that a conceptualization can be suggested, or all the collecting of facts that is possible would have little hope of convincing the reader.

The physical and medical reasons against using some of the presently illegal drugs are valid only for the impure street variety drug. The current, regular intravenous use of heroin, the stimulants, or any drug is clearly dangerous and frequently leads to hospitalization and/or death. Used orally and on an occasional basis the potent hallucinogens sometimes result in hospitalization, but with moderate doses of pure drugs there are only infrequent adverse effects. Marijuana, up to now, appears to be as safe (and as dangerous) in moderate social use as alcohol.

Drug-taking behavior seems to belong in the same category of personal freedom as does sexual behavior. It is probably easier, though, for nondrug users to understand and accept the motivations behind increased individual rather than societal responsibility for one's sexual behavior than to understand or accept personal freedom in drug use. Nevertheless, it seems unlikely that the area of personal rights and freedoms can be increased much further without the right to use certain now-illegal drugs becoming an open question for society and the law.

Among those individuals who are satisfactorily integrated into the present culture, there is a low incidence of use of most illegal drugs. *There is extensive use of a drug only when the drug meets unfilled needs of the individuals in a society.* It seems clear that to diminish drug use or to prevent its further increase, the needs of individuals must be satisfied in a nondrug setting. Society must offer attractive alternatives to a drug-using life style if there is to be a decrease in drug use.

Evidence has been frequently presented that, historically, *drug use has initially altered society and then functioned as one of the stabilizing and supporting forces of the altered culture.* Changing patterns of drug use do change society. Once the change has occurred the behaviors that develop around the use of the drug oppose additional change. The more unique the drug and the behaviors associated with its use, the more difficult the drug is to assimilate into a society and the greater the change required by society. It is debatable whether the legalization of marijuana would greatly alter today's culture. On the other hand, general use of the more potent hallucinogens most likely would result in considerable changes in today's society.

One of the major differences between today and previous periods is that the stabilizing social institutions have lost some of their stability as well as their influence. *In every previous period of high drug use there have been potent forces countering the extensive use of drugs.* This assured a relatively slow spread of usage and some rational social debate on the meaning of the use of the drug. Today, even the federal government has not thought through the question of widespread drug use and, as such, is not an effective counteragent to recreational drug use.

There seems little debate over the fact that *for every psychoactive drug in use, legal or illegal, there will be a certain percentage of the users who are abusers.* It does not seem possible for a drug to be used without it also being abused by some. This seems a fact of life. As new psychoactive drugs are developed, their abusers will spring up. What is not known is whether each new drug will add to the total number of abusers or whether the number of abusers will remain constant, with only the specific drug being used changing.

One of the amazing things is the almost magical belief many people have that the law and law enforcement are something separate from and independent of society. Failure to appreciate that the law is but one of the reflections of the culture is one of the points of contention in the drug scene today. *Law enforcement works as a social control only when the society wants it to work, and that occurs only when the law is in agreement with the major themes and beliefs of the society.* This is the difficulty with considering the drug problem to be a law-enforcement problem. Until a resolution is reached in society about the role of drug-taking behavior in our culture, the role of law enforcement will be ambiguous.

A final premise is that *education can change patterns of drug use.* Much of the difficulty over so-called educational programs is that they do not present facts, only opinions. The opinions expressed are not set in a context, a framework, so that the underlying assumptions can be considered. The anticigarette campaign is effective because there is good evidence that that form of drug use is medically dangerous, and almost everyone agrees with the basic assumption that it is better to be healthy than ill. Perhaps educational programs that clearly point out the possible personal and social implications of various forms of drug use will also alter consumption patterns. For this to occur, though, the assumptions on which the implications are based must be clearly identified.

CONCLUDING COMMENT

The difficulty today in obtaining a clear picture of the changing patterns of drug-taking behavior seems primarily to be a result of viewing drug use as an isolated phenomenon. The facts about the actions and behavioral effects of psychoactive drugs are meaningful only when considered in the context of social history. It is necessary to identify and debate those cultural trends that foster and oppose the current increase and diversification of drug-taking behavior if society is to understand and resolve the present crisis in drug use.

PRECEDING QUOTES
1. Bergel, N. F., and Davies, D. R. A.: All about drugs, London, 1970, Thomas Nelson & Sons, Ltd., p. 141.
2. Huxley, A.: The history of tension, Annals of New York Academy of Sciences 67:683-684, 1967.
3. Wall, J. H. Quoted in Hodgins, E.: The search has only started, Life, October 22, 1956, p. 140.
4. Cover, R. M.: Hallucinogens, Columbia Law Review 68(3):560, 1968.

General references

Blum, R. H., and others: Society and drugs, Drugs I, San Francisco, 1970, Jossey-Bass, Inc., Publishers.

Blum, R. H., and others: Students and drugs, Drugs II, San Francisco, 1970, Jossey-Bass Inc., Publishers.

Clark, W. G., and del Giudice, J., editors: Principles of psychopharmacology, New York, 1970, Academic Press, Inc.

DiPalma, J. R., editor: Drill's pharmacology in medicine, ed. 4, New York, 1971, McGraw-Hill Book Co.

Efron, D., editor: Psychopharmacology, a review of progress, 1957-1967, Proceedings of the Sixth Annual Meeting of the American College of Neuropsychopharmacology, San Juan, Puerto Rico, December 12-15, 1967, Public Health Service Publication No. 1836, Washington, D. C., 1968, U. S. Government Printing Office.

Goodman, L. S., and Gilman, A., editors: The pharmacological basis of therapeutics, ed. 4, New York, 1970.

Goth, A.: Medical pharmacology, ed. 5, St. Louis, 1970, The C. V. Mosby Co.

Harris, R. T., McIsaac, W. M., and Schuster, C. R., editors: Drug dependence, Austin, 1970, University of Texas Press.

Lennard, H. L., and others: Mystification and drug misuse, San Francisco, 1971, Jossey-Bass, Inc., Publishers.

Nowlis, H. H.: Drugs on the college campus, New York, 1969, Doubleday & Company, Inc.

Wittenborn, J. R., and others: Drugs and youth, Proceedings of the Rutgers Symposium on Drug Abuse, Springfield, Illinois, 1968, Charles C Thomas, Publisher.

List of drugs

Medical uses, symptoms produced, and their dependency potentials*

Name	Slang name	Chemical or trade name	Classification	Medical use
Heroin	H, horse, scat, junk, smack, scag, stuff, Harry	Diacetyl-morphine	Narcotic	Pain relief
Morphine	White stuff, M	Morphine sulfate	Narcotic	Pain relief
Codeine	Schoolboy	Methylmorphine	Narcotic	Ease pain and coughing
Methadone	Dolly	Dolophine Amidon	Narcotic	Pain relief
Cocaine	Corrine, gold dust, coke, Bernice, flake, star dust, snow	Methylester of benzoyl ecgonine	Stimulant, local anesthesia	Local anesthesia
Marijuana	Pot, grass, tea, gage, reefers	*Cannabis sativa*	Relaxant, euphoriant, in high doses hallucinogen	None in U.S.
Barbiturates	Barbs, blue devils, yellow jackets, phennies, peanuts, blue heavens	Phenobarbital, Nembutal, Seconal, Amytal	Sedative-hypnotic	Sedation, relieve high blood pressure, epilepsy hyperthyroidism
Amphetamines	Bennies, dexies, speed, wake-ups, lid poppers, hearts, pep pills	Benzedrine, Dexedrine, Desoxyn, Methamphetamine, Methedrine	Sympatho-mimetic	Relieve mild depression, control appetite and narcolepsy
LSD	Acid, sugar, big D, cubes, trips	d-Lysergic acid diethylamide	Hallucinogen	Experimental study of mental function, alcoholism
DMT	AMT, businessman's high	N,N-Dimethyl-tryptamine	Hallucinogen	None
Mescaline	Mesc	3,4,5-Trimeth-oxyphenethylamine	Hallucinogen	None
Psilocybin		3-[2-(dimethylamino) ethyl]indol-4-ol dihydrogen phosphate	Hallucinogen	None
Alcohol	Booze, juice, etc.	Ethanol, ethyl alcohol	Sedative-hypnotic	Solvent, antiseptic
Tobacco	Fag, coffin nail, etc.	*Nicotinia tabacum*	Stimulant-sedative	Sedative, emetic (nicotine)

*Adapted from Resource book for drug abuse education, National Institute of Mental Health, October, 1969, pp.
†Question marks indicate conflicts of opinion.

ow taken	Usual dose	Effects sought	Long-term symptoms	Physical dependence potential	Mental dependence potential
ected or niffed	Varies	Euphoria, prevent withdrawal discomfort (4 hrs.)	Addiction, constipation, loss of appetite	Yes	Yes
allowed r injected	15 milligrams	Euphoria, prevent withdrawal discomfort (6 hrs.)	Addiction, constipation, loss of appetite	Yes	Yes
allowed	30 milligrams	Euphoria, prevent withdrawal discomfort (4 hrs.)	Addiction, constipation, loss of appetite	Yes	Yes
llowed injected	10 milligrams	Prevent withdrawal discomfort (4 to 6 hrs.)	Addiction, constipation, loss of appetite	Yes	Yes
fed, jected, or wallowed	Varies	Excitation, talkativeness (varies, short)	Depression, convulsions	No	Yes
ked, vallowed, sniffed	1 to 2 cigarettes	Relaxation, increased euphoria, perceptions, sociability (4 hrs.)	Usually none	No	Yes?
lowed injected	50 to 100 milligrams	Anxiety reduction, euphoria (4 hrs.)	Addiction with severe withdrawal symptoms, possible convulsions, toxic psychosis	Yes	Yes
lowed injected	2.5 to 5 milligrams	Alertness, activeness (4 hrs.)	Loss of appetite, delusions, hallucinations, toxic psychosis	Yes?	Yes
owed	100 to 500 micrograms	Insightful experiences, exhilaration, distortion of senses (10 hrs.)	May intensify existing psychosis, panic reactions	No	No?
ed	60 to 70 milligrams	Insightful experiences, exhilaration, distortion of senses (less than 1 hr.)	?	No	No?
wed	350 milligrams	Insightful experiences, exhilaration, distortion of senses (12 hrs.)	?	No	No?
wed	25 milligrams	Insightful experiences, exhilaration, distortion of senses (6 to 8 hrs.)	?	No	No?
wed	Varies	Sense alteration, anxiety reduction, sociability (1 to 4 hrs.)	Cirrhosis, toxic psychosis, neurologic damage, addiction	Yes	Yes
d, ed, ved	Varies	Calmness, sociability (time varies)	Emphysema, lung cancer, mouth and throat cancer, cardiovascular damage, loss of appetite	Yes?	Yes

Index